Bodily Matters

A BOOK IN THE SERIES

Radical Perspectives

A *Radical History Review* book series

Series editors:

Daniel J. Walkowitz, New York University

Barbara Weinstein, University of Maryland

at College Park

NADJA DURBACH

Bodily Matters

THE ANTI-VACCINATION

MOVEMENT IN ENGLAND,

1853–1907

Duke University Press Durham and London   2005

© 2005 Duke University Press

All Rights Reserved

Printed in the United States of America

on acid-free paper ∞

Designed by C. H. Westmoreland

Typeset in Scala with Octavian display

by Keystone Typesetting, Inc.

Library of Congress Cataloging-in-Publication

Data appear on the last printed page

of this book.

TO MY MOTHER AND FATHER

WITH LOVE, AFFECTION, AND GRATITUDE . . .

History, as radical historians have long observed, cannot be severed from authorial subjectivity—indeed, from politics. Political concerns animate the questions we ask, the subjects on which we write. For over thirty years, the *Radical History Review* has led in nurturing and advancing politically engaged historical research. Radical Perspectives seeks to further the journal's mission: Any author wishing to be in the series makes a self-conscious decision to associate her or his work with a radical perspective. To be sure, many of us are currently struggling with what it means to be a radical historian in the early twenty-first century, and this series is intended to provide some signposts for what we would judge to be radical history. It will offer innovative ways of telling stories from multiple perspectives; comparative, transnational, and global histories that transcend conventional boundaries of region and nation; works that elaborate on the implications of the postcolonial move to "provincialize Europe"; studies of the public in and of the past, including those that consider the commodification of the past; and histories that explore the intersection of identities such as gender, race, class, and sexuality with an eye to their political implications and complications. Above all, this book series seeks to create an important intellectual space and discursive community to explore the very issue of what constitutes radical history. Within this context, some of the books published in the series may privilege alternative and oppositional political cultures, but all will be concerned with the way power is constituted, contested, used, and abused.

Fears of anthrax, smallpox, and other forms of biological attack in the aftermath of the events of September 11, 2001, and controversial calls for compulsory vaccination make *Bodily Matters*, Nadja Durbach's study of the anti-vaccination movement in late Victorian and Edwardian England, a timely contribution to this series. As Durbach points out, major issues in the current debate—about the effectiveness and safety of vaccines, government abuse of power, and calls for alternative health practices—echo concerns from the anti-vaccination campaign of a century earlier. *Bodily Matters* locates the English anti-vaccination movement at the center of a series of broad assaults by the liberal state on the private lives of its citizens. Foreshadowing the global reach of contemporary health crises, the book also places this movement in the context of international debates about the role of the modern state and the regulation of the body. Few today may question the value of immunization against smallpox, but *Bodily Matters* demonstrates that vaccination, the development and implementation of medical technologies, and the anti-vaccination movement they spawned, must still be understood as political acts.

Contents

☞

Acknowledgments xi

Introduction 1

1. The Parliamentary Lancet 13

2. Fighting the "Babies' Battle" 37

3. Populism, Citizenship, and the Politics
of Victorian Liberalism 69

4. The Body Politics of Class Formation 91

5. Vampires, Vivisectors, and the Victorian Body 113

6. Germs, Dirt, and the Constitution 150

7. Class, Gender, and the Conscientious Objector 171

Conclusion 199

Notes 209

Bibliography 243

Index 269

Acknowledgments

☞ This book has been a labor of love and has brought me into contact with an array of exceptionally kind and intellectually curious individuals. It is a pleasure to be able to thank all of those who made the research and writing of this book not only possible, but exceedingly enjoyable.

I thank the Department of History and the Frederick Jackson Turner Fund, Johns Hopkins University; the Social Sciences and Humanities Research Council of Canada; the Midwestern Victorian Studies Association; and the Charlotte Newcombe Foundation for funding this project.

I am grateful to the staff of many libraries and archives. In the United States and Canada I thank the staff of the National Library of Medicine; Ed Mormon and Christine Ruggere, Institute for the History of Medicine, Johns Hopkins University; Katherine Donahue and Teresa Johnson, University of California, Los Angeles, Biomedical Library; Lee Perry, Woodward Library, University of British Columbia; and Zach Jaffe and the staff of the Interlibrary Loan division of the Milton S. Eisenhower Library, Johns Hopkins University. In England I thank the staff of the British Library and its Picture Library, the Colindale Newspaper Library, the Public Record Office, the Wellcome Library, the Wellcome Trust Medical Photographic Library, the London School of Hygiene and Tropical Medicine, the Tower Hamlets Library, the London Metropolitan Archives, the Fawcett Library (now Women's Library), the Mary Evans Picture Library, the Bodleian Library, the Corporation of London Records Office, the Tameside Local Studies Library, Brunel University, the Modern Records Centre at the University of Warwick, the Gloucestershire Record Office, the Greater Manchester Record Office, the Jewish Studies Library at University College London, the Southwark Local Studies Library, the Bishopsgate Institute, the Bromley Central Library, the Keighley Library, Julie Anne Lambert at the John Johnson Collection at the Bodleian Library, Anne Wheeldon at the Hammersmith and Fulham Archives and Local History Centre, and Tim Boon at the Science Museum, London.

Over the many years that I have been fortunate to know them, Chris and Michele Kohler, antiquarian book dealers extraordinaire, have provided me not only with rare books and pamphlets but with an even more precious gift: their friendship. Denis Vandervelde generously shared his passion for medical ephemera with me, allowed me to reproduce many of his images here, and kindly welcomed me into his family.

Academic work is always a collaborative effort and I have benefited greatly from my discussions with Sascha Auerbach, Gillian Calder, Melanie Clews, Geoff Crossick, Nadav Davidovitch, Jim Epstein, David Feldman, Sue Ferry, Stuart Hogarth, Robert Johnston, Susan Lederer, Marjorie Levine-Clark, John McKiernan, Rohan McWilliam, Katy Rashid, Ruth Richardson, Sonya Rose, Alan Sinel, Stephen Straker, Jennifer Tucker, Luise White, and a former employee of the National Anti-Vaccination League (who prefers to remain unidentified).

Many people have read parts of this book in its various incarnations, and it is much better for their input. I am very grateful to Tim Alborn, Sally Alexander, Amanda Anderson, David Barnes, David Bell, Antoinette Burton, Felicity Callard, Mary Fissell, Alison Fletcher, Julie Kimmel, Lara Kriegel, Anna Krylova, Harry Marks, James Mokhiber, Mary Catherine Moran, John Plotz, Mick Worboys, and the assorted members of the Nineteenth Century Studies Group at Johns Hopkins University.

Joy Dixon read the entire manuscript at a critical stage and gave much needed encouragement and sage advice. I am equally indebted to George Behlmer, whose willingness to read and reread and keen eye for detail made all the difference. Logie Barrow's enthusiasm and his valuable insights have made him an ideal companion on my anti-vaccination adventure, and I thank him wholeheartedly for his kindness to me over the many years that we have both been engaged in this research.

I am profoundly grateful to Judith Walkowitz, who has been with this project from the beginning. Seamlessly weaving together the roles of adviser, colleague, and friend, she challenged and supported me throughout the process of writing my Ph.D. dissertation and helped immensely with the transition from dissertation to book.

My colleagues and friends at the University of Utah have provided me with the ideal intellectual environment in which to work and more than enough food and wine to allow me to relax. Many of them have read parts of this book, and I am extremely grateful for their feedback. I particularly thank Megan Armstrong, Beth Clement, Ben Cohen, Bob Goldberg, Eric Hinderaker, Becky Horn, Jim Lehning, Tracy McDonald, Bradley Parker, Susie Porter, and Janet Theiss.

Working with Duke University Press has been a pleasure. I thank Valerie Millholland, Miriam Angress, Mark Mastromarino, the series editors Daniel Walkowitz and Barbara Weinstein, the external referees, and the staff of the press, all of whose time and energy has made this a painless process.

I dedicate this book to my mother and father, whose love and support have meant more to me than I can adequately express, and who, like the anti-vaccinationist parents in this book, have only ever wanted their children to be healthy and happy.

A version of chapter 4 appeared previously as " 'They Might as Well Brand Us': Working-Class Resistance to Compulsory Vaccination in Victorian England," *Social History of Medicine* 13(1) (2000): 45–62. It is reproduced here by permission of Oxford University Press. A shorter version of chapter 7 was published as "Class, Gender, and the Conscientious Objector to Vaccination, 1898–1907," *Journal of British Studies* 41(1) (2002): 58–83. It is reproduced here by permission of the University of Chicago Press, © 2002, and by the North American Conference on British Studies. All rights reserved.

Bodily Matters

Introduction

☞ In 1876, seven of the Poor Law Guardians of the Yorkshire industrial town of Keighley were imprisoned in York Castle. While they had fulfilled their obligation to oversee the distribution of poor relief, the guardians had refused to enforce the vaccination acts that mandated the vaccination of all infants against smallpox within the first three months of life. Since the guardians had been elected the year before on an anti-vaccination platform, their imprisonment made them both local and national heroes for their very public defiance of such a controversial law. Indeed, the "Seven Men of Keighley" did not go quietly to jail. "The streets were soon thronged by a dense mob," reported *The Times*, "with so menacing an appearance that it was soon evident that a rescue of the prisoners was intended." The guardians were taken to the railway station, bound for their incarceration in the debtor's prison at York, some forty miles away. At the station the vehicle was surrounded by the crowd, who released the horses and then dragged the carriage, along with the prisoners and the police officers, back to Keighley. "Several of the officers," declared *The Times*, "were maltreated and had their clothes torn from their backs." The police were ultimately obliged to allow the guardians to return to their homes, having promised to surrender once the commotion had subsided. The town, however, "continued in a state of excitement till late in the evening." The following day, the guardians surrendered, and a number of well-known local anti-vaccinators escorted them to the train station, where they departed for the jail "amid the cheers of a large crowd of sympathizers." The Keighley guardians remained imprisoned in York Castle for a month before being released on bail. When they appeared in court several months later, they refused to renounce their beliefs but agreed nevertheless to refrain from obstructing the machinery of compulsory vaccination.[1]

The imprisonment of the Keighley guardians was a unique event, although the protest and tensions that surrounded it were typical of the contest over compulsory vaccination. Under the Vaccination Acts of 1853, 1867, and 1871, the Poor Law Guardians were responsible for ensuring that all infants born within their districts were vaccinated against smallpox. The Keighley guardians were not alone in refusing to enforce what many considered tyrannical legislation. However, Keighley had been an anti-vaccination stronghold since the 1860s, and by 1875 it not only had a majority of anti-vaccinators serving as guardians, but was in the throes of a smallpox epidemic. The Keighley guardians were thus a convenient scapegoat for the government's frustration with the inefficiency of its vaccination administration, which relied heavily on local enforcement. Keighley was to serve as an example to the nation. While the conservative *Times* declared that "the campaign of the Keighley Guardians against the Vaccination Acts has ended in an unconditional surrender," the incident in fact dramatically highlighted tensions within the state itself and fueled an anti-vaccination movement that was gaining momentum in the 1870s.[2]

While historians have often seen anti-vaccinationism as anti-progressive, how well nineteenth-century vaccination actually worked is a complicated historical question. There can be little doubt that most people who were properly vaccinated did not acquire smallpox. However, nineteenth-century smallpox statistics are problematic, at best. The field of statistics developed in Britain in the late eighteenth century, and by the 1830s statistical societies had been formed to collect and categorize data on social and economic subjects. Statistics quickly became a tool of public policy, for numbers had the appearance of objectivity and added scientific weight to otherwise subjective opinions.[3] The state thus frequently mobilized statistical "facts" to counter anti-vaccination rhetoric. These data, the government maintained, clearly demonstrated that the unvaccinated died more frequently of smallpox than the vaccinated. Government administrators gathered the statistics at isolation hospitals, which treated only a fraction of the cases. There, doctors routinely classified those with no visible vaccination marks as "unvaccinated." A patient pitted with smallpox rarely had vaccination scars that could actually be seen. Those who did have such scars and caught smallpox nevertheless often were classed as "imperfectly vaccinated," which in some cases was incorporated into the "unvaccinated" category. Vaccination statistics are therefore highly unreliable. Anti-vaccinationists, like other Victorian pressure groups, attempted to beat the government at its own numbers game, deploying only the data that would support their position and inflame their publications' readership. Thus, it was disingenuous at best for George Gibbs, the organized anti-vaccination campaign's prime statistician, to claim that it was "statistically demonstrated that Vaccination causes very many more deaths than, even in the worst times, result from Small-Pox."[4]

Even if vaccination did protect one against smallpox, this was only one element of whether or not it worked. The technology used to control smallpox in the nineteenth and early twentieth centuries was neither a painless nor a minor intervention. Victorian public vaccinators used a lancet (a surgical instrument) to cut lines into the flesh in a scored pattern. This was usually done in at least four different places on the arm. Vaccine matter, also called lymph, would then be smeared into the cuts. While some private practitioners preferred to use calf lymph supplied by the National Vaccine Establishment, the government urged public vaccinators to vaccinate from arm to arm to keep the supply of vaccine flowing in the community. This meant that vaccinators required infants to return eight days after the procedure to allow lymph to be harvested from their blisters, or "vesicles." This matter was then inserted directly into the arms of waiting infants.[5] After 1871, a fine of up to 20 shillings could be imposed on parents who refused to allow lymph to be taken from their children for use in public vaccination. By this time, infants had become not only recipients of vaccine matter but its incubators.

This invasive, insanitary, and sometimes disfiguring procedure seemed to many to be potentially more harmful than beneficial. Indeed, those who promoted compulsory vaccination failed to take into account the operation's side effects on the bodies of urban working-class children in particular, the prime target of public vaccination. The relatively poor nutrition of working-class children made them more vulnerable to adverse reactions; thus, some babies responded badly to the vaccine, no matter how pure its source. Others fell victim to a range of blood-borne diseases that could be passed via the arm-to-arm method. The difficulties inherent in caring for vaccination wounds compounded these problems, for limited water supplies and the insanitary condition of cities meant that serious infections, such as gangrene, could follow even a successful vaccination.

Whether or not children could survive a vaccination both immune from smallpox and relatively unscathed, however, is only part of the issue. The procedure was clearly incompatible with many shared cultural attitudes toward disease and its prevention. Vaccination could "work," therefore, only insofar as it could be incorporated into an already available medical cosmology.[6] As we shall see, many Victorians believed that health depended on preserving the body's integrity, encouraging the proper circulation of pure blood, and preventing the introduction of any foreign material into the body. The enforcement of a procedure that blatantly undermined these principles was unacceptable, especially to those unused to this degree of state interference in matters of an intimate bodily nature. Throughout the nineteenth and early twentieth centuries, compulsory vaccination was at odds with both popular understandings of bodily economy and assumptions about the boundaries of state intervention in personal life. A history of anti-vaccinationism therefore suggests that it is the success of vaccination itself—as a medical and a social practice—that requires further explanation.

Indeed, resistance to vaccination was not unique to Victorian England. From its invention in the 1790s in rural Gloucestershire to its role in the South Asian Smallpox Eradication Program in the 1970s, vaccination provoked fear and suspicion throughout the world. Anti-vaccinationist movements were organized across Europe and North America in the late nineteenth and early twentieth centuries, as riots, acts of civil disobedience, and other forms of resistance erupted around the globe.[7]

When the British Raj attempted to impose vaccination on the Indian population, it was met with marked resistance. The imperial state replaced the indigenous practice of variolation, which had an important ritual component, with vaccination, which was practiced not by familiar members of the community but by those rightly seen as agents of the colonial state. In addition, vaccination entailed incorporating the cow, an animal sacred to Hindus, into the body. Compulsory vaccination thus disrupted local religious and healing practices.[8] Similar attempts to vaccinate the Ugandan population also proved unpopular, as the Baganda feared that they were being deliberately poisoned by European settlers. Vaccination, alongside other technologies of Western biomedicine, came to be seen as an insidious "weapon of intimate colonial domination" as the imperial state exercised its authority not only on, but from within, the bodies of its subjects.[9] The colonial context made these cases particularly fraught. American vaccination policy, however, also provoked significant tensions on the Texas–Mexico border in the early twentieth century. That Mexican nationals were vaccinated with or without their consent when crossing the border, while American bodies were left literally unmarked, highlighted the contested relationship between citizenship, ethnicity, and bodily control.[10] In Brazil, class rather than ethnic or racial tensions took center stage in debates over state-enforced vaccination. In 1904, compulsory vaccination became a flash point for larger working-class concerns around the process and direction of Rio de Janeiro's modernization project. For the urban working class, mandatory vaccination was the last straw in a "renovation–sanitation–civilization plan" that served the needs of rich Brazilians and foreign capitalists while systematically discriminating against the masses.[11]

In each of these cases, who wielded the needle or lancet and whose body was marked governed how vaccination was experienced and the meanings attached to it. While each instance of resistance grew out of its own, unique social circumstances and took a distinct form, the often violent reactions to vaccination reveal widespread and cross-cultural concerns about the role of the state, the rights of the individual, and the health and safety of the body. These comparative cases suggest that vaccination is a particularly polysemic medical technology, and its enforcement is always a political act. For according to a nineteenth-century English anti-vaccinationist, "[T]he very moment you take a medical prescription and you incorporate it in an act of Parliament, it passes beyond the confines of a purely medical question and becomes essentially a social and political one."[12]

Bodily Matters contends that the British anti-vaccination movement is particularly historically significant not only because it was arguably the largest medical-resistance campaign ever mounted in Europe, but because it clearly articulated these anxieties around the safety of the body and the role of the modern state. This book locates anti-vaccinationism at the very center of wider public debates over the extent of government intervention in the private lives of its citizens, the values of a liberal society, and the politics of class that were taking shape at a key moment in the reconfiguration of the meanings, forms, and boundaries of the nation and the polity.[13] Who controlled the body was a highly charged political issue precisely because pro- and anti-vaccinators had very different ideas about how human bodies worked and how best to safeguard them from disease. Anti-vaccinators saw their bodies not as potentially contagious and thus dangerous to the social body, but as highly vulnerable to contamination and violation. Their sensationalist images of bodies polluted and mutilated by state-sanctioned doctors were produced in a dynamic relationship to medicalized models that were themselves shifting in response to new developments in disease theory. These contests over access to, and knowledge about, the body played an important role in the production of class, gender, and racial identities and in negotiations over the relationship between the individual and society. Resistance to compulsory vaccination was therefore not a marginal movement, but central to nineteenth- and early-twentieth-century body politics.

While the meanings invested in the body are historically contingent, according to Michel Foucault, the modern body operates as a, if not *the*, key site of political contestation.[14] Building on Foucault's theory of "biopolitics," historians and sociologists have theorized the role of modern states in regulating and disciplining the body. Analyzing the discourses of science, medicine, and sexuality as technologies of the modern state, these scholars have investigated bodies as "the matrix in which are written the rights a society allots to people of various genders, races, and classes."[15] This relationship between the body and the state is perhaps starkest in its colonial form. But the bodies of metropolitan British citizens were equally crucial to the state's "construction of its own authority, legitimacy, and control."[16] For as the Victorian state expanded, its reach extended into previously private realms as the government increasingly sought to regulate the bodies of its citizens.

During the period between the 1832 Anatomy Act, which sanctioned the dissection of paupers who died unclaimed in a workhouse, and the 1916 Military Service Act, which conscripted British bodies to defend the nation, Parliament consistently introduced, local authorities enforced, and the judicial system upheld legislation that focused on bodily issues. From acts dealing with the laboring bodies of women, children, and, later, adult men through legislation surrounding prostitution and homosexuality to the introduction of maternal and child health programs, the British state became intimately involved in bodily matters as never before.

Indeed, by the 1880s the feminist social reformer Mary Hume-Rothery was insisting that neither "the persons of women nor the cradles of infants, nor the sick-room itself" were safe from the tyranny of state-sanctioned doctors.[17] Three pieces of legislation connected infants, women, and the sick: the contagious diseases acts, the notification of infectious diseases acts, and the vaccination acts. The Contagious Diseases Acts of 1864, 1866, and 1869 subjected the bodies of all those suspected of being prostitutes to medical inspection for venereal disease. A woman found to be infected could then be confined in a hospital for the treatment of venereal diseases, with or without her consent. Similarly, the Notification of Infectious Diseases Acts of 1889 and 1899 required that all contagious diseases—though, significantly, not tuberculosis, which was common enough among the middle classes—be reported to the local medical officer of health, who could then forcibly remove the patient to a hospital. Opponents argued that these were blatant examples of class legislation that targeted the poor and working class. These acts, protesters maintained, infringed on individual rights and subjected vulnerable bodies to invasive and inhumane medical treatments by doctors intent on exercising their own professional authority. That the British government, unlike some of its European counterparts, did not articulate these initiatives in the language of "medical police," preferring the terms *state medicine* and *public health*, did not mean, therefore, that it did not participate in "the enforcement of health," as some historians have implied.[18]

The vaccination acts, as Hume-Rothery made clear, were closely related to these other legislative efforts to contain dangerous (and particularly working-class) bodies in the name of public health. Compulsory vaccination was first introduced in England and Wales in 1853 in an attempt to protect the population against smallpox, which intermittently attacked both urban and rural communities throughout the nineteenth century.[19] Pro-vaccinationists argued from empirical evidence that cowpox inoculation was an effective means of warding off smallpox and should be made mandatory to protect not only each individual but the nation as a whole against this deadly contagious disease. The 1853 legislation was targeted at the poor and working classes and made vaccination both mandatory and free. It failed, however, to devise a strategy for enforcing the compulsory aspect of the law. In the 1850s, most Poor Law unions charged with overseeing vaccination lacked the staff to pursue defaulters, as well as the funds to pay for prosecutions and, perhaps, the motivation to do so. *The Times* reported in 1859 that a laborer named George Fry was fined the maximum penalty of 1 pound, 18 shillings, and 6 pence for non-vaccination plus steep court costs, but few other prosecutions took place before 1867.[20]

In 1867, a new vaccination act introduced several of the necessary mechanisms for enforcing vaccination more efficiently. In addition to mandating the appointment of public vaccinators for each district, it clarified the nature and extent of penalties for noncompliance. Section 29 imposed a fine of up to 20 shillings for the non-vaccination of a child within the first three months after birth. More significantly, Section 31 allowed the repeated prosecution of parents of children up to fourteen years old who refused to obey the order to vaccinate. This meant that as long as one's child remained unvaccinated, a fine could be levied at any time. This legislation overturned the landmark case *Pilcher v Stafford*, which had determined in 1863 that only one penalty could be obtained for default of vaccination. Under this new legislation, Poor Law Guardians were required to keep a register of vaccinations, which they compiled by comparing vaccination certificates against the semiannual reports provided by local registrars of births and deaths. This made tracing defaulters much easier, and after 1867 prosecutions became more frequent.

In the early years of compulsion, the duty of enforcing vaccination often fell by default to the public vaccinator. By 1871, it had become clear that tracing cases of noncompliance was not only crucial to the success of compulsory vaccination but a job unto itself. To this end, the 1871 Vaccination Act mandated the employment of vaccination officers for each district. Vaccination officers were not medical practitioners but public servants who were directly responsible to locally elected Poor

Law Guardians, many of whom, as in Keighley, were sympathetic to the anti-vaccinationist position. This meant, much to the central government's frustration, that practice differed, often quite radically, from district to district. These new vaccination officers took over the supervision of vaccination registers and issued warnings to parents who did not obtain certificates of successful vaccination, of insusceptibility, or of medical unfitness for vaccination, or who did not send in the certificates. If this warning went unheeded, the vaccination officer was responsible for taking the parents to court. If found guilty, parents could be fined up to 20 shillings plus court costs and ordered to vaccinate. Often the parents could not, or refused to, pay these fines, as court costs sometimes amounted to more than the fine itself. This generally resulted in the issue of a distress warrant for the family's goods, which were seized and auctioned to generate funds. If the family had no appropriate goods (bedsteads, linens, and artisanal tools were exempted), or if enough money could not be garnered from the sale, one of the parents (generally, but not necessarily, the father) was then imprisoned for a period of up to two weeks. The process could be repeated almost indefinitely under Section 31 of the 1867 legislation.

While similar to other state attempts to police the public health, the vaccination acts occupy a unique place within the nexus of body–state relations, for they applied to all infants and were the only government initiatives to intervene in direct and invasive ways with apparently healthy bodies that posed no immediate risk to the social body. Indeed, this legislation was denounced as even more draconian than the contagious diseases acts because it involved the most vulnerable, and presumably least dangerous, members of society. They call "our smiling healthy babes 'nuisances,' 'explosive material,' [and liken] them to 'nitro-glycerine,'" complained one campaigner.[21] By mandating a medical procedure for its newborn citizens, the government had crossed an important line, setting a precedent for state interference with all British bodies, healthy or otherwise.

The vaccination issue, however, complicates the narrative of the progressive growth of state power and its relationship to developments in medical, scientific, and bureaucratic expertise. The vaccination administration has served historians as an example of the nineteenth-century "revolution in government."[22] But the story of vaccination policy is equally bound up in local politics and in tensions between and within government agencies. The success of the national program relied heavily on a "varied palimpsest of local bureaucracies" that in the end failed to provide the basis of a coherent policy.[23] As the case of Keighley demonstrates, the vaccination system was hopelessly inefficient precisely because of its lack of centralization and its reliance on locally elected Poor Law Guardians, who often felt more responsible to their constituents than to a central administration. Far from being shut out of the "new, knowledge-based form of governance,"[24] men and women from across the social spectrum—even though many remained unenfranchised—participated in public-policy debates and forced the government to accede to their demands by actively campaigning against compulsory vaccination.

In 1889, in response to widespread noncompliance and open hostility to the vaccination laws, Parliament appointed a Royal Commission to investigate the vaccination administration and to draft recommendations for a more efficient system. The Royal Commission on Vaccination sat for seven years, releasing its sixth and final report in 1896. During this period, hundreds of communities across Britain suspended all prosecutions for noncompliance, eagerly awaiting a definitive answer as to the value of the compulsory clauses. This led to a marked decrease in vaccination. In the late 1890s, Leicestershire was reporting that approximately 80 percent of births were unvaccinated; Bedfordshire, 79 percent; Northamptonshire, 69 percent; Nottinghamshire, 50 percent; and Derbyshire, 48 percent. The commission's conclusions, while underscoring the need for compulsory vaccination, also validated the anti-vaccinationist position. The final report recommended the introduction of exemptions for conscientious objectors, which was passed into law in 1898. This provision proved contentious, however, and certificates were only rarely conferred. To remedy the problems posed by the inconsistent administration of the 1898 act, an amendment passed in 1907 forced magistrates to grant exemption certificates to all parents who made a statutory declaration that they conscientiously believed vaccination to be injurious to their children's health. After 1907, magistrates were granting between 150,000 and 200,000 exemptions annually, representing approximately 25 percent of all births.[25] In this case, widespread popular beliefs about both the body and the limits of state intervention overrode the authority of medical expertise.

By focusing on both the events of the resistance campaign and the richness of its rhetorical strategies, *Bodily Matters* provides a complex account of anti-vaccination agitation over the fifty years that saw the vaccination debate at its most heated. Chapter 1 situates the first Compulsory Vaccination Act within the political and medical context of the 1850s, revealing the 1853 legislation's relationship to the professionalization of medicine, the rise of a bureaucratic state, and the politics of alternative medicine. The first vaccination act provoked outrage from heterodox medical practitioners and was blatantly disregarded by many parents; organized and widespread resistance to vaccination, however, emerged largely after the more stringent 1867 act was passed. Chapter 2 locates the anti-vaccinationism of this later period within the context of a broad range of dissenting movements, arguing that this campaign was integral to a vibrant culture of political protest and social reform that was characteristic of the second half of the nineteenth century. Chapters 3 and 4 focus on the politics of compulsion, revealing the centrality of the vaccination question not only to other reform campaigns, but also to larger nineteenth-century debates over the meanings of liberalism, the rights of parents, and the nature of citizenship, as well as to the production and politicization of the English working class. As these chapters illustrate, anti-vaccinators consistently appealed to the logic of rights and participated in informed political debate. But their language also revealed deep social anxieties. Chapters 5 and 6 explore the meaning of resistance not just to state interference in private life, but also to vaccination itself, highlighting the dread of contagion and contamination that reached its peak toward the end of the nineteenth century. The first of these chapters examines the range of fears and fantasies generated around blood purity and bodily integrity by analyzing the gothic tropes of the vampire and the vivisector that anti-vaccination propaganda consistently invoked. Extending these concerns for the health of the individual into the realm of the social body, the following chapter maps the interplay between scientific and popular ideas about contagious disease in the context of shifts in medical understandings of disease processes and social concerns over urban poverty. Finally, chapter 7 investigates the debates surrounding the

1898 and 1907 legislation, which effectively ended compulsion by allowing parents who "conscientiously objected" to vaccination to obtain exemption certificates. By interrogating the classed and gendered assumptions about the nature of the conscience, this chapter argues that anti-vaccinationists provoked significant public discussion of the nature of modern subjectivity and set an important precedent for conscientious objection during World War I. *Bodily Matters* thus positions anti-vaccinationism not as a fringe movement of eccentric Victorians, but as a widespread popular phenomenon that was central to the problematics of both the body and the state in nineteenth- and early-twentieth-century England.

1

The Parliamentary Lancet

[W]ho could receive with cordiality and respect the Doctor of Physic

who should burglariously thunder at the door, armed with scab and

lancet, feloniously threatening to assault the inmates therewith, and, no

matter how loudly he should protest that he was bent upon a mission

of mercy, who could avoid suspecting that his real objects were

power and gain?—John Gibbs, 1854[1]

☞ "Are we to be leeched, bled, blistered, burned, douched, frozen, pilled, potioned, lotioned, salivated . . . by Act of Parliament?" demanded an outraged John Gibbs in 1854.[2] This graphic image of a body medically tortured by government decree was a direct attack on the Compulsory Vaccination Act of 1853, which mandated the vaccination of all English infants against smallpox. That the state could impose medical procedures on the"free-born Briton" seemed to usher in a new and dangerous era in which the individual had no right to his or her own body. Are "the intelligent people of this free realm," Gibbs challenged, merely to become "abject slaves to the medical profession"?

For Gibbs, a hydropath, and his community of heterodox practitioners, compulsory vaccination represented the epitome of an already pervasive system of medical despotism. Indeed, the 1850s were a critical moment for conflicts over medical access and authority as orthodox medicine emerged as a profession and as heterodox practitioners vigorously opposed their exclusion from the medical marketplace. The Compulsory Vaccination Act of 1853 played a particularly important role in these larger debates, for compulsory vaccination quickly became a flash point for contests over state authority, professional control, and the meanings of "medical liberty."

The Growth of Professional Medicine

Historians have consistently demonstrated that Georgian medicine favored and encouraged pluralism in the medical marketplace, permitting consumers to purchase the services of a variety of practitioners. In search of remedies, the sick often moved freely from one type of practitioner to another, employing, among others, surgeons, bonesetters, and patent-medicine vendors. This meant both that treatments were often negotiated between patient and practitioner and that the sick could be active in orchestrating their cure.[3] In theory, a structured system of medical provision still existed within the larger marketplace, as orthodox practitioners were hierarchically divided into physicians, surgeons, and apothecaries. However, these boundaries remained fluid, as medical roles could not always be clearly demarcated.[4] Methods for training varied widely even within each category, and degrees could be purchased freely and openly. Until the middle of the nineteenth century, there existed no uniform regulation of medicine, no single licensing body, and no nationally recognized and agreed on standards or criteria against which one could measure legitimacy and illegitimacy in medical practices. In fact, before 1858 nineteen different licensing bodies existed in Britain.[5] The most prestigious, the Royal College of Physicians (RCP), was more an aristocratic club than a professional association, as it accepted only Oxbridge graduates. Admitting only 168 fellows between 1771 and 1833,[6] the RCP had neither the base of support nor the clout to prevent nonmembers from practicing medicine. Divisions within medicine, therefore, were as much social markers as descriptors of actual practice.

By the end of the eighteenth century, these traditional divisions within medicine appeared increasingly outdated. Doctors—especially those practicing outside London—performed varied medical roles, being at one and the same time physician, surgeon, apothecary, and midwife. Throughout the nineteenth century, the tripartite system slowly disintegrated, leaving a dichotomy of general practitioner and consultant (a doctor with a hospital appointment) in its place.[7] If the clientele of the orthodox physician in the eighteenth century was generally the social elite, in the nineteenth century regular medicine expanded its mandate and sought increasingly to provide treatment to many more people by way of the general practitioner. The general practitioner's reach extended into the working classes, for his practice was no longer highly specialized. In the early nineteenth century, medicine began to take on a much more significant social role. No longer merely a service rendered for profit, it gradually became an institution with exclusive rights to control medical knowledge and, by extension, the health and bodies of the entire population. This process of professionalization involved both a move toward scientizing medicine and an attempt to strengthen ties with an expanding and increasingly bureaucratic state.

The changing relationship between doctors and the state became evident in the 1830s. The 1832 Anatomy Act bolstered the relationship between medicine and the state at the expense of the destitute. It specified that the bodies of those who died in a workhouse or charity hospital and went "unclaimed" by their kin would be turned over to anatomists for dissection. Bodies for dissection were difficult to obtain before 1832, and grave robbers abounded as anatomy became an increasingly important component of medical education. The sensational true story of Burke and Hare, who murdered the poor in order to sell their bodies to anatomists, contributed to a climate of fear among the laboring population. The 1832 act did little to mitigate this anxiety. Opponents of the act claimed that it objectified the bodies of the poor, allowing them to be probed and penetrated for the use of middle-class doctors and medical students. While the bodies of criminals had been dissected for centuries, those of the innocent poor had not. Although paupers' graves were generally the first to be robbed, until 1832 the state treated this practice as immoral. It was not, however, illegal, as the dead body did not constitute property. The new act sanctioned the dissection of the poor; in doing so, critics insisted, the state confounded the "unclaimed" pauper with the criminal. In effect, the Anatomy Act made poverty a crime and the destitute dead body property of the state.[8] Not surprisingly, this only provoked working-class anxieties about the relationship between medicine and the state.

According to Ruth Richardson, the Anatomy Act "was in reality an advance clause to the New Poor Law." The 1834 New Poor Law represented an important move away from humanitarian approaches to the problems of poverty and toward a regime that privileged utilitarian economics over charitable impulses.[9] With its doctrine of "less eligibility" and its emphasis on institutionalization, the New Poor Law radically reformulated the philosophy of relief, attempting to force all recipients of Poor Law benefits into the workhouse. There administrators segregated the sexes, separated families, and outlawed personal belongings. These increased regulations made more severe the standard workhouse experience of grueling labor, poor food, and squalid living conditions. Rumors abounded regarding cruelty and cannibalism, tales that were passed along well into the late twentieth century, imprinting themselves on workhouse buildings long after they had ceased to serve the Poor Law.[10] Ironically, many of the myths that circulated about the terrors of the workhouse were encouraged by the Poor Law commissioners themselves.[11] Because the workhouses were intended to be the place of last resort, administrators rendered the workhouse regime undesirable and nurtured resistance to institutionalization to keep the number of those dependent on relief as low as possible. To the poor, these "bastiles" seemed little better than prisons, which, like the Anatomy Act, served to criminalize poverty.[12]

While the New Poor Law denied outdoor relief to the able-bodied pauper, it kept a system of outdoor *medical* relief in place, presided over by Poor Law medical officers who treated the sick poor out of the rates. By 1847, medical services had become a standard component of poor relief; by 1871, the Poor Law itself had "developed into the State medical authority for the poor."[13] However, some unions refused to provide this type of relief altogether, and many found the poor resistant to the pauperizing nature of Poor Law medicine. State medicine was born and nurtured, then, within a context already invested with contentious meanings. It was by definition pauperizing, and, its critics maintained, it shamed and punished precisely those whom it was intended to serve.

By the middle of the nineteenth century, the government was not only providing medical services, but also regulating those offered by private practitioners, for medical reform had become an ardent concern for many practitioners and parliamentarians. Although calls for improvement came from a number of directions, the most active agitators were general practitioners who felt unrepresented by any of the corporations. They opposed the power of the colleges and denounced the tripartite division as unrepresentative of medical practice. Despite internal conflicts, by the 1850s most medical practitioners could agree that change was necessary. Exactly what these reforms would look like was the subject of heated debate, but practitioners intent on making medicine more professional lobbied for a definition of a legally qualified practitioner as well as a centrally kept medical register. It would take a Select Committee in 1847, followed by fourteen medical-reform bills, before anything specific could be agreed on.[14]

The 1858 Medical Act emerged out of this debate. It established a General Council of Medical Education and Registration that united representatives of medical corporations into a single body to oversee medical education and licensing. It published a general register of qualified practitioners, meaning those with licenses from any corporation, although it did not distinguish between different types of practice. The Medical Act also restricted unregistered practitioners from government employment and from using titles such as physician, surgeon, doctor, and apothecary, without the corresponding license. Its reforms were limited, however, as it did not establish a uniform system of education or examination, and it continued to allow each corporation to grant its own licenses. Perhaps most significantly, it did not prevent unregistered practitioners from plying their trade.[15] The Medical Act was a compromise; it went only partway toward professionalizing medicine. But it was an important step in what was to be a long process of consolidating this authority, a process in which vaccination was to play a vital role. For vaccination, a technology of orthodox medicine, was the first medical intervention to be enforced by British law. The Compulsory Vaccination Act was thus crucial to the development of the field of state medicine, and thus to the rise of medical authority.

Compulsory Vaccination and the Medicalization of Public Health

Vaccination, as the first continuous public-health activity undertaken by the state, ushered in a new age in which the government began to provide health care to the general public.[16] Significantly, the policy of universal compulsory vaccination also marked an important shift away from sanitary approaches to the persistence of dirt and disease and toward preventive medicine. Compulsory vaccination was therefore central to the new state emphasis on scientific medicine as the key to public health.

THE SANITARY IDEA   The sanitary programs that Edwin Chadwick pioneered in the 1830s were essentially an institution of local government administered not by doctors but by bureaucrats. Their intent was to combat the urban problems of dirt and disease, but the solutions they offered were not primarily medical. Chadwick, former secretary to the Poor Law Commission, focused on reforming municipal and household technologies. Chadwick's "sanitary idea" became institutionalized in state-sponsored projects that culminated in the 1848 Public Health Act. This act established the General Board of Health, charged with administering local boards in the promotion of municipal sanitation. Since the establishment of local boards was entirely voluntary, few towns applied for a board, and fewer still could be encouraged to, as the General Board of Health seemed to be merely another "coercive central interference with local government."[17] According to Christopher Hamlin, this approach to public health concealed the relationship between disease and poverty, substituting toilets and sewers for any larger efforts to deal with social conditions. Public health took shape in Britain largely within discourses around sanitation that engaged with neither medical responses to disease nor the larger issue of poverty. An emphasis on sewers and public works does not necessitate a denial of the importance of food, work, and disease. But a decision to pursue the former was in this case also a conscious choice not to pursue the latter. Chadwick, Hamlin argues, suggested that "sewers and water were to end famine fevers, Chartist threats, drink, despair, and discontent, and to produce disciplined industrial laborers and happy proletarian families."[18]

Despite their emphasis on a seemingly apolitical plumbing infrastructure, the sanitary reforms of the early Victorian period deliberately exposed the bodies of the working classes to greater scrutiny and regulation. During the cholera and fever epidemics of the 1830s, '40s, and '50s, poor neighborhoods were labeled "fever dens." Sanitary bureaucrats perceived these areas as squalid and poorly ventilated and associated them with other sites of disease: prisons, charity hospitals, workshops, and workhouses. By implication, these administrators saw the

bodies of the working classes themselves as contagious and, like prisoners, patients, and paupers, in need of surveillance and control. This
manifested itself, among other ways, in the policing of poor neighborhoods by state-sanctioned medical officers of health, who quarantined
cholera patients and destroyed their property. For all the disinterested-
ness of sanitary-engineering schemes, public health in this period also
had a decidedly moral element, as it identified and tracked the "great
unwashed."[19]

Although highly influential, Chadwick's policies were not enough in
and of themselves to combat the enduring problems of urbanization.
While Chadwick and his sanitary technologies dominated the public-
health movement of the 1830s and '40s, it was John Simon, medical
officer of health for the City of London and then medical officer to the
Privy Council, and his epidemiological coterie who were to be the public face of public health in the 1850s and '60s. During the 1850s, medical doctors and their institutions, such as the Association of Medical
Officers and the British Medical Association, began to play more active
roles in turning the public's health into a scientific, and decidedly medical, pursuit.[20] Some practitioners even proposed that the safety of the
public depended on medical men obtaining seats in Parliament.[21] The
Public Health Act of 1858, which abolished Chadwick's Board of Health
and instead transferred Simon and certain health responsibilities to the
Privy Council, was passed in the same year as the Medical Act. By the
late 1850s, then, Parliament had helped to create a medical profession
and endowed it with the authority to superintend the health of the
nation. But it was the Compulsory Vaccination Act of 1853 that really
initiated—and, indeed, continues to epitomize—the medicalization of
public health.

THE COMPULSORY VACCINATION ACT OF 1853   When mandatory
infant vaccination was introduced in 1853, the practice was almost sixty
years old. Prior to the discovery of vaccination in the 1790s, the British
public had practiced variolation, or what was more commonly called
inoculation. Variolation was imported from Turkey by Lady Mary Wortley Montagu in the 1720s and was quickly absorbed into both elite and
popular healing practices.[22] It was a method of creating an immunity to
smallpox by artificially introducing, or "inoculating," the disease into

the system. The inoculated caught a mild case of smallpox but would be able to resist more severe attacks in the future. While many people condemned inoculation, by the early nineteenth century the practice had become embedded within popular medical culture. Roger Langdon, a station master and self-taught astronomer, recalled being "knockle-headed" in 1829 by Nanny Holland, the local "oracle," "quack doctor," midwife, bonesetter, and owner of the only bread oven in the village. Armed with an old knife, a razor blade, and a stocking needle, she created a hinged hole in the skin of his arm, which she then filled with smallpox matter as "a painter stopping a hole in a board with putty."[23] Clearly, inoculation had been understood by the laboring population as their own response to epidemic disease. Some inoculators, such as the father of the circus showman George Sanger, even produced their own medicine to accompany the procedure.[24] Inoculation was thus part and parcel of the vibrant self-help culture of healing that characterized the first half of the nineteenth century.

Vaccination was invented in the 1790s by Edward Jenner, a country surgeon. He observed that milkmaids who regularly came in contact with cows infected with vaccinia, more commonly called cowpox, rarely contracted smallpox. Jenner thus modified the practice of variolation by substituting cowpox for smallpox. His experiments revealed that inoculation with cowpox—or what he termed *vaccination*—provided the individual with a similar ability to ward off smallpox. Cowpox, however, caused only a mild reaction in humans and unlike smallpox is not transmissible from person to person. The practice of vaccination was thus based entirely on empirical evidence rather than on any theoretical understanding of immunity, for the science of the immune system was still a century away and depended, as chapter 6 will reveal, on the emergence of bacteriology. While vaccination quickly replaced variolation among medical practitioners, smallpox inoculation continued to be practiced by lay healers, not only because smallpox matter was much easier to obtain than vaccine, particularly in times of epidemic, but also because many people preferred to use what they considered "the real thing."[25]

By the early nineteenth century, supporters of vaccination among the medical community had embraced it to such a degree that they believed it was essential that it be encouraged and practiced by medical professionals. The 1840 report of the Provincial Medical and Surgical Association's Vaccination Committee alerted the association's members that vaccinations were being performed by "itinerating quacks, petty tradesmen of an inferior order, blacksmiths, excisemen, druggists, &c; the poor, one with another."[26] While the "safety and well-being of the community" may have been at the forefront of the minds of this committee, issues of professional control were equally important. As vaccination was a medical procedure, medical practitioners wanted to control it, not least because it could be a lucrative part of a practice. However, practitioners did offer their services free to the poor, including vaccination. Despite the efforts of the medical community, the report continued, "a very great proportion of poor remain unvaccinated."[27]

In 1840, in response to this report and similar pressure from medical practitioners, the British Parliament introduced free, voluntary vaccination targeted at the poor. The following year it criminalized variolation, as the government feared that the practice could contribute to, rather than arrest, the spread of smallpox. Significantly, however, inoculation was generally performed by paramedical personnel such as Nanny Holland, who were in direct competition with vaccinating doctors. Indeed, doctors consistently depicted inoculation as a feminine, foreign, folk practice in contrast to vaccination, which they construed as masculine, English, and expert.[28] This effort to encourage the poor to be vaccinated by governmentally employed practitioners, while at the same time criminalizing inoculation, proved largely unsuccessful. The laboring population generally preferred paying "a dissenting minister, a blacksmith, a miller, [or] an old woman" to inoculate them to seeking out the services of a Poor Law medical officer.[29] As F. B. Smith has argued, "Inoculation among neighbours, performed by a local house doctor, wise woman, preacher or itinerant quack, was a shared, understood procedure. Incision by a barely known person with superior status was neither shared not reassuring."[30]

The 1840 act was thus a resounding failure. In an 1851 letter to Viscount Palmerston, who was to become Home Secretary the following year, Edward Seaton lamented that the "lower and uneducated classes" were not taking advantage of the free service. While he registered their vehement prejudice against the operation, Seaton, a doctor and an epidemiologist, insisted that their excuses stemmed merely from "indolence and indifference." Whenever the alarm of epidemic was raised, he declared, they ran straight to the vaccinators.[31] Seaton followed this report with another in 1853 that warned that in certain districts, vaccination was being carried out at "dispensaries, at iron-works, in clubs, and so on where other than the public vaccinators are employed."[32] Seaton expressed, then, both a social concern with the spread of disease and a professional concern with control of the procedure.

Seaton was a member of the Epidemiological Society of London, which Simon and other notable medical men had founded in 1850 to bring public health more in line with the "teachings of science." As its name suggests, the society's object was to "endeavour by the light of modern science to review all those causes which result in the manifestation and spread of epidemic diseases."[33] While the society was initially formed in response to cholera, which reached epidemic proportions in 1848–49 and again in 1853–54, it also assembled committees on fever and epizootic diseases. But its most public concern remained smallpox. Although a disfiguring and often fatal disease, smallpox had been on the decline since the late eighteenth century, due in part to the practices of inoculation and vaccination but also to variations in the virulence of the virus strain.[34] It trailed far behind measles, scarlet fever, whooping cough, enteric fever, diarrhea, dysentery, and cholera as a leading cause of death.[35] But if cholera was more problematic than smallpox in 1853, it was also more confusing. The medical journal *The Lancet* demanded satirically that year: "Is it a fungus, an insect, a miasma, an electrical disturbance, a deficiency of ozone, a morbid off-scouring from the intestinal canal? We know nothing; we are at sea in a whirlpool of conjecture."[36] Although little could be done to arrest the spread of cholera,[37] medical experts and their parliamentary allies believed that compulsory vaccination could be an effective way of attempting to reduce smallpox morbidity.

The Epidemiological Society's Smallpox and Vaccination Committee was chaired by Seaton, who was soon to become a world-renowned expert on vaccination. For pro-vaccinationists such as Seaton, the issue was clear: Smallpox posed a serious danger to the national community, as it was extremely contagious and, if not fatal, certainly disfiguring. Vaccination, the Epidemiological Society argued, had proved to be an effective preventative and was therefore the best way to arrest the spread of disease, thereby protecting society from its ravages. Since the diseased individual was "a centre of contagion," and every unvaccinated population a "nidus for the disease to settle in and propagate itself," only compulsory vaccination could ensure the health of the social body.[38] Nobody, the Epidemiological Society argued, should be able to jeopardize the lives of others. They proposed, therefore, a compulsory vaccination act, applicable to all infants in England and Wales and carrying penalties for noncompliance.

While Seaton's committee had been investigating the workings of the 1840 act, Lord Lyttleton, an advocate of Poor Law reform and working men's clubs, had independently been drafting a compulsory vaccination bill. The Epidemiological Society's report persuaded him to reconsider his initial formulation, and in consultation with Seaton's committee he "very materially altered" the bill.[39] In spring 1853, at a poorly attended late-night session of Parliament, Lyttleton's bill passed with little debate, although he admitted to relying solely on information provided by the society, having no knowledge of vaccination himself.[40] In short, the Epidemiological Society, staffed by Seaton and Simon (who was also to be heavily involved in formulating the Medical Act), was authority enough.

This act, while introducing mandatory universal infant vaccination, nevertheless explicitly targeted the poor and working classes. Lyttleton claimed that in introducing the bill he sought to increase the facilities for vaccination among "the poorer classes."[41] The poor, Seaton maintained four years later, needed to be compelled to vaccinate, as they were apathetic, indifferent, and neglectful parents. Implicit in the professional and institutional desire "to protect children from negligent parents," therefore, was the assumption that it was the poor who were the most likely to spread disease and the least likely to vaccinate, being too "engrossed in procuring bread" to think about the health and safety of their children, let alone of the wider community.[42] The Compulsory Vaccination Act of 1853 thus aimed to secure the vaccination of those children whose parents were not taking advantage of the free service provided by the Poor Law medical officers. For this reason, despite the fact that all babies were now required to be vaccinated, public vaccination continued to be administered by the Poor Law and targeted at the lower classes.

PROFESSIONALIZING VACCINATION   As the first medical technol-ogy that could claim to prevent the spread of infectious disease, vaccina-tion embodied the promise of scientific medicine as the route to public health. While the Compulsory Vaccination Act was not the first health legislation passed by Parliament, no other laws were as wide-reaching or invasive, and none had so clearly been brokered by doctors. By mak-ing vaccination mandatory, and delivering it by way of government employees, the Compulsory Vaccination Act wedded preventive medi-cine to the state. Eager to defend their new role in preserving the pub-lic's health, doctors became highly concerned about their institutional authority in these years. The provision of vaccination thus became em-broiled in larger debates over professionalization.

While general practitioners in particular widely agreed that vaccina-tion was a medical preserve, the details of its provision left much to be desired. The *Associated Medical Journal* (precursor to the *British Medical Journal*) argued that compulsory vaccination meant more work without proper remuneration. In the months before and after passage of the bill, the *Associated Medical Journal* received many letters from irate med-ical practitioners who objected, among other things, to filling out forms without compensation. Initially, it was unclear who would be autho-rized to serve as a public vaccinator. Some doctors worried that they would be compelled to vaccinate an unwilling public and in the process lose their clientele to those not associated with the procedure. A corre-spondent to *The Lancet* in 1853 expressed a prescient concern that the operation would be seen as "an act of oppression and tyranny on the part of the vaccinator, and will convert the practitioner . . . into an agent of aggression." Others feared the opposite—that they themselves would lose business to these new government employees, insisting, to little avail, that all general practitioners also be appointed public vaccina-tors.[43]

In the end, while permitting all practitioners to vaccinate, the law limited the number of public vaccinators who could bill the state for their services and stipulated that these government employees must be "legally qualified medical professionals."[44] The irony of this lay in the fact that, in 1853, exactly what a legally qualified medical professional *was* remained under negotiation. It was not until the Medical Act was passed five years later that any attempt was made to define this term. Furthermore, even licensed practitioners may not have been able to claim any more knowledge or skill in this area than the "unqualified." As a correspondent to *The Lancet* noted in 1853, "[T]here is no such thing as either authoritative teaching or requisite examination on the theory and practice of vaccination" at any hospital or medical school.[45] No matter how one defined a professional, none would be technically qualified to perform the procedure. Not until 1867 was a certificate of proficiency in vaccination required from all public vaccinators, and even then exemptions were granted to those who had already demonstrated this as a component of their medical degree.

Having the technical skill to vaccinate, however, was less troublesome to doctors than having the professional authority to do so. Since the 1840s, doctors had been threatened by the variety of lay and heterodox medical practitioners who also performed vaccinations. They supported making vaccination a service of the state precisely because this allowed it to be more closely regulated and restricted exclusively to so-called medical professionals. In November 1853, a Dr. Watts complained to the Poor Law Board that the public vaccinator for his Staffordshire town was a Mr. Kettle, "a Druggist who has not a single qualification, and who is performing the duties to the disgust of everyone." But since Kettle had been employed since 1844, the Poor Law Board saw no reason to intervene. The following year, a surgeon in Glossop protested that a male midwife was vaccinating a steady stream of children; his only qualification was a diploma from Giessen, "obtained by fraud and with a forged apothecaries certificate."[46] Doctors' ongoing concern thus remained how to squeeze "clergymen, amateurs, druggists, old women, midwives" out of the vaccination trade and, in the process, out of the business of medicine entirely.[47]

Medical Resistance at Midcentury

At the moment that compulsory vaccination was passed into law, it was unlikely that the laboring classes routinely consulted regular orthodox practitioners. The "sick poor" were relieved by Poor Law medical officers. The more fortunate sought the advice of herbalists, chemists, and druggists or consulted the local midwife. Some may also have used a voluntary hospital or public dispensary, institutions largely funded through charitable donations and accessible to those with a letter of recommendation from a benefactor. But most medical care, at least, until World War I, happened within the home. Mothers pulled teeth with thread and used paraffin to destroy lice and nits. They practiced home remedies and dosed their children with licorice powders and cod-liver oil to maintain regularity. Even for those on limited budgets, a degree of choice in medical matters remained in the 1850s, and the Victorian laboring classes were often able to consult a variety of practitioners, as did their Georgian counterparts. But with the professionalization of orthodox medicine and its attempt to control the provision of medical services, many people felt that their health-care choices were becoming limited and decried the disappearance of the medical marketplace.

THE RISE OF ALTERNATIVE MEDICINE   From the 1840s, the drive toward professionalization had stimulated a parallel rise in medical theories and therapies belligerently opposed to orthodox medicine. Alternative medicine—such as medical botany, hydropathy, homoeopathy, and mesmerism—flourished in the 1850s. While strands of homoeopathy, mesmerism, and water cure did have a decidedly middle-class following, many forms of alternative medicine specifically catered to a plebeian audience. Medical botany, hydropathy, hygieanism, and other hybrid sects that promoted natural remedies and self-medication spoke directly and self-consciously to a working- and lower-middle-class public.[48] These practitioners and their followers invoked the doctrines of laissez-faire economics, arguing that medicine was a service to be traded freely on the open market.[49] While laissez-faire was a decidedly middle-class liberal doctrine, it also had wider resonance. The Medical Act appeared to the working class as an extension of the reforms of the 1830s that privileged middle-class practitioners who seemed to be seeking control over all types of health care, and thus over all kinds of bodies. It was these medical reformers who publicized the concept of "medical liberty" and furnished anti-vaccinationism with its earliest support.

As orthodox medicine was attempting to assert its legitimacy and monopoly over medical practice and theory, so alternative medicine challenged and resisted this dominance. The 1850s mark only the very beginning of orthodox medicine's consolidation of its authority. What the British system for the provision of medical care in the modern period would look like remained open to debate. Alternative medicine attracted a large following by promoting a self-help culture of healing and by offering its patients a different and generally more holistic approach to sickness and health. More to the point, alternative medicine, unlike quackery, was self-defining in that it consciously constructed itself in belligerent opposition to orthodox doctors.

Although Victorian heterodox medicine was not a unified movement, many of these sects had common features. Their medical philosophy tended to reduce all complaints to one particular and fundamental problem that usually involved the balance of one or more vital fluids. Thus, they treated the body as a whole system, seeking to redress this imbalance. In addition, these practitioners generally sought the active participation of patients in the healing process.[50] Significantly, these movements also shared a combative relationship to allopathic orthodox medicine. The similarities between these sects encouraged them to form a supportive community of medical dissenters who communicated through the pages of a vibrant alternative medical press. In the 1850s, anti-vaccination sentiment helped to cement these alliances, drawing these movements together by providing a single issue around which to agitate.

Like some forms of religious dissent, medical dissent appealed largely to the ranks of laborers, artisans, and tradesmen and attracted an already politicized following.[51] Many Chartists and Owenites turned to medical reform in the years after 1848 as their own movements saw a rapid decline. The medical botanist John Skelton, a former shoemaker, had been an active Chartist leader; his Six Propositions of vegetable medicine echoed the six points of the People's Charter.[52] These reformers not only were radicals, a political position shared by a somewhat diverse group of nineteenth-century activists, but often defined themselves in classed terms. Skelton maintained that his followers were "generally of the working class"; so, too, a water-cure journal claimed that hydropathy had taken hold among the "London Working Classes."[53] But exactly what it meant to belong to a working class was something still being negotiated (or, more precisely, renegotiated) in this period, in part in relation to medical dissent. In fact, as chapter 4 will argue, these movements helped to shape the production of a working-class identity by locating class consciousness in shared bodily experience.

Alternative medical practitioners consistently claimed that orthodox medicine was a tyrannical system of state-sanctioned interference with the lives and health of an oppressed people. Practitioners of alternative medicine fought loudly for medical pluralism. "Shall GOVERNMENT decide the particular method which shall be adopted in the cure of disease," queried *Dr. Skelton's Botanic Record and Family Herbal,* or should each person have the right "to select for himself whatever medical attendant he may think proper to employ agreeable with *his own views,* desires, feelings, and convictions"?[54] While most sects promoted their medical theories and practices as the best route to health, none suggested that their system retain a monopoly. Alternative practitioners understood access to medical care as a political issue on par with that of the Corn Laws, an earlier radical cause: "let us say with this as we have with corn, FREE TRADE and no monopoly."[55] Since medicine, like corn, was a consumer good, heterodox practitioners insisted that it should remain unregulated. If this appeal reflected a commitment to the ideology of laissez-faire, it also revealed their investment in the commerce of medicine. Even alternative practitioners, who generally sought to make medical practice easier and cheaper, could not resist the opportunity to profit from the ills of others by selling patent pills and anti-venereal powders. Regulation, they feared, would certainly put a swift end to the lucrative trade in medicines.

It was not only that their preferred medical attendants and products were disappearing from the marketplace, but also that patients, particularly working-class patients, were losing the ability to negotiate the appropriate treatment. Primitive man, argued the *Botanic Eclectic Review and Medical Tribune,* was not "bound to employ a medical tyro, to bleed, blister, cup, salivate with mercury, (a direful poison), and lacerate his system against his own inclination."[56] Orthodox medicine in the 1850s was still based largely on heroic therapies and thus seemed threatening and intrusive. While medical science in the early nineteenth century was "progressing at an unprecedentedly rapid rate," therapeutics—what the physician could actually do for a patient—was at a standstill.[57] Bloodletting and drugging remained the norm, and toxic medicines such as opium and mercury were standard prescriptions. This meant that the side effects of the treatment could be as bad as the disease itself, and patients were constantly at risk of a lethal dosage. The medical botanist Albert Isaiah Coffin attacked the use of these medications as ludicrous: "Twice two will not make five is a fact not more evident than that which will kill cannot be expected to cure."[58]

While the pharmacopoeia of alternative medicine was often as purgative as that of orthodox practice, alternative practitioners appealed to the healing powers of nature in an effort to contrast gentle herbs with damaging minerals. For these reformers, medicine was essentially a healing art rather than a scientific pursuit. It was not that the heterodoxies attacked science per se, for they also staked a claim to scientifically provable therapies. Rather, they objected to scientific experimentation on the human body. "Our object is to cure," Coffin claimed, "and not to delight ourselves in torturing experiments upon our fellow creatures."[59] Death was more valuable than life to regular doctors, medical dissenters maintained, because scientific medicine had become preoccupied with performing autopsies. "What sensible man," demanded Coffin, "can admire the policy of cutting up a body after death, in order to ascertain the nature of the malady of which the patient died?"[60] As we shall see, this was particularly resonant in an age that saw heated controversy over the use of animals for scientific experimentation. In light of the Anatomy Act, these fears seem understandable, for as the hygiest John Morison argued in 1833, "There has been no end to [doctors'] fruitless tortures, trials, and experiments on the human body."[61]

Doctors were able to carry out these "impositions," dissenters argued, by keeping the public both ignorant and in awe of their scientific expertise. For Coffin, science was no more than "a tissue of incongruities, interwoven with the obsolete and unmeaning language of the schools of antiquity." Its sole purpose was to "confer wealth on a few individuals" while "throwing dust into the eyes of the people."[62] Coffin identified mystification as the backbone of the orthodox monopoly that sought not to educate the people but, rather, to keep the secrets of the body "inviolate." While heterodox medicine was openly critical of the practices of its orthodox counterpart, it also maintained that all should have access to this knowledge.

The language of alternative medicine was not unlike that of other radical reform movements of the early nineteenth century. It expressed a "democratic epistemology," which included a fervent belief that knowledge should be available to all.[63] "To mystify, shut up in the schools, and make private property of that knowledge, which of all others ought to be universally taught is a wrong the deepest and most injurious to society," argued Skelton.[64] Access to education was key to this movement, for knowledge lay at the root of all political action. Since orthodox medical terminology was based on Latin, its use was necessarily reserved for the classically educated elite. For alternative practitioners, this language was unnecessarily esoteric and served merely as obfuscation. It had no purpose, they argued, other than to undermine the intellectual authority of the people to prevent them from acting as their own physicians.

For these reasons, heterodox medicine presented its followers with an easily explainable etiology of illness and sought remedies that seemed gentler and more "natural." As members of an early "nature cure" movement, these health reformers, though followers of distinct sects, shared a belief that disease is not a foreign entity to be suppressed but, rather, the body's attempt to throw off impurities derived from unhealthy habits such as intemperance or a flesh-based diet.[65] Most alternative philosophies of health and sickness proposed that disease had a sole root cause, generally relating to the circulation of the blood. For medical botanists, disease was caused by an obstruction in the blood that cooled the body. Cures could be found in herbs such as cayenne pepper and *lobelia inflata*, which produced heat to dislodge the obstruction. Similarly, both hydropathy and hygeianism proposed that health was directly related to the purity of the blood.

To make bodily processes easier to understand, the heterodoxies generally used vernacular language and self-consciously accessible analogies drawn from the experiences of laboring life. Coffin compared the stomach to a gristmill, arguing that "to obtain good flour it is necessary in the first instance the corn be good."[66] Alternative medicine's language and its generalized theories of disease served a political purpose, for they were easy to understand and thus available to all. It was through self-help—particularly collective self-help, these reformers maintained—that the poor and laboring classes would inevitably throw off the "yoke of medical bondage."[67]

Alternative medicine was physic for the people. It insisted that every man and woman could and should be his or her own doctor. The idea of self-help was not new or novel. Self-help had been advocated since the Reformation and re-emerged in the nineteenth century not only as a middle-class principle, but also as a working-class response to their own needs and goals.[68] The doctrine of self-help was central to most types of alternative medicine. Medical botany fiercely promoted self-medication and self-diagnosis, and hydropaths, hygiests, and the like encouraged their patients to become heavily involved in their own treatment. According to the veteran water-cure practitioner Mary Nichols, the first object of hydropathy "is to teach patients to cure themselves—to make them independent of us."[69]

Alternative medicine seemed less invasive precisely because it was often self-administered. Thus, it contrasted sharply with orthodox medicine, which was practiced by members of another class who appeared to be bent on demonstrating their social rank. While regular doctors in the mid–Victorian period were overwhelmingly middle to lower middle class, the rhetoric of alternative medicine imagined them as aristocratic tricksters. Skelton maintained that physic was a "genteel profession" practiced by "compounds of *cigars* and *cognac*."[70] These "emancipated Barbers," he argued, were bent not only on swindling, but on torturing and murdering their poorer patients with the tacit approval of Parliament. The medical reformer John Stevens openly criticized the violence of orthodox therapies and the difficulty of resisting treatment. "The tax-gatherer," he argued "raps at your door" and demands his due. But "the licensed to kill" enters the home and exercises "his exclusive right over the prostrate victim, whose blood he draws, whose frame he tortures, whose bowels he secretly poisons, and whose disease he cures, or, at his will, prolongs." The doctor, Stevens claimed, was exempt from the "charge of murder or manslaughter." It was this professional "monopoly," he maintained, that prevented people from "administering to each other" in times of illness, "a violation of the first impulse of domestic love and the most important dictates of christian duty."[71] According to Stevens, then, orthodox medicine was worse than taxes. It was not only dangerous, but certainly fatal. Indeed, he argued, it was precisely by enacting horrific therapies that doctors could display their privilege. General resistance to orthodox medicine drew support by articulating the vulnerability of the body in relationship to an increasingly powerful "State-nursed-corporation-protected-faculty."[72]

ANTI-VACCINATIONISM AND ALTERNATIVE MEDICINE Anti-vaccinationism was thus easily absorbed into this alternative medical ideology. For many practitioners, it epitomized the "despotism" not only of state-sanctioned but also of state-enforced medicine. The first public protest against the Compulsory Vaccination Act came from John Gibbs, the teetotal son of an Irish captain, in an 1854 pamphlet entitled *Our Medical Liberties*. From 1843 to 1847, Gibbs had trained as a hydro-path in Silesia under Vincent Priessnitz, the father of water cure.[73] When he returned to England to open a hydropathic establishment at Barking, Gibbs brought with him more than specialized training. His stay in central Europe contributed to his patriotic appreciation of the rights of the "British freeman" and the glories of English justice.

Our Medical Liberties denounced the 1853 act as the "*first direct aggression upon the person of the subject in medical matters*, which has been attempted in these kingdoms."[74] Vaccination was an attack on the physical person, the conscience, and the religious beliefs of British citizens, Gibbs argued. The "lower classes" were particularly vulnerable under this legislation, for, he maintained, the compulsory clauses were aimed at and affected chiefly the laboring population. Gibbs complained that the "Profession" denied the "masses" access to any knowledge of the procedure, preferring "mystery and concealment" over attempts "to popularise medical science." Our "rulers," he argued, "deem it easier to coerce than to convince." Vaccination legislation, Gibbs concluded, was tyrannical, unchristian, and decidedly un–English. It smacked not of English liberty but, rather, of the centralization and regulation of continental nations. "Has England become an Austrian province," Gibbs demanded, "or have our rulers imported an Austrian police?"[75]

Gibbs's attack on the Compulsory Vaccination Act circulated quickly through alternative medical circles. The following year, he transformed it into a letter to Parliament. *Compulsory Vaccination Briefly Considered in Its Scientific, Religious, and Political Aspects* was addressed to Sir Benjamin Hall, president of the General Board of Health. Released in pamphlet form in 1856, *Compulsory Vaccination*'s critique of government medicine reached a large audience both inside and outside the Houses of Parliament. In fact, Gibbs's letter was influential enough to contribute to the defeat of two more vaccination bills introduced in 1856 and 1857 by stoking the ire of parliamentarians who were already resistant to anything emanating from the General Board of Health.[76] For a brief moment it seemed that many politicians agreed with Thomas Slingsby Duncombe, radical M P for Finsbury, that it was time to "take the Parliamentary lancet out of the national arm."[77]

During the 1850s and '60s, the anti-vaccination cause was taken up by many alternative practitioners, for, as Gibbs declared, "a belief in vaccination is at variance with the theories of all the 'pathies' and 'isms.' "[78] That said, anti-vaccinationism was the intellectual property of no one heterodoxy and in fact failed to establish itself among middle-class mesmerists and homoeopaths. The former seemed largely uninterested in the debate while the latter often adopted vaccination as perfect proof of their own theory that like cured like. Nevertheless, opposition to compulsory vaccination helped consolidate ties between alternative sects and gave medical dissent in this period a discrete and focused goal.

Compulsory vaccination provoked heated discussions in the pages of the heterodox press. Alternative medical journals provided a forum for members of varied sects to debate the issue, to advertise anti-vaccination meetings, and to sell their pamphlets. The *Hydropathic Record*, a water-cure journal, heavily supported the campaign and in the 1860s publicized the activities of the first anti-vaccination league.[79] Skelton often reprinted letters from Gibbs in his *Botanic Record* revealing that, though they may have differed on points of medical theory, they shared each other's larger commitment to free trade in medicine and considered themselves "co-worker[s] in the cause."[80] It was a "tyrannical oppression," argued the *Botanic Eclectic Review*, to be forced to "lacerate" one's system.[81] Skelton's son, also named John, lectured in the late 1850s on the evils of compulsory vaccination and started another short-lived journal to which Gibbs became a frequent correspondent.[82]

To promote a series of letters on anti-vaccinationism, the hygiest John Morison produced an illustration titled, "John Bull in His Medical Fetters" (see Figure 1). In the illustration, a plump and portly John Bull is tied up by doctors and bound by the straps of "vaccine poison," "pharmaceutical poisons," "medical despotism," and "fees." The graphic clearly illustrates the centrality of anti-vaccinationism to Morison's larger critique of orthodox medicine. The *Hygiest or Medical Reformer*, the journal of Morison's movement, was subtitled "Defender of Liberty of Conscience and Private Judgment," a direct reference to the coerciveness of state vaccination. Every issue devoted several articles and letters to compulsory vaccination. Here medical reformers suggested that vaccination benefited only doctors as it produced a sicklier population.[83]

Alternative practitioners opposed both the politics of compulsion and the technology of vaccination itself. Vaccination, they insisted, was a blood poisoner. Since these forms of alternative medicine stressed the importance of good blood to a healthy body, the introduction of any foreign material into the system was immediately suspect. Cowpox, they maintained, disrupted the blood and threatened to corrupt the system; thus, Coffin denounced vaccination as a "mysterious nostrum."[84] Correspondence and editorials to the *Hygiest* warned that vaccination led to the "degeneration of the human race" through blood pollution.[85] In addition, vaccination not only polluted the blood with animal material, they maintained, but spread dangerous diseases such as scrofula and syphilis.

Heterodox practitioners argued that vaccination was not only dangerous but unnecessary. Smallpox, they proposed, could be prevented by alternative means: Keep the body clean, eat wholesome foods, and breathe plenty of fresh air, they advised, and health would follow. Toward the end of the century, these practitioners also began to offer curative remedies. Disciples of James Morison at the British College of Health claimed in the 1860s that "Mr. Morison's Medicines" could keep the body in health and serve as a natural preventive against smallpox, while the homoeopath J. J. Garth Wilkinson endorsed the use of cream of tartar.[86] Hydropaths, like Gibbs himself, proposed that water cure could treat smallpox by drawing the poison out through the skin. During the Gloucester epidemic of 1895–96, the hydropath John Pickering successfully treated over 100 smallpox victims free of charge, most of whom had previously been vaccinated.[87] Thus, to alternative practitioners, vaccination was not only dangerous but entirely unnecessary.

By focusing medical debate on a single issue, then, anti-vaccinationism brought discrete but intellectually similar movements together. It did

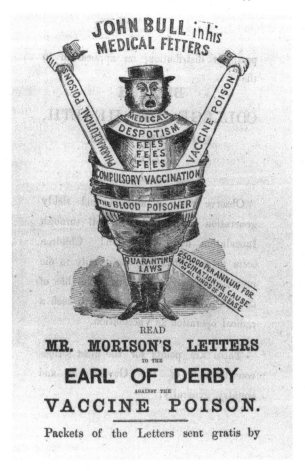

1. "John Bull in His Medical Fetters," c. 1866.
By permission of the Bodleian Library, University of Oxford,
John Johnson Collection, Societies Box 5.

so by uniting them behind a cause that was part and parcel of a wider concern with the power of both professionalizing medicine and the expanding Victorian state. This early resistance is crucial to understanding the intellectual and social roots of later protest and reveals an alternative genealogy for the anti-vaccination campaign. Anti-vaccinationism was adopted by middle-class reformers in the 1870s as part of philanthropic and social-reform efforts; however, working- and lower-middle-class involvement in the campaign has a different history. It grew out of these well-established traditions of medical dissent that pitted the people against the alliance of orthodox medicine and a bureaucratic state.

The 1850s was a crucial decade, then, both for the formulation of vaccination policy and for its early opposition. It was at this moment that the field of state medicine began to develop and thus that alternative healers felt most professionally threatened, and the public most physically vulnerable. But a national and enforceable program of compulsory vaccination was still over a decade away. It was not until the late 1860s that the state actually compelled the public to vaccinate through threat of fine and imprisonment, and thus that opponents launched an organized anti-vaccination campaign.

2

Fighting the "Babies' Battle"

Our cause is the cause of the suffering

little ones, the cause of the oppressed poor,

the sacred cause of freedom in the home. No

nobler fight is being fought than this our babies'

battle: no appeal more tender than that of the

boundless pathos of an infant's trust.

— *Vaccination Inquirer*, 1899

☞ While vaccination had been compulsory since 1853, it was not regularly or consistently enforced until the late 1860s, when the administrative machinery for policing it was set into place. With more effective means of implementing vaccination came an increase in public resistance, both to the procedure itself and to the principle of compulsion. The anti-vaccination movement, while born in the 1850s, took shape in the late 1860s and early '70s as resisters responded to what they considered an increasingly coercive vaccination policy. The anti-vaccination campaign was an organized national movement with a leadership who coordinated events and the dissemination of propaganda. But its success depended on grassroots resistance that took the form of local demonstrations and individual acts of civil disobedience. Anti-vaccinationism was thus both a coherent campaign for the repeal of the vaccination acts and a series of local and individual initiatives aimed at circumventing the law and disrupting the proper functioning of the vaccination administration.

The Organized Campaign

Historians of anti-vivisection, the temperance agitation, and the campaign against the contagious diseases acts have all recognized anti-vaccinationism as a similar and typical political pressure group built, like the others, on the foundation laid by the abolitionist cause.[1] Anti-vaccinationists also capitalized on the success of Victorian friendly societies and spiritualist, vegetarian, Owenite, Chartist, and temperance associations, forming leagues to organize against the vaccination acts. These leagues distributed membership cards and organized debates, concerts, conversaziones, tea parties, and mass meetings in Temperance Halls and Corn and Cotton Exchanges. By the 1860s, anti-vaccinationism was a national movement; over the course of the next three decades, almost 200 of these local anti-vaccination leagues were formed from Newcastle to Plymouth. The movement's strongest support came from the industrial North, particularly the cluster of Lancashire factory towns in the square bounded by Blackpool, Leeds, Sheffield, and Liverpool. While these societies were not all operative at the same time, and some may have lasted only a few years, the sheer numbers of people involved in these organizations was significant, and their geographical distribution impressive.[2]

The earliest leagues were branches of the Anti-Compulsory Vaccination League (ACVL), the first anti-vaccination society. The ACVL was formed at Finsbury in 1866 under the direction of Richard Butler Gibbs, the noted vegetarian and food reformer.[3] Members of the ACVL included, among others, the rest of the Gibbs family—Richard's wife, who formed the Mothers' Anti-Compulsory Vaccination League; his brother George, an accountant and statistician; and their cousin John, author of the first anti-vaccination pamphlet. By 1870, the ACVL had 103 branch leagues, and the following year it claimed 10,000 members, which was optimistically raised to 200,000 if one included sympathizers.[4] However, the death of Richard Butler Gibbs in 1871, and the cessation of the *Anti-Vaccinator and Public Health Journal* in 1873, a periodical devoted to the campaign, caused a lull in the movement.

Organized anti-vaccinationism was soon revived by Mary and William Hume-Rothery. Mary Hume-Rothery was the daughter of the Benthamite Liberal MP Joseph Hume; her husband, William Hume-Rothery, was an Anglican minister, although he divested himself of his orders in 1876.⁵ The Hume-Rotherys were typical Victorian reformers active in the repeal of the contagious diseases acts, the campaign against compulsory education, and the Anti-Mourning Society, which was aimed at reducing the excesses and expense of Victorian funerals and mourning practices. In 1874, they established the National Anti-Compulsory Vaccination League (NACVL) at their home in Cheltenham. In the same year, they began to issue an *Occasional Circular*, which eventually became the monthly *National Anti-Compulsory Vaccination Reporter*. While the Hume-Rotherys established several branch leagues throughout England, the tone of their protest alienated much of the working-class anti-vaccination constituency that came to the cause from an interest in alternative medicine or through other dissenting movements.

In fact, the Hume-Rotherys often patronized and disparaged precisely the constituency they claimed to serve. While Mary Hume-Rothery argued that the vaccination acts were framed in the interests of the "luxurious classes" as against "the mass of intelligent working classes," elsewhere she rebuked the laboring classes. "[O]ur working classes," she complained in 1882, would happily strike and sacrifice their families' income, for a shilling more in pay or an hour less work, but would not donate even a trifle to the NACVL. "Are beer and tobacco more precious to them than the health and lives of their children?"⁶ The Hume-Rotherys pleaded for funds from the working classes but at the same time denied the unenfranchised any meaningful role in the campaign, for they argued that the vote was the best, and perhaps only, means for change. While the 1867 Reform Act had incorporated many more voters into the polity, many working men in both urban and rural districts, and all women, did not have the vote. Even with the passage of the Third Reform Act in 1884, some working-class men and all women remained unenfranchised. According to the NACVL, then, real political change could come only from middle- and lower-middle-class male voters. In addition, the NACVL did nothing to materially help its fellow resisters. In 1873, the *Anti-Vaccinator and Public Health Journal* characterized the more radical Anti-Compulsory Vaccination and Mutual Protection Society (ACVMPS), run by the pharmaceutical chemist William

Young, as a "Working Men's Club," as it agreed to pay the fines for noncompliance imposed on the poor. The Hume-Rotherys refused to do the same. This proved especially problematic as the ACVMPS frequently received donations intended for the NACVL.[7]

In the end, Young's marriage of sympathetic engagement and practical financial aid enabled his new league, the London Society for the Abolition of Compulsory Vaccination (LSACV), to compete successfully with the NACVL for control of the movement. The LSACV was established in February 1880 under the leadership of William Tebb, an abolitionist and merchant; William White, a Swedenborgian bookseller; and Young. The LSACV took over production of the *Vaccination Inquirer*, which had first appeared in 1879 under the editorship of White and which soon became the organ for the national repeal campaign. The LSACV's troika of Tebb, White, and Young was more socially diverse than the firmly middle-class Hume-Rotherys, who fiercely resisted the LSACV's independence and tried unsuccessfully to incorporate it into their own organization. Tebb was a wealthy merchant, and White and Young seem to have belonged to a growing and socially mobile lower middle class. This enabled the LSACV to attract a wider following, but ultimately its leaders had little in common with the working class they sought to represent. While it was relatively successful in cultivating working-class support, the LSACV nevertheless shifted focus away from local and thus popular agitation toward national and parliamentary solutions. Under Tebb's guidance, the LSACV lobbied for a government inquiry and focused its initial attention on the recruitment of influential parliamentarians, administrators, and doctors to the repeal campaign.[8] In 1896, as the Royal Commission on Vaccination—charged with investigating the value of vaccination and its compulsory clauses—was releasing its final report, the LSACV dissolved to form the National Anti-Vaccination League (NAVL). The NAVL was an alliance of local leagues across the United Kingdom that sought to combine their funds and efforts to present a united front at a key moment in the anti-vaccination campaign.

While the importance of these national leagues and their leadership cannot be overlooked, resistance to compulsory vaccination was mobilized by a much broader public than that represented by either the leagues or their leaders. If anti-vaccinationism was a national move-

ment, it operated as a series of largely local and not necessarily organized initiatives and thus involved many more people than league
membership may at first suggest. Looking back from the 1940s, the
medical officer of health for the anti-vaccination stronghold of Leicester
from 1901 to 1935 maintained that "it would be a mistake to regard this
widespread hostility to vaccination as merely the result of organized
agitation." Instead, he argued, it was primarily due to the personal
experiences of many individuals who believed that vaccination had injured their children.[9]

A Community of Dissent

Anti-vaccinators were largely drawn from the ranks of laborers, artisans,
and small shopkeepers. They were grocers and clerks, factory operatives
and journeymen artisans, tradesmen and travelers, sectarian ministers
and shoemakers, wage laborers and their wives.[10] Anti-vaccinationism
flourished among the working class and members of both the labor aristocracy and the lower middle class, groups whose boundaries in this
period were permeable and fluid.[11] The movement appealed to this
plebeian public who already felt vulnerable to exploitation within Britain's industrial economy and garnered support from causes with similar concerns. By the 1860s, anti-vaccinationism had not only cemented
its relationship to alternative medicine, but it had also firmly established
itself within a larger culture of dissent. It found allies within other
movements by tapping into concerns over working-class exploitation,
and it was seized on as a resource by an enthusiastic group of progressive and humanitarian activists who added the anti-vaccination cause to
their social and political agendas. Working-class autobiographies at-
test to the strength of these relationships. Frank Goss remembered that
at the turn of the century, his father, a piano maker, supported "Vegetarianism, anti-vivisectionism, spiritualism, anti-vaccination, teetotalism, and a host of other humanitarian, altruistic and abstract tribu-
taries of thought." Similarly, Ifan Edwards recounted that his father was
committed to food reform, anti-vaccination, and the Swedenborgian
religion.[12]

Edwards, however, dismissed his father's enthusiasms as "cranky," as did many who feared the strength of popular pressure groups who, while committed to single-issue campaigns, also united together to champion a range of related causes. Indeed, anti-vaccinators were often attacked as anti-everything "cranks." "They are anti-alcoholists, anti-tobaccoists, anti-opiumists, vegetarians, homoeopaths, Matteists," maintained one such critic. "[They] have a natural taste for theosophy, hypnotism, and spookism, and are generally of fads and fancies all compact."[13] Similarly, the journalist Blanchard Jerrold critiqued anti-vaccinationists as victims of "public opinion," manipulated into fighting for any cause. The anti-vaccination leagues, he proclaimed in 1883, belonged in the company of "The Association for the Total Suppression of White Hats! The Anti-Flower-in-the-Button-Hole League! The Society for the Abolition of Green-Tea Drinking! The Association for the Restriction of Glove-Fastenings to One Button! The Local Option Snuff Confederation!"[14] There must be countless societies whose sole raison d'être, echoed a pro-vaccinationist as late as 1902, is "to be anti-something—against some constituted authority."[15] These accusations of eccentricity struck rather close to home. In 1884, Walter Hasker, a one-time member of the Executive Council of the NACVL, was detained for eight weeks in Bethlehem Royal Hospital, the infamous Bedlam asylum, as a "dangerous lunatic." One of the charges leveled against him was that he was an anti-vaccinator.[16] Victorians thus easily dismissed the anti-vaccination campaign as part of a tiresome anti-authoritarian and heretical fringe, in much the same way that George Orwell famously condemned socialist hangers-on as fruit-juice-drinking, sandal-wearing, nudist sex maniacs in pistachio-colored shirts.[17] Despite the condescension of their contemporaries—and, indeed, of subsequent historians—anti-vaccinationists must nevertheless be positioned as part of a vibrant culture of medical and social reform that was intensely meaningful to its participants.

Anti-vaccinationism forged its earliest alliance with the co-operative movement. Co-operation was a self-help strategy that sought to overcome consumer exploitation by establishing co-operative stores that sold high-quality goods at reasonable prices to members who shared in its profits. The first anti-vaccination periodical, called simply *The Anti-Vaccinator*, was conceived initially in August 1869 by Henry Pitman, a co-operator, Owenite, and temperance advocate in Manchester who preached anti-vaccinationism to the Northern working classes. After eighteen weeks, Pitman incorporated *The Anti-Vaccinator* into his other journal, *The Co-operator*. A self-described "Reporter, Teacher of Phonography, Lecturer on Co-operation, Phonography, and Anti-Vaccination," Pitman (brother to Sir Isaac Pitman, the inventor of shorthand) saw a clear relationship between his allied interests. "Co-operation is increasing the people's power and independence," he argued, "and thereby enabling them to resist tyranny and stupidity." He also asserted that "[m]any a Co-operator has used part of his 'dividend' to aid the anti-vaccination movement. Small-pox is caused by foul living: Co-operators go in for fair living, and are building healthy pox-proof houses for themselves."[18]

If the co-operative and anti-vaccination movements were linked by a shared commitment to independence of thought and action, so, too, were these movements intertwined with other mutual self-help strategies. Anti-vaccinationism quickly found support among trade unionists. Lewis Watson, a bricklayer from Stalybridge, a town just outside Manchester, was heavily involved in trade unionism and came to the anti-vaccination campaign through an interest in union politics.[19] Similarly, Ben Turner, a cotton-mill worker, popular poet, and renowned Yorkshire trade-union activist, became a strident anti-vaccinator. He devoted a chapter of his autobiography to his "Anti-Vacc Days," where he fondly remembered defending many a parent, appearing in court in his work smock and clogs.[20] In some areas by the late nineteenth century, anti-vaccinationism seemed to have clear alliances with specific trades. In the Enfield district of Middlesex, countless noncompliers were manual laborers at the local gun factory—specifically, machinists, filers, and fitters.[21] As Turner recounts, he and other mill workers had to be "passed" by the factory surgeon, since vaccination was a prerequisite of employment. Anti-vaccination sentiment thus may have developed in some industrialized areas as a reaction to the impositions of factory life, growing out of the same political environment that nurtured trade unionism.

In 1885, a lecturer who visited the mess rooms of the three largest works in Lincoln to address the workers during their breakfast half hour found that, when he spoke on vaccination and polled the men as to their opinions, only 4 out of 750 were in favor of the procedure. In Leicester in 1885, some of the factories had to shut down during a large anti-vaccination demonstration to accommodate workers attending the event.[22] By the early twentieth century, over twenty trade unions opposed an attempt to render vaccination and revaccination a condition of employment in shops, warehouses, and factories. In 1904, the Durham Cokemen's and Labourers' Association declared defiantly that "when vaccination interferes with the employment of labour it is going a step too far."[23]

Support for the anti-vaccination campaign came not only from the labor movement. It was also found among a variety of religious dissenters. Medical and religious dissent were intertwined in the mid-nineteenth century as religious nonconformity provided a pattern and base for other modes of social reform.[24] Medical dissenters often expressed their relationship to orthodox medicine through religious metaphors. Alternative medicine, they claimed, stood in the same relationship to orthodoxy as nonconformists vis-à-vis the Church of England. But religious dissent was more than just a rhetorical device. Many who resisted vaccination did so for deeply held religious, as well as for political or medical, reasons. William Hume-Rothery, who had been an Anglican minister, testified that while anti-vaccinationism was political, it was also "a religious movement," for religion and politics, he maintained, were "always united as soul and body." If it were not a religious movement, he argued, he would have nothing to do with it.[25] Nonconformists had been actively involved in political and social reform throughout the nineteenth century, from anti-slavery movements through campaigns for religious toleration to debates over education and moral reform.[26] Many, though certainly not all, anti-vaccinationists were affiliated with some sort of dissenting religious community: They were Quakers, Baptists, Methodists, Congregationalists, Wesleyans, Unitarians, and members of the Salvation Army or other chapel-based sects.[27]

Nonconformist anti-vaccinators were deeply opposed to the alliance between the state and the established Church of England and likened vaccination to a sacrament zealously enforced on the people. Compulsory vaccination seemed little different from compulsory baptism, these anti-vaccinators argued; if they would not be force-fed religion, then they would also resist this "medical baptism." A favorite anti-vaccination joke involved the child who confused vaccination with baptism, circumcision, or the crucifixion, all seemingly comparable religious rites or sacraments.[28] A correspondent to the *Personal Rights Journal* in 1887 compared compulsory vaccination to "compulsory salvation" through the domination of Catholicism. He implied that the anti-vaccination movement operated as a type of medical Reformation. It is our duty, he proclaimed, to "resist the presumption of these would-be saviours of our bodies as our fathers resisted the would-be saviours of our souls."[29]

If there was religious freedom, anti-vaccinators argued, there should also be medical liberty. The Reverend Hugh Price Hughes, "the most celebrated Methodist divine of the century,"[30] argued that vaccination was much like transubstantiation. "We do not doubt the sincerity of our opponents, any more than a Protestant doubts the sincerity of the Roman Catholic priest," he wrote. However, he continued, "[T]hat is no reason why I should submit to what I consider is totally mistaken and utterly wrong."[31] This analogy was strengthened by the very real relationship between established religion and vaccination. In its early years, vaccination was frequently practiced by itinerant preachers and members of the clergy. The station master Roger Langdon recalled that, in the 1830s, his mother had been encouraged to vaccinate by the village curate.[32] The *Church Sunday-School Magazine* maintained in 1884 that all babies must be registered, vaccinated, and christened before they could be considered English Christian children. Indeed, some Anglican clergymen reminded parents of their duty to vaccinate when they baptized their babies.[33]

Anti-vaccinationism had ties to an established tradition of Protestant dissent, but it also appealed to those involved in relatively new alternative spiritual movements that were unrelated to (or only tangentially associated with) Christianity. Theosophists supported the cause, and lecturers on spiritualism, such as Chandos Leigh Hunt, soon began to incorporate anti-vaccinationism into their own movement.[34] Followers of the Swedish mystic Swedenborg, such as J. J. Garth Wilkinson and William White, were drawn to the campaign because vaccination was discordant with their own theories of the relationship between physical and spiritual health. For Swedenborgians, damaging the body could also endanger the soul. Significantly, this type of esoteric spirituality was an important sphere for middle-class women's involvement with the cultural fringe, not least because these religious movements embraced an "occult body politics" that imagined bodies to be fluid and permeable and thus interconnected. This "immanentist theology" linked all bodies as part of the unity of life and thus lent itself to new feminist approaches to humanitarian and animal-rights issues.[35] Particularly toward the end of the nineteenth century, these kinds of female social reformers began to absorb anti-vaccinationism into their feminist platform.

Anti-vaccinationism appeared alongside anti-vivisectionism, vegetarianism, and related physical- and social-purity movements in feminist periodicals such as *Shafts* and the *Women's Penny Paper*, for, as chapter 5 will discuss in greater detail, these movements were linked through common, and particularly female, fears surrounding bodily vulnerability.[36] The relationship between anti-vaccinationism and the campaign against the contagious diseases acts was even more pronounced, as there was significant overlap in personnel and support. Josephine Butler, the force behind the repeal of the contagious diseases acts, was also a vice-president of the LSACV. As Mary Hume-Rothery, who was active in both campaigns, declared, under these acts "freeborn Englishwomen can no longer call their bodies or their babies their own."[37] The issue in both cases was bodily autonomy, for agitators argued that both the contagious diseases acts and the vaccination acts violated the bodies of those most vulnerable and thus stripped women of their rights to protect themselves and their children.

Just as working-class men connected anti-vaccinationism to industrial reform, so working- and middle-class women's-rights activists such as Jessie Craigen, Millicent Garrett Fawcett, Elizabeth Wolstenholme Elmy, and Ursula Bright, drew links between anti-vaccinationism and other explicitly feminist political agitations. Anti-vaccinators were involved in the women's suffrage campaign, for both movements made claims to women's ability and right to participate in national debate and political life. What bound the campaigns together was an understanding that women of all classes would vote against compulsory vaccination. John Bonner, a paid agent of the NAVL, maintained that women should demand the vote precisely to vote out pro-vaccination legislators.[38] Bright, a member of the Women's Franchise League and treasurer of the Married Women's Property Committee, advised the Women's Suffrage Association to agitate for the enfranchisement not only of spinsters and widows but of all women, since the "oppression of little children" was at stake. For this reason, explained *The Anti-Vaccinator* as early as 1871, the women's suffrage movement has our "hearty support."[39] By engaging with these other feminist, labor, and social causes from the late 1860s, the campaign against compulsory vaccination established its important place not only within alternative medical circles, but also within a wider cross-class and heterosocial culture of reform and dissent.

Popular Protest and Popular Culture

Anti-vaccinationists' attempt to repeal the compulsory clauses of the vaccination acts was a highly politicized campaign that involved public protest and the production of massive amounts of propaganda. Resistance to compulsory vaccination drew on older traditions of popular culture and protest still extant within Victorian society, while at the same time incorporating elements from an expanding commercial culture. While anti-vaccination activities were largely local initiatives, their forms were not necessarily regionally specific. Rather, protest manifested in similar ways in cities and towns across England and Wales. This was due in part to the strength of the anti-vaccination press, which provided models for agitation and a national audience for otherwise local events.

PROPAGANDA AND PRINT CULTURE   Since the campaign hoped to reach a broad public, it generated a mass of propaganda. Indeed, anti-vaccinators used the resources of an increasingly print-oriented Victorian culture to their best advantage. The campaign's publicists produced hundreds of handbills and pamphlets of various shapes, sizes, and genres aimed at the popular reader, some with runs of 100,000. These relied not only on sensationalist stories and dramatic events but also on reports of routine acts of civil disobedience and on statistical data. Not only did they engage in a spirited letter-writing campaign to national and local newspapers, but they produced three periodicals of their own that cover the movement from 1869 through the 1970s: *The Anti-Vaccinator* and its various incarnations (1869–73), the *National*

Anti-Compulsory Vaccination Reporter (1874–84), and the *Vaccination Inquirer* (1879–1971). Little detailed evidence about the circulation of these journals remains, although letters from readers indicate that they were widely distributed across England and into Wales, as well.[40]

Anti-vaccinationists made the most of an ever widening public sphere, using visual as well as literary forms of propaganda. Graphic representations of the horrors of vaccination were a frequent and innovative way to raise public awareness. Anti-vaccinators hung posters in shop windows and sold prints to adorn parlors, intending to provoke conversation on the topic of vaccination. Some made a habit of photographing cases of injury and death from vaccination and used these images in lectures. The Birmingham Anti-Variole League's magic-lantern show was so successful that multiple copies of the slides were circulated among Northern audiences.[41] Anti-vaccinators also produced these photographs for inspection in court cases and hearings. The president of the Yorkshire Anti-Vaccination League sent a packet of photographs of injured children to the Royal Commission on Vaccination. A Leicester father who testified before the commission brandished a photo of his child suffering from cancer of the eye, for which he blamed vaccination. Another employed the same tactic when tried in court for noncompliance. Photographs of this nature were available on request, and some local societies kept a photograph archive precisely for these purposes. Professional photographers may even have traded in this type of propaganda. The *Vaccination Inquirer* advertised that photos of bad cases of vaccinal injuries could be obtained from a local photographer.[42]

W. J. Furnival, an anti-vaccinator from Staffordshire, collected these photographs into an album of "vaccination disasters," which he published himself. The photos depicted not only healthy-looking children who had later died after vaccination but also babies in coffins, children's arms nearly rotting out of their sockets, and those severely disfigured by useless limbs and festering tumors. These images were in many ways not unlike Victorian postmortem memorial photography, which frequently did not try to disguise the brutality of death.[43] While they were deployed publicly to shock and to raise sympathy for victims of vaccination, they were also mementos—perhaps the only photograph of the child a family might own. The photographs served, then, as grim but sentimental reminders of children lost to the lancet (see Figure 2).

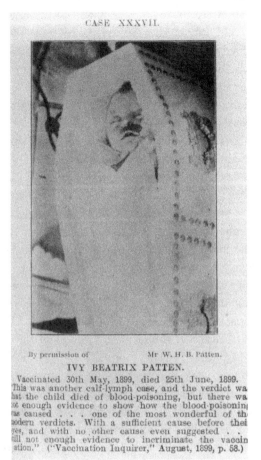

CASE XXXVII.

By permission of   Mr W. H. B. Patten.

IVY BEATRIX PATTEN.

Vaccinated 30th May, 1899, died 25th June, 1899.
This was another calf-lymph case, and the verdict wa
hat the child died of blood-poisoning, but there wa
ot enough evidence to show how the blood-poisonin
as caused . . . one of the most wonderful of th
modern verdicts. With a sufficient cause before thei
yes, and with no other cause even suggested . .
till not enough evidence to incriminate the vaccin
ation." ("Vaccination Inquirer," August, 1899, p. 58.)

2. "Ivy Beatrix Patten," in W. J. Furnival,
Professional Opinion Adverse to Vaccination
(Stone: W. J. Furnival, 1906). *By permission of the*
National Library of Medicine, Bethesda, Maryland.

Not only did they produce an abundance of propaganda, but anti-
vaccinationists also mobilized a distribution system that put their opponents to shame. Campaigners handed out leaflets at meetings and debates, sent them to supporters through the mail, distributed them at
vaccination stations, and made them widely and freely available through
anti-vaccination societies and their lending libraries. Anti-vaccination
societies also targeted new parents, sending postcards to those who

placed birth announcements in major newspapers, warning them that vaccination would only "Welcome Early Death!"[44] While pro-vaccinationists contrived equally alarmist material to counter the anti-vaccinationist position, they were much less effective at disseminating it. Anti-vaccinators, lamented Ernest Hart, editor of the *British Medical Journal*, have "an extremely energetic system of distributing tracts, inflammatory postcards, grotesquely drawn envelopes, and other means of disseminating their views." There is nothing on the other side, he complained, using a distinctly medical analogy, as "an accessible antidote to these productions."[45]

POPULAR PROTEST AND PUBLIC SPACE   Campaigners also carried on older traditions of protest and demonstration by regularly laying claim to public space. Anti-vaccinators marched up the High Street of many an English town and occupied countless public squares, market-places, and meeting halls throughout England and Wales. A common anti-vaccination demonstration involved driving a newly released anti-vaccination prisoner, often still in prison dress, around town in a cart adorned with ribbons and banners and accompanied by a brass band. Banners were typical of Victorian popular and radical reform movements, and brass bands had been an integral part of working-class culture in Lancashire, Yorkshire, and the colliery districts since at least the 1830s.[46] In Banbury in 1876, although a band could not be found, the cart was followed through the streets by two cornet players tooting, "Oh, dear, what can the *matter* be?" This was a popular parlor song and a play on words, for *matter* here referred to vaccine lymph.

The Leicester Demonstration in March 1885 was a tour de force of anti-vaccination organization, perhaps the best example of "the perfect carnival of common merriment" that anti-vaccination protest often produced.[47] As Thomas Cook had done for the temperance rallies, anti-vaccinators made traveling arrangements with the railway companies to provide cheap excursions to the Leicester meeting.[48] Here a giant parade converged on the marketplace with banners and babies, "a well-appointed hearse, with a child's coffin, inscribed 'Another victim of vaccination,'" and trolleys with furniture "seized for blood money." A model of a prison cell, complete with oakum, and "doctors riding cows and holding on by the tail, and mothers at upper windows clasping their infants, while policemen were trying to commit a legal burglary at the keyhole in the street below, were also conspicuously enjoyed." Of particular delight was a dummy of the inventor of vaccination, Edward Jenner, who was hanged in effigy, then tossed around, only to be decapitated and removed to the police station. The 80,000–100,000 participants were well entertained and treated this demonstration as little different from a local fair such as those held on Easter and Whitsun.[49]

As this symbolic beheading of Jenner makes clear, anti-vaccination demonstrations, like most forms of popular and political protest, involved a degree of "folk violence." In Dewsbury in 1880, the effigy of a vaccination officer was thrown to a crowd of 10,000 people and was "torn to pieces." Four years earlier, an "anti-vaccination Guy" representing a particularly harsh magistrate was incinerated in a Somerset Guy Fawkes bonfire.[50] From midcentury, Guy Fawkes effigies frequently represented local employers, policemen, and other "moral offenders."[51] Some anti-vaccinators clearly enjoyed brutalizing the symbolic bodies of these state agents who, they felt, violated their infants, and they did not always stop at these ritualistic acts of violence. While anti-vaccinators prided themselves on being respectable and otherwise law-abiding citizens, their meetings and demonstrations intermittently devolved into small-scale riots where they pelted Poor Law and vaccination officials with eggs, stones, cayenne pepper, or rotten fruit.[52] Some went as far as to assault the vaccination officials. In Brighton, the public vaccinator was shoved around, emerging with cuts and blows to his body and with his clothes "considerably mauled." A witness to the Brighton riot reported that the people "would smash [the vaccination station] and tear the vaccination officers to pieces with the slightest encouragement."[53]

Fearing this type of confrontation, local authorities generally mobilized a police force to supervise these events. But while the police were present at demonstrations to keep the peace, and sometimes attempted to collect fines or to distrain goods, they had no formal role in the policing of the unvaccinated. In the second half of the nineteenth century, the provincial police acted as Poor Law relieving officers and inspectors of nuisances and common lodging houses.[54] These were the same positions that vaccination officers often held to supplement their income, yet there is no evidence of any crossover between vaccination

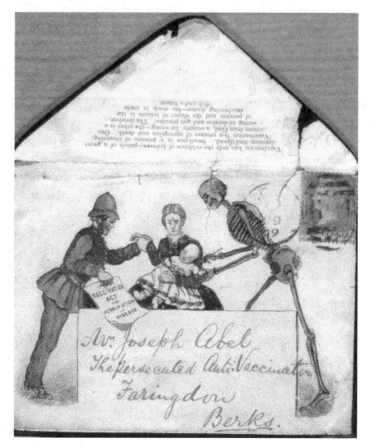

3. Anti-vaccination caricature envelope, 1879.
By permission of Denis Vandervelde.

officers and policemen. Anti-vaccinators used the image of the police in their propaganda, but this was a symbolic reference to the state and its agents rather than to actual police officers (see Figure 3). Ironically, a number of policemen seem to have been anti-vaccinators themselves— or, at least, sympathetic to the cause.[55]

The most contentious site both for anti-vaccinationists and the police who monitored them was the distraint sale. If one could not afford to pay the fine for noncompliance with the vaccination act (or simply chose not to), one's goods could be seized and sold at auction to raise funds (see Figure 4). Distress warrants were generally issued only to the working class. A clerk to the justices at Derby admitted that the man in "poorer circumstances" was "compelled to submit to the judgment of the Court, whereas his neighbour who is in a better position, and able to pay the penalty, defies the magistrates," as the police would not dare to seize his goods.[56] Distraint sales provided a perfect opportunity for protest, and anti-vaccinators took full advantage of this by using these auctions as meeting sites. When an anti-vaccinator's goods were distrained, the local anti-vaccination league mobilized its members and supporters to demonstrate at the sale by placarding the town with incendiary posters (see Figure 5).[57] Their goal was to prevent the auction from taking place or to purchase the goods themselves. In 1889, the *Sheffield Telegraph* reported that a Mr. Cockroft had covered his distrained furniture—a dresser and a wringer—with anti-vaccination literature to make them unfit for sale. Cockroft, after an argument, purchased his own furniture back.[58] A resister in Charlbury screwed a cherished table to the floor, claiming to the auctioneer that it "grew there, and we built the house around it."[59] Since local anti-vaccination leagues regularly ended up purchasing or replacing the furniture, the sale was often no more than a joke at the auctioneer's expense.

If distraint sales provided comic opportunities to shame the auctioneer and undermine the process, they were also the primary site of anti-vaccination violence. In 1887, Robert King, a resident of Leicester, was prosecuted for noncompliance with the vaccination acts. It seemed to make little difference that King's child, while admittedly unvaccinated, had been dead for over a year. Since King refused to pay the fine, the police proceeded to seize and auction his goods to raise the equivalent sum. No local auctioneer could be found to "incur the odium of conducting the sale," reported *The Times*; one had to be imported from Birmingham, some fifty miles away. The auctioneer was conveyed to King's house inside a furniture van, "driven by police and strongly guarded." Sixty uniformed and a large number of plainclothes policemen were present. A "great crowd" gathered near King's house, which the police "attacked" with crowbars "amid the hooting of the crowd." The door was "shattered to pieces," and the policemen removed King's furniture and placed it in the van, "where the auctioneer was sheltered behind a strong guard of police." The van proceeded to a vacant piece of

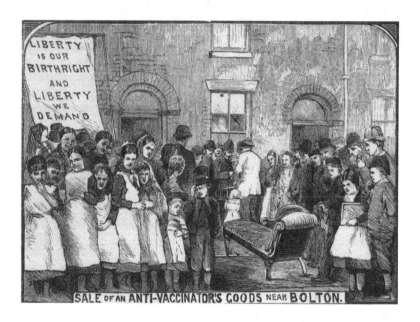

4. (above) "Sale of an Anti-vaccinator's Goods near Bolton," *Illustrated Police News*, 2 October 1886. *By permission of the British Library.*

5. Distraint sale poster, Stalybridge, c. 1880s. *By permission of Tameside Local Studies and Archives.*

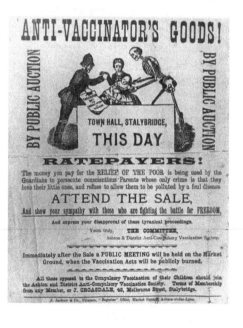

ground for the auction, but instead of bidding, the crowd pelted the
auctioneer with stones and eggs. The auctioneer took shelter in the
police station, and two men were apprehended for stone throwing. The
police, reported *The Times*, were "very roughly handled." During the
afternoon, another sale took place during which the auctioneer was
again "hooted and pelted with eggs."[60]

At a similar sale in Gravesend, the crowd grew menacing. The hall
was "packed like a sardine tin," and the auctioneer and his assistant
quickly became "the objects of abuse and derision." The protesters
"indulged in a Highland fling and made a deafening din with heavily-
nailed boots" while the auctioneer cowered behind a cordon of police.[61]
At Stroud in 1893, the sixteen constables sent to guard the auctioneer
were "tossed about like cockle-shells, and finally were rushed together
with the object of the hostile demonstration from the marketplace into
the High Street." The superintendent was forced to wire to Gloucester
for its police force.[62] Not surprisingly, as the agitation escalated, it became increasingly difficult to find auctioneers willing to officiate at a
sale of this nature.[63]

The Gender of Resistance

While anti-vaccination violence seems largely to have been initiated by
men, both men and women were involved in all aspects of the movement, including its riotous dimension. Indeed, anti-vaccinationism was
a successful heterosocial campaign, as there was little tension between
the sexes as to their duties and goals. The movement nevertheless
identified different if complementary roles for male and female agitators and relied on explicitly gendered rhetoric that appealed to Victorian
ideals of masculinity and femininity.

Francis T. Bond, medical officer of health for Gloucester rural district
in the 1890s and an enthusiastic proponent of compulsory vaccination,
characterized the archetypal anti-vaccinator as male. Mothers objected
to vaccination primarily, Bond argued, because it was mandated within
the first three months of life, when babies still had "fair" and "unspot-
ted skin" and were doted on and "lavished" with "sympathy." If the
period were extended, to compel vaccination only at the point of entry

into school, Bond proposed, nine out of ten mothers would eventually give in: By this time, the angelic baby would have become a "brat" so "troublesome" that the mother would "gladly get it off to school," vaccinated or not. Fathers, Bond suggested, were another matter. While mothers were all the same, there were "fathers and fathers," he theorized—three kinds, to be precise: those who objected to vaccination because they were ignorant, those who were "Radical" and thus resisted everything that is "established," and those who claimed to be "conscientiously" opposed to the practice after careful consideration. It was this last group of "militant" fathers who for Bond posed the greatest threat to compulsory vaccination.[64]

Bond may have imagined the extremist anti-vaccinator to be male, but anti-vaccinators expected and encouraged committed and fervent resistance from both men and women. Campaigners maintained that refusing vaccination was part and parcel of the duty of good parenting. However, they often insisted that mothers and fathers had different, if complementary, roles to play in the movement. In an anti-vaccination newsletter, Mrs. S. J. West spoke to mothers and fathers in quite distinct languages. "Mothers!" she trumpeted, "you who know and mourn over hundreds of cases of children injured by Vaccination—you who nurse and tend them during the unnatural illness inflicted upon them by vaccination—you who wring your hands in impotent agony at the sight of your darling little ones suffering from the effects of vaccination—you who having carried them, with aching hearts, to the blood-poisoner to have them vaccinated under the threats of the Vaccination Inspector." Here, West spoke to mothers as sentimental nurses overcome by emotional attachment to their children: women grieved, nursed, and agonized. This rhetoric valorized the feminine and domestic; indeed, West went on to critique vaccination for perverting the true meaning of motherhood. Vaccination, she argued, was "conceived in ignorance, born in corruption, brought forth in cupidity, and nurtured by falsehood, fraud and bribery." By describing vaccination as something "conceived," "born," and "nurtured," West drew on the imagery of birth and development to underscore that the risks inherent in this procedure made a mockery of women's maternal duties to their children. Vaccination, West stressed, was not the product of a woman's womb or a mother's care; it "stalks through the land—a hideous thing—spreading disease, desolation, and death in its path!" Compulsory vaccination was like Frankenstein's monster, she implied—the creation of heartless scientists and bureaucrats more interested in their own brainchild than in "darling" suffering children. Women thus had important roles to play in the movement as true guardians of their children's welfare. They were, however, to act on the local level, opposing the vaccination officials. As such, women were largely to be helpmates to their crusading male counterparts.[65]

To fathers, West directed a different message and deployed a different rhetoric. "Fathers!" West argued,

> ascertain for yourselves, by enquiry in your own neighbourhood, that Vaccination sows the seeds of disease and death; that it is child-murder to an incalculable extent. Is it not then a burning shame that doctors should thus curse the country; that the clergy and ministers of religion should look coolly on whilst this wickedness is being perpetrated; that Whigs and Tories should maintain the infernal laws which enforce this detestable quackery; that guardians and magistrates should so disgrace humanity as to administer the Vaccination law; and that the country should tolerate the injustice and misery inflicted upon many of the best people in the land, under its infamous sanction.[66]

In speaking to fathers West deployed the language of public life, encouraging men to act independently, to "ascertain" for themselves the value of vaccination. Identifying the medical profession, the church, political parties, and local administrators as culprits, she placed the male sphere of anti-vaccination resistance within a larger public and political realm. Here she implied that men could act by influencing politicians and other figures of authority and in turn effect national change. West was not alone in these distinctions. Most anti-vaccinators shared her views of male and female spheres of influence. But anti-vaccinators also demonstrated that the roles and duties of mothers and fathers were wider-ranging and more complex than a simplistic separate-spheres ideology would suggest. By publicly campaigning as mothers and fathers, anti-vaccinators challenged the division between public and private itself, illustrating that parents had political roles to play within the public sphere.

A FATHER'S DUTY   For the men involved in the anti-vaccination cause, their protest was part of much larger working-class campaigns for political rights. As the next chapter will argue in greater detail, they repeatedly drew on the rhetoric of citizenship that was also central to the agitation for manhood suffrage. Male anti-vaccinators claimed their rights on the basis of being good men and critiqued the government for undermining their masculinity by propping up working-class independence with one hand and removing it with the other. "Shall I thank him for Manhood Suffrage," inquired a correspondent from Brooklyn in the wake of the 1884 Reform Act, "although he steals my manhood?"[67] This agitator suggested that the vote was only one essential component of working men's claims to both citizenship and masculinity; equally important was the authority of the husband and father within his household.

Male anti-vaccinators constantly affirmed their masculinity, claiming to be "Manly" men. A demonstrator's call to "Quit you like men" and to agitate against the compulsory clauses fed the idea that anti-vaccinationism was essentially a masculine enterprise.[68] "Where is the father who submits his child to the operation without feeling that he sacrifices his dignity as a man?" proposed one agitator.[69] The vaccination laws were despicable, anti-vaccinators argued, precisely because they "trampled" on "manhood."[70] In part, compulsory vaccination threatened masculinity because it removed "the sovereignty of a father in his family."[71] But it also endangered the lives of children, who for many men represented both the preservation of family blood lines and their virility. An 1880 cautionary tale that first appeared in the *Weekly Times*—a periodical with a decidedly working- and lower-middle-class readership— advised mothers to yield to their husbands' desires regarding nonvaccination of children. Here the wife of a respectable South London working man vaccinated her child against her husband's wishes while he was away. The child fell sick and died. "Joe" eventually forgave his wife after the funeral, but she was haunted by her actions, for she knew "how much of the hope and promise of his manhood lay buried in the tiny grave."[72]

Fathers often constructed the campaign as a battle or crusade in which a man's physical strength and mental convictions could be tested and publicly demonstrated. One protester proclaimed that the vaccination acts waged "war on infancy," while another declared he was proud to be fighting the "babies' battle."[73] Anti-vaccinators maintained that to win this "war" they must stand "shoulder to shoulder."[74] This was not mere rhetoric, for as we have seen, anti-vaccination agitation could devolve into brutal outbursts. Anti-vaccinators rationalized this behavior by arguing that "the working man must fight for his manhood and his freedom."[75] Ironically, the imprisonment of these "martyrs" revealed how susceptible the male body actually was to physical trials, for, as chapter 4 shows, anti-vaccination prisoners repeatedly complained about the harshness of the penal regime.

While claims to masculinity encouraged these public acts and displays of strength and conviction, anti-vaccinators also appealed to domestic manhood. The anti-vaccination movement provided a rare opportunity for men in general, and working-class men in particular, to articulate their identities as loving, nurturing fathers. Anti-vaccinators were forced to work against Victorian critiques of the working-class father that frequently portrayed him as a stupid brute who cared little for his offspring. In a poem satirizing conscientious objection to vaccination, the poet maintained that the male anti-vaccinator knew neither his child's name nor its sex.[76] Some even proposed that it was to the father's advantage to keep the family small and implied that anti-vaccinationism was merely a form of infanticide.[77] Anti-vaccinators were outraged at this suggestion and objected to being dragged into court in the "midst of culprits" being tried for "wife-beating" or child abuse. The *Anti-Vaccinator and Public Health Journal* expressed its disgust that an anti-vaccinator could be found guilty of a crime while a child abuser could be dismissed because of insufficient evidence although the child was black and blue. The district nurse Margaret Loane described the indignation of a working-class family forced to appear in court for noncompliance. What the family objected to was being "jostled in along o' them Adlams" who had been accused of cruelty and neglect of their children by the National Society for the Prevention of Cruelty to Children.[78]

Male anti-vaccinators routinely expressed an emotional and selfless devotion to their children. In describing the arrest of a Leicestershire anti-vaccinator, the LSACV portrayed him as a martyr "seated, with his four children kneeling round him, engaged in their evening prayers." Holding this resister up as a model of respectable fatherhood, the society inquired rhetorically, "Is this the kind of man whose body you want for an English gaol?"[79] Mr. Emery, a ham and tongue dealer, denounced compulsory vaccination "with much feeling, as was not unnatural," declaring, "I would rather allow my legs to be chopped off, than I would allow another child of mine to be vaccinated."[80] This father claimed that he would rather endure bodily violence than allow the equivalent to be performed on his own child. Similarly, a "working man" proclaimed, "I would rather eat dry bread all my life, than allow my child to be 'poisoned' by vaccination."[81] These fathers illustrated not only their tenderness but also their commitment to the protection of their offspring. "At the peril of his life," argued the water-cure practitioner T. L. Nichols, "a good father would protect his child from poison, from disease"[82] One activist argued that this was the true test of masculinity: "No crime can sink a man so low in the scale of manhood, or so brand him as an arrant coward, as a refusal to protect his helpless offspring."[83] It was this kind of devotion that prompted a sympathetic doctor to testify before the Royal Commission that anti-vaccinators were "excellent fathers."[84]

A MOTHERS' CRUSADE   Although male anti-vaccinators were over-represented in public, women from all social classes wrote pamphlets, contributed letters to newspapers, and were vocal activists at meetings, distraint sales, and other public protests. Indeed, according to Pitman, who was instrumental in generating working-class support for the cause, women were even more opposed to the "filthy practice" than men.[85]

While feminists joined the campaign, anti-vaccination propaganda returned repeatedly to images of a decidedly domestic, emotional, and instinctual femininity that was at odds with feminist representations of the modern woman. Vaccination was understood by men and women alike to be undoubtedly "a mother's question."[86] While not all women involved in the campaign were mothers, "woman" and "mother" became synonymous terms for agitators, as it was assumed that women by their very natures were maternal. Mothers' rights, anti-vaccinators argued, were "natural rights" to care for their children as they saw fit;

"the cradle is the mother's birthright," argued one agitator, "no law can override it."[87] These rights derived from mothers' instinctual ability to know what was best for their children. Female anti-vaccinators, proclaimed the *Hackney Express* in 1896, are "obeying the highest instincts of motherhood." These "maternal instincts," anti-vaccinators insisted, were "great teachers," and thus it was to women's special knowledge that one should turn for enlightenment.[88] Women attacked the notion that a doctor could evaluate the health or sickness of their children better than they could. Mothers could tell which children were healthy and which were not, and which had been corrupted by vaccine "poison," anti-vaccinators maintained. For no "doctor watches over the life and health of any person, like a mother over her child," declared the short-lived Society for the Suppression of Compulsory Vaccination, and no "*male* being" could care for a "three-months babe in the same way as the mother" who bore it.[89] Thus, compulsory vaccination appeared to a "Loving Mother" to be a "gross outrage on our maternal rights."[90] Women's rights, these anti-vaccinators suggested, were biological, not political.

Mothers made claims based largely on an emotional attachment to their children and on the basis of maternal love. At the great Leicester Demonstration of 1885, a banner with a cartoon "demon" trying to entrap a child proclaimed, "Maternal love says hands off."[91] The love of a mother was a force to be reckoned with, anti-vaccinators argued, as it was perhaps the strongest emotion. In a public-health pamphlet that masqueraded as a gothic tale, it was the "Love of Womankind" who was disease's greatest foe. "The Love of a Mother," a "Measles-Fiend" declared, "has often made me shrink."[92] This rhetoric of maternal love was intimately linked to the symbol of the desperate domesticated mother, which appealed to sentimental sensibilities. "Who has to nurse the sick child day and night," proclaimed Mary Hume-Rothery, "and see its agonies and hear its moans? The mother."[93] Often these descriptions were part of moralistic fictional tales of sacrificing mothers who either lost their babies to vaccination or refused to submit them to the lancet. Inevitably, the appeal of these characters, whether fictional or not, was an empathetic one.

In anti-vaccination literature, maternal love was frequently linked to suffering, for vaccination was considered a torment to loving mothers who were forced to watch their babies sicken or die from vaccinal injuries. "What can exceed a mother's love, and what can satisfy a mother's sorrow," proclaimed a pamphlet promoting healthy skin as a preventative for smallpox.[94] Anti-vaccinationist mothers regularly invoked their broken, bleeding, or aching hearts. In an "appeal to women," Mrs. Longman, wife of a well-known agitator so committed to the cause that he named his children after the anti-vaccination leadership, spoke as a "mother, and a wife" to future "victims" of the vaccination acts, which, she claimed, had nearly "broken" her heart.[95] An anonymous pamphleteer sympathized with mothers whose "hearts have sickened and almost bled at the sight of the loathsome blotches and the running sores" of children poisoned by the lancet.[96] In a letter to the *Vaccination Inquirer*, Annie Beaton, who claimed to have lost a child to vaccination, pleaded for the repeal of the acts. "Is there no mercy for mothers," she implored, "nor pity for their broken hearts?"[97]

Anti-vaccinationists frequently gestured to archetypes of suffering motherhood, drawing on biblical matriarchs. Campaigners of both sexes regularly hailed anti-vaccinationist women as "Rachels of the day," proclaiming that, like the mother of Joseph and Benjamin, they were "weeping for their children all over the land."[98] An anti-vaccination caricature envelope featured the biblical verse, "In Rama was there a voice heard, lamentation and weeping, and great mourning, Rachael weeping for her children, and would not be comforted because they are not."[99] Rachel, maternal ancestor of two of the ten tribes of Israel, served as a symbol to the prophet Jeremiah of suffering motherhood in the days of Jewish exile from the holy land. In Matthew, Rachel's lamentation was used to prefigure the slaughter of the newborns under King Herod, and it was to this reference that anti-vaccinators repeatedly turned. "Like the mother of Moses," maintained a schoolmistress, "I have 'hid' my little one. Hers was in danger from the execution of a senseless and murderous law; mine *now* is; but no ark of bulrushes would avail me, and there is no Pharaoh's daughter to interpose." Anti-vaccinationists suggested, then, that like the Jews in Egypt their children were being slaughtered by a "Herodian Decree."[100]

Anti-vaccinators staged mothers' marches to draw attention to their cause. These mock funeral processions provided women with an opportunity to display themselves publicly as grieving mothers. In 1885, in response to the death of a Hackney infant from vaccinal injuries, a parade of women traversed London from east to west. "There was a brass band playing appropriate music, an open hearse with the child's coffin, a number of mourning coaches filled with women in black, and a banner inscribed, 'In memory of 1,000 children who have died this year through vaccination,'" reported the anti-vaccination press. The "funeral" apparently "excited much attention, much sympathy, and much indignation."[101] A similar protest the year before, which marched to the House of Commons, paraded along the Old Kent Road, an ancient pilgrimage route. A band played the Dead March, and participants carried banners proclaiming, "Murdered by Compulsory Vaccination." This "respectable company" was dressed in mourning attire to publicize its anguish and distributed black-bordered handbills that incited "working women" to "join us in our appeal to the legislature."[102]

Anti-vaccinationist women frequently appealed to the state and to the nation for reform in their role as grief-stricken and wronged mothers. The mother, anti-vaccinationists maintained, was not merely a domestic role but also a public position. Particularly in the years after the Boer War, motherhood gained national significance, for mothers produced the next generation, and "population was power."[103] Hence, John Bonner suggested in 1907 that women should "strike against motherhood."[104] Although there is no evidence that women actually attempted to restrict births as a protest against compulsory vaccination, the idea of a strike against motherhood gestured to the growth of maternalist politics and suggested that women could use their bodies as political tools by controlling their fertility.[105] This positioned anti-vaccinationists as part of a tradition of female body politics. From the 1860s through the 1880s, campaigners against the contagious diseases acts had used the bodies of women violated by the speculum as a powerful political symbol of the excesses of a regulatory state. In ensuing years, suffragists would use their bodies to political ends by engaging in hunger strikes in prison.[106]

As "Mothers of the nation," anti-vaccinationist women claimed that they had both a right and a responsibility to defend their helpless children. Banners from the Leicester Demonstration proclaimed that the "mothers of the people"—or, alternatively, that the "mothers of England"—demanded repeal of the vaccination acts.[107] "Women of England!" railed one agitator, "You can speak at home—speak before the bench. Ask for justice! Plead your claims! Demand your rights! Tell your neighbours."[108] Women's vocal participation in the campaign prompted some to dub the agitation a "mothers' rebellion," which one editor characterized as a "new political phenomenon," although radical motherhood had been modeled at least since the French Revolution.[109]

Female anti-vaccinationists often invoked the symbolic mother of the nation, Queen Victoria, who was represented—and indeed represented herself—as a wife and mother. It was to this domesticated queen, whom anti-vaccinators hailed as "a tender-hearted mother," that campaigners frequently turned.[110] Ann Turnell, a working woman, petitioned the queen, speaking as an "English mother and wife whose heart cries aloud to your majesty under a cruel wrong." Her husband, she claimed, was a "good citizen" who she requested be released from prison, lest she herself be obliged to enter a workhouse.[111] The intention of the petition was to draw a relationship between this mother of seven children and the fecund queen, who, it was assumed, shared her motherly and womanly feelings.

Queen Victoria was unresponsive. She vaccinated her own family and showed little interest in the debate. This enraged Mary Hume-Rothery, who considered both the vaccination acts and the contagious diseases acts an "indelible blot" on the "fair fame of Queen Victoria." As a "Woman and a Mother," the queen should never have assented to policies that "violate all the best feeling of motherhood and womanhood," Hume-Rothery maintained. It was even more degrading and cruel, she continued, that women should suffer at the hands of a woman who had ascended the throne as a young girl and who had enabled other women to feel "their own sex and maidenhood exalted and honoured as true womanhood deserves to be honoured." If royalty in the person of a woman could not save women from preserving "their bodies" and "their babies" as "their own," she complained, "what is Royalty worth to us?"[112]

As historians have increasingly noted, working women understood motherhood not only as the expression of domesticated maternal love but also as a duty that involved working for their children. Working-class women thus often represented the family in court when prosecuted for noncompliance, as their schedules were generally more flexible than their husbands'. While many more men were prosecuted under the vaccination acts than women, 150 women were tried in court for default of vaccination from the beginning of 1875 to the end of 1878. Almost half of these cases were discharged, but the rest received fines or were occasionally imprisoned.[113] In Lincoln, a woman appeared regularly before the court, and she was not afraid to give the magistrates "a twenty minutes' lecture."[114] Some even went to prison to defend their position. Mrs. Blanchard, the widow of an Andover grocer and confectioner in "humble circumstances," was imprisoned twice for noncompliance. When she spoke at a meeting, Mrs. Blanchard was cheered "vociferously" by a crowd who gave her a standing ovation.[115]

Working women had for some time incorporated resistance to the state and its allied agents into the practices of good mothering.[116] Indeed, some women had no qualms about rejecting outright any state interference with the family. Although she eventually vaccinated her child, a Hammersmith mother told a vaccination officer that she "would have it done when she pleased" and was apparently both "abusive" and "insulting."[117] Many mothers took their roles as guardians of the home literally. They refused to open their doors and regularly hid from vaccination officers, shielding their homes and their children from intruding officials. In 1872, a Leeds woman maintained that she knew "dozens of mothers" who hated vaccination, and when the inspector "comes into the neighbourhood, we shut our doors, pull down the blinds, and go upstairs till he's gone; that's how we trick him."[118] In the early 1890s, a vaccination officer noted in his report book that he had called several times at one house but had been unable to gain admittance as he could make no one hear him.[119] Women were often encouraged in this obstructive behavior by their husbands. "When the vaccination inspector calls round 'seeking whom he may devour,'" suggested the father of four "unvaccinated laddies," "raise a hue and cry after him, cry shame on him, and both you and your neighbours hoot him out of the neighbourhood; drive the wolf from the door and let the authorities know that mothers are mothers still, and that it is a mother's duty to protect her child."[120]

Some mothers called their children only by pet names in public so as not to let anyone know their real names and thus be able to inform on them to the vaccination officer. In 1892, defiant Kentish parents chris-

tened their daughter Annie Antivaccinator Austin.[121] Others endeavored to safeguard their children from vaccination by not registering the
birth in the first place, although the nonregistration of birth was itself
an offense.[122] Alternatively, mothers gave false addresses on registration so that they could not be found.[123] The vaccination officer's report
book for a Southwark district in South London reveals that most of the
cases that needed following up had either given a false address or
completely disappeared. In Fulham, the same was true, as many cases
were listed as "not known," "removed," or "gone away."

"Moving house" was a common tactic for avoiding vaccination. Frank
Goss distinctly remembered having two birthdays, a "real" and a "statutory" one, and moving house frequently. His mother, a dressmaker, had
delayed the registration of her children's birthdays to avoid the vaccination officer. My mother, Goss explained,

> having a new baby on the way, waited to make sure of its safe arrival
> before putting her law avoidance tactics into operation. Dad, with fore-
> knowledge of what was required of him, in whatever spare time he had
> available would be looking for a new home for his family in a district
> not covered by the same local officer of health as the area in which the
> child was expected to be born. Came the birth, and with it the pro-
> gramme of avoidance came into action. Within six weeks after the
> registration of birth the doctor would be along to carry out his vaccina-
> tion job. The get-away had, therefore, to be made a certainty before the
> registration of birth was actually made. When the arrangements for
> moving house were decided, the birth was registered and six clear
> weeks still remained to get well clear of the menacing poisoner.

It is difficult to confirm how widespread these tactics were, but the
number of false addresses in vaccination officers' report books suggests
that this was a relatively common practice. The frequent appearance of
these types of stories in anti-vaccination literature also indicates that
they were imagined to be common strategies. At the very least, stories
of women's subversive actions serve to demonstrate the role anti-
vaccinationism played within the culture of working-class motherhood.
While his father had carried out the relocation plan, Goss was certain
that the impetus for "coking a snoot [sic]" at the law came from his
mother's profound distrust of both medical science and the state.[124]

Women also used their position as primary caregivers in the family to counteract the impact of vaccination on the child's body. While they may not have been able to prevent the vaccination, mothers could nevertheless attempt to impede its effects. Stories circulated widely throughout the anti-vaccination press about mothers sucking, steaming, or wiping the vaccine matter out of their children's arms after a visit to the vaccinator as one extracts the poison of a snake. This allowed them to obtain a certificate of vaccination with, they hoped, none of the ill effects of the operation. A pamphleteer reported that mothers sucked the virus out of their children's arms, "spitting it out on the steps" of the vaccination station. Others wiped out the lymph with a handkerchief or removed the virus using a poultice at home. Anti-vaccinators also recommended using borax to scrub the vaccine pus out of the arm and neutralize its effects. As one agitator noted, there was no law yet "to prevent a mother disinfecting her child of pollution."[125]

Alternatively, a substitute for vaccine matter could be employed to create the look of a vaccination without the results. Mothers who could afford to sometimes paid medical men to give certificates of successful vaccination but to perform the operation without using vaccine matter. "It is well known that tartar emetic," proposed T. R. Allinson, medical practitioner and whole-meal bread industrialist, "produces a vesicle and leaves a cicatrix scarcely distinguishable from those described and illustrated by Jenner in his 'inquiry' without risk of syphilis or other contaminations." A physician living in a fashionable London suburb, Allinson reported, administered vaccine as an oral dose and then proceeded to fill out certificates of vaccination.[126] Technically, this was not actually illegal, as no definition of what constituted "vaccination" existed. If a legally qualified medical man, argued Alfred Milnes, a political economist and editor of the *Vaccination Inquirer* in the 1890s, "chose to present an infant with an effigy of a cow, in wood, and called that vaccinating the child, there is no law of England to prevent him."[127]

Just as their male counterparts had appealed to their need to fight, female anti-vaccinators demonstrated that maternal love and duty could also manifest itself in a violent defense of the child. "Get the blood of the Northallerton mother well up," claimed the *Vaccination Inquirer*, and she would soon induce her husband to action. Riots in Brighton and the Midlands, claimed W. J. Collins, an ophthalmologist and progressive politician, were a direct result of women in the "humbler class of life . . . stirring up their husbands."[128] Women were also directly involved in demonstrations that often resulted in a violent outburst. In 1892, John Pickering, former editor of the *Anti-Vaccinator and Public Health Journal*, recounted the story of the wife of a provisions dealer in Leeds. While serving a customer sliced meat, she was interrogated by the vaccination officer. On ascertaining his identity, she chased him through the streets with the knife in hand, proclaiming that, had she caught him, she would have "taken a bigger sweep of flesh out of his back than that covered by any five cicatrices" the public vaccinator ever saw. She was never bothered again.[129] Another woman in the East End of London in 1881 was reported to have assaulted the doctor after losing a child to vaccination: She "shook her fist in his face, laid hold of him, gave him such a shaking, and such a lecture that the fellow looked quite foolish."[130] Similarly, in a production of a Roman play at the Westminster School, an original monologue was introduced to comment on contemporary events. A "mother" delivered the threatening lines: "If he dare scratch baby with his lancet / I'll scratch his face—yes, that I will—and chance it!"[131] Indeed, a man brought before magistrates at Bow Street Police Court in central London in 1873 warned: "If I consented to have my child vaccinated, my wife would not. If I could not persuade her, I am certain no one else would."[132]

Mothers' and fathers' roles in the movement were thus complex and complementary, as both men and women actively participated in and shaped the culture of anti-vaccinationism. Men promoted themselves as archetypes of virile masculinity, crusading against tyranny and defending their families. But they also took great pains to portray themselves as tender, loving fathers. While this discourse of respectable manhood was already in play from the 1860s in relation to parliamentary debates over an expanded male franchise, anti-vaccinators emphasized how significant this emotional attachment to their children was to working men's identities. Women also campaigned as domestic sentimental parents. But in addition, they staked out their role as militant defenders of their homes, their children, and their own political and biological rights. Thus, while participating in the Victorian construct of separate spheres, anti-vaccinators also challenged this division—and, indeed, the distinction between private and public. For, as chapter 3 will demonstrate, they argued that parental rights were political rights and thus the entitlement of all respectable English citizens.

3

Populism, Citizenship, and
the Politics of Victorian Liberalism

I would rather see England pock-marked than without the personal
independence which is the basis of everything worth having in our
national character—Millicent Garrett Fawcett, 1899[1]

☞ The anti-vaccination movement was a cross-class campaign that
often drew on populist discourses to unite agitators against what they
interpreted as the coercive policies of an increasingly interventionist
state. Campaigners from all social classes claimed their rights to govern
their homes and families. These rights, they maintained, derived from
their English citizenship. Both working- and middle-class agitators
used the discourse of citizenship to argue that the state had no right to
compel them to vaccinate their children. While this populist language
of the rights of the freeborn Englishman bound campaigners together,
middle-class activists did not actually experience the indignities of compulsory vaccination firsthand, as they were rarely pursued by the vaccination administration. For middle-class anti-vaccinationists, then, the
issue of compulsion was largely bound up not in intimate experiences
of the state's exercise of its authority, but in broader political debates
over the nature of liberalism and the trajectory of the Liberal Party.

Populism and the Cross-Class Alliance

The anti-vaccination movement, like the anti-vivisection campaign and
the agitation against the contagious diseases acts, seems to represent a
successful cross-class alliance. Campaigners were drawn from the mid-

dle, lower middle, and working classes, as well as from the gentry. In many respects, this alliance suited most of the parties involved, as it furnished a large group of protesters to back the campaign. When it suited their crusading or pragmatic purposes, most anti-vaccinationists were quick to assert that the movement successfully integrated campaigners from different social and economic groups. Testifying before the Select Committee on the Vaccination Act of 1867, Aaron Emery, a provisions dealer, was asked which classes of people opposed vaccination. "They're all classes," he replied, "well-to-do and middle-class men, working-class men and the very poor."[2] William Hume-Rothery, the firmly middle-class president of the NACVL, concurred. He argued that it was the responsibility of all "true men, in every class" to rise up and oppose the vaccination acts.[3] The *Co-operator and Anti-Vaccinator*, which catered primarily to a working-class readership, echoed this sentiment in a vaccination poem, but drew on an older language of social divisions: "Come, parents, help us in our work, / from every rank and station, / that widely we may spread the cause / of Anti-Vaccination."[4]

To unite campaigners across the social spectrum, anti-vaccinators often drew on a populist rhetoric. Alfred Milnes argued that this law "was never demanded by the people."[5] "The people are with us," echoed the LSACV.[6] When they adopted this populist vision, anti-vaccinators pitted "the people" against doctors as a "class." This was not a proletarian discourse but an older usage of the term that emphasized the need for the masses to fight the power of the privileged few.[7] The vaccination acts "are class laws," argued William Hume-Rothery in *Vaccination and the Vaccination Laws: A Physical Curse and a Class-Tyranny*, "inasmuch as they benefit only the doctor class."[8] Like Josephine Butler's attack on those "terrible aristocratic doctors," who more often than not actually came from an expanding middle class, this rhetoric enabled a disparate group of activists to unite as an oppressed people against the privilege of the "medical monopoly."[9]

Populist language was exceedingly flexible and could be used by different kinds of campaigners for a variety of ends. For the middle class, this discourse operated as an emotive gesture to long-standing traditions of political protest and allowed them to envision and position themselves as an integral part of the struggle. For workers, it was used interchangeably with a new and equally powerful language of class conflict that, as chapter 4 will argue, reveals profound class tensions within the movement. But, significantly, it also enabled plebeian anti-vaccinators to ally themselves with the middle-class repeal campaign and thus to claim "the equal rights of English citizenship."[10] The populist discourse of the anti-vaccination campaign thus served an important political purpose, blunting the class tensions inherent in the movement. It found its clearest expression in the language of citizenship that emphasized the rights of the freeborn Englishman.

The Politics of Parenthood

The government's emphasis on the vaccination of children was consistent with its efforts in the last three decades of the century to incorporate them into the state as citizens in need of governmental protection. In the 1870s and '80s, Parliament not only tightened the vaccination laws but also passed legislation pertaining to compulsory education and child protection, revealing the state's increasing concern with legislating for the welfare of children as future citizens of the nation. Anti-vaccinators from all social classes vehemently objected to this interference in their private lives and accused the state of usurping the parental role. This policing of parents, they argued, deprived freemen of their "civil rights and privileges as citizens of an otherwise free country."[11]

Campaigners against compulsory vaccination maintained that the rights of citizens involved not only political rights to the franchise and equality under the law, but also domestic rights to control over family and home. Hence, Walter Hadwen, a pharmaceutical chemist and one of the movement's greatest orators, declared that he agitated "as a father and a citizen."[12] For Milnes, the "guardianship of [his] own children" was in fact "the first right of citizenship."[13] Anti-vaccinators campaigned thus as "enlightened citizen-parents" against the "invasion of personal and parental rights."[14] For they maintained that their "parental, conjugal, and domestic rights" included "the right to be pure and unpolluted."[15]

While anti-vaccinators, as we shall see, readily embraced the nation, they saw vaccination as a technology of the Victorian state, which they

denounced for interfering in family affairs. Middle-class anti-vaccinators in particular contended that their own domestic structure was being replaced by a new governmental family, the product of the marriage
of "Papa Medicine" to a "meddling foster-mother" state.[16] They warned
of the dangers of, in the words of the future Home Secretary William
Harcourt, a "grand-maternal Government which ties nightcaps on a
grown-up nation by act of Parliament."[17]

Anti-vaccinators demanded the right to parent as they saw fit and to
control over their children. The state, they contended, was usurping the
parental role. I will never "give up my child, who am its proper guardian,
to the guardianship of any other person or persons whatever," maintained a father.[18] At an inquest in Battersea in 1883, convened to investigate the death of a child from vaccinal injuries, the coroner allegedly
turned to the father on completion and declared, "You can take away that
corpse; it belongs to you now." As Milnes was quick to note, living
children did not belong to their parents. But when "the doctors had done
with them, and when the vaccination fee had been earned, then came in
the inalienable right of the father—to pay the undertaker."[19] Pro-vaccinators, such as John Makinson Fox of the National Health Society, argued
that English law had "never placed the child's life at the disposal of the
parent. Every child rather belongs to the law and to the nation."[20] Anti-
vaccinators stridently opposed this position, claiming, in the words of a
Scottish father, that children "are not children of the State, but of their
parents."[21] In 1883, Mary Hume-Rothery used the feminist campaign
for married women's property rights to assert that there was "no property belonging to Married Women one-half so precious to them as their
babes."[22] Appealing to traditions of radical individualism—and to a liber-
tarian and, more recent, feminist—concern for property rights, anti-
vaccinators maintained that their children were literally their property
and as such were not to be tampered with.

How best to raise a family, they insisted, was a domestic issue and a
parental right over which the state had no authority to interfere. "What
right has that Law, or any Law, to step between you and your child,"
asserted the ACVMPS, "and force you to do what you believe to be fatal to
its health and happiness?"[23] Mary Hume-Rothery feared that compulsory vaccination was a slippery slope that could eventually result in
Parliament's prescribing or prohibiting certain diets or drugs. She cau-

tioned that the state would soon be subjecting mothers to a "compulsory nursing drill," or forbidding them to "rock their infants lest (according to fashionable modern theories) it should injure their brains." These governmental interventions were particularly troubling, for, as William Gladstone admitted, the state was "a very bad nurse."[24]

Anti-vaccinators often gestured to the hypocrisy of a state that maintained the right of "puncturing babies" but claimed no responsibility for the outcome.[25] If the government could not guarantee the success of the procedure, anti-vaccinators argued, then they should not be able to compel parents to take such a risk. In a letter to *The Pioneer*, a father raised concerns about the spread of syphilis through vaccination. "It becomes a question of choice of risks," he reasoned, "and I am only one amongst thousands of fathers in this country who are determined, at any cost and at any trouble to themselves, to insist upon the right of a parent to decide *what* risks his child shall run."[26] Thus, anti-vaccinators consistently argued for the freedom to govern themselves and their families. Their critiques suggested that, while vaccination was a passing fad, the rights of parents were a long-established English privilege. The "rights of parents," argued Milnes, are the Englishman's birthright, "derived from our ancestors."[27]

If the rights of parents were to be protected, then the home needed to be made safe from governmental scrutiny and control. In one of the earliest critiques of compulsory vaccination, John Gibbs maintained in 1856 that this new legislation not only infringed on the rights of the parent but "invade[d]" the "sanctity of the home." This rhetoric persisted in anti-vaccination propaganda throughout the century, for campaigners insisted that there could be no true liberty "where the home-life is invaded."[28] Compulsory vaccination, warned one agitator, introduces "vexatious interference into the hitherto sacred privacy of your homes and families."[29] Anti-vaccinators returned to the oft-repeated epigram that the Englishman's home is his castle and complained bitterly that compulsory vaccination ensured that this was no longer the case: " 'An Englishman's house is his castle' no more. / For foul Persecution lays siege to his door," chimed an anti-vaccination poem. To compel a man to vaccinate his child against his better judgment, proclaimed a campaigner, "is to infringe on the sacred right of an Englishman to reign supreme in his own household."[30]

The extension of the long arm of the state into the previously private and domestic realm of child care was not only a symbolic violation of the home. It was also experienced as a physical invasion of private space. When the homoeopath J. J. Garth Wilkinson warned parents to "insist on new frontiers to your homes, frontiers of fortified right over your persons," he meant quite literally that compulsory vaccination transgressed the boundaries of the home to gain access to the person.[31] Working-class noncompliers were routinely seized from their houses and dragged to jail. As chapter 2 described, in 1887 a "crowbar brigade" attacked the door of the vaccination defaulter Robert King. Similarly, J. A. Picton, the anti-vaccinationist M P for Leicester, reported that the police had "assailed" the house of Mr. Eagle, "climbing over the garden wall for the purpose, at 1:30 A.M. on Whit Monday morning."[32] Vaccination officers, inspectors routinely considered medical police, were renowned for calling at home while the father was at work, attempting to intimidate the mother into compliance. It was preferable, argued a correspondent to the *Vaccination Inquirer*, "to find a burglar in the house than an inspector, as he departs at once, is rather cheaper, and does not pretend to be acting for the 'common good.'"[33]

It was not only law enforcement officers and government inspectors who invaded the working-class home, but also medical personnel themselves. The expansion of district nursing and health visiting in the late nineteenth and early twentieth centuries meant that many medical personnel attempted, in the words of the district nurse Margaret Loane, to launch "flank or frontal attacks upon the Englishman's Castle."[34] Some public vaccinators made illegal rounds, forcibly vaccinating unsupervised children.[35] After 1898, when domiciliary vaccination replaced public vaccination stations, vaccinators were authorized to enter the home to perform their duties. Although anti-vaccinators objected to vaccination stations, they were equally opposed to this new practice, which the former mayor of Leicester denounced as a "house to house inquisition."[36] In 1899, the *Vaccination Inquirer* advised fathers to leave a note at home when going off to work, instructing the "Peripatetic Cowpox[er]" that he was forbidden to vaccinate.[37] Anti-vaccinators thus felt that the sanctity of the home was quite literally under attack and defended their individual rights to their property and their privacy.

The Language of Citizenship

Anti-vaccinators maintained that their rights as parents were political rights that derived not only from a biological imperative to protect their infants but, perhaps more significantly, from their status as English citizens. From the 1860s, crusaders on both sides of the vaccination debate used the language of citizenship to forward their causes. For those who promoted vaccination, the procedure was part of the duty of good citizenship, for it protected the entire community from disease. Pro-vaccinationists attempted to incorporate working people into the national community as citizens through participation in maintaining the public's health. In an address to Manchester workers in 1878, the medical officer of health for Southport appealed to his audience as "sanitarians, as citizens, and as parents" to do "our duty" in reducing infant mortality. Similarly, a Ladies' Sanitary Association tract from the 1860s argued that "we are all members of one body." If one member suffers, it argued, all the others must suffer with it. "If we, as fellow citizens, allow our prejudices or our ignorance—when we have the means of knowing better—to interfere with the general good," it concluded, "on ourselves individually rests the guilt."[38]

While many anti-vaccinators argued that "the State" had no right to compel "a father to jeopardise the health and lives of [his] children in the name of the public weal," they also mobilized the rhetoric of citizenship and used it to their own advantage.[39] "I speak as a citizen to citizens," announced F. W. Newman, brother of the cardinal and an ardent social reformer.[40] Anti-vaccinators consistently maintained that they were good, law-abiding citizens and demanded to be treated with respect. Henry Pitman, editor of the *Co-operator and Anti-Vaccinator*, defended a vaccination defaulter by arguing that he was "as meritorious a citizen as ever lived."[41] Robert Stobbs, a factory worker and pharmaceutical chemist, insisted that he was a "peaceable citizen and loyal subject of the British Crown."[42] In fact, anti-vaccinators maintained that their resistance in and of itself demonstrated good citizenship. Good citizenship, Mary Hume-Rothery held, did not mean enforcing public-health measures. Rather, it entailed respecting the bodies of one's neighbors. It is not "*decent*, in a free country, even to talk of legalising bodily assault and possible murder on the bodies of a fellow-citizen's children," she contended.[43] Not only should one personally resist vaccination, but, agitators proposed, "[I]t behooves every good citizen to endeavour by every constitutional means . . . to get these laws completely and permanently extinguished."[44] This discourse of citizenship was marshaled by working and middle-class campaigners alike, as anti-vaccinators sought to claim their rights as members of a just and free nation.

CITIZENSHIP AND THE NATION   If anti-vaccinationism operated in practice as a series of local initiatives, its vision was national in scope and nationalistic at heart. It was to Englishness, rather than to local or regional affiliations, that anti-vaccinators consistently turned. Occasionally, anti-vaccinators appealed to the people of the "United Kingdom" or the "three kingdoms," but the focus remained on English rights and English resistance.[45] The vaccination acts of 1853, 1867, and 1871 applied only to England and Wales, although Wales lagged far behind England in its ability to mobilize support for the anti-vaccination cause. In the 1860s, similar acts were passed for Scotland and Ireland, but they were less stringent and less vigorously enforced. Encouragement for Scottish anti-vaccinators was more forthcoming, but Irish victims of compulsory vaccination received little sympathy from their English counterparts. In fact, the Irish question served as an impediment to English anti-vaccinators. They claimed not only that the treatment of English anti-vaccinators was more draconian than that of Irish political prisoners, but also that the issue of Home Rule stood in the way of parliamentary debate over vaccination. It was not until the twentieth century, when the movement waned and the English campaign scrambled for supporters, that the plight of the Irish was taken up.[46]

Anti-vaccinators' appeals for their rights rested on nationalistic claims that unified campaigners under the banner of English patriotism. They repeatedly drew on "the narratives of the nation" so central to popular politics before the passage of the 1867 Reform Act,[47] perpetuating this rhetoric into the twentieth century. "The feeling of nation is being aroused from end to end," argued the Reverend A. T. Guttery in 1889; the anti-vaccination movement "will win the increasing adherence of all faithful and patriotic people in this land."[48] Propagandists repeatedly invoked the national symbols of John Bull and the British Lion and appropriated "Rule Britannia" for their own purposes. Compulsory vaccination, anti-vaccinators warned, undermined this patriotic spirit; it made one "ashamed almost of being an Englishman."[49]

Appealing to the popular constitutionalism so crucial to the populist politics of the first half of the nineteenth century, anti-vaccinators maintained that their rights to have control over themselves and their property were historically rooted in the English constitution. Although England's constitution was unwritten, anti-vaccinators used the nostalgic language of the Norman Yoke and the Magna Charta to defend their rights as parents.[50] Compulsory vaccination, argued a pamphleteer, is "repugnant to the spirit of our constitution."[51] "Englishmen were wont to boast that their constitution assured the *inviolability of the person*," argued John Gibbs in 1856. "That security no longer exists. *The constitution is daily violated in the person of the most innocent*."[52] The word *constitution* here had a double resonance, referring to a charter of rights and to a physical bodily system, both of which were being "violated," anti-vaccinators insisted, by a "despotic" law. Similarly, in addressing a demonstration in Northampton, Councillor Thomas Purser proclaimed anti-vaccinationism's place in a historical, patriotic, and literary narrative. He linked the persecution of the "citizen . . . who would not have his children's blood poisoned" to that of "Bunyan, and those who fought for right 100 years ago."[53]

To be English, anti-vaccinators asserted, also meant to have a sense of "duty" toward one's fellow subjects and to possess a certain "national character." "John Bull," argued Mary Hume-Rothery, "is stolid, but at bottom justice-loving, and child-loving."[54] Above all else, Englishness, as an anti-vaccination song made clear, was synonymous with freedom: "Men of England, claim your freedom, / Make a noble stand / Sweep the unjust law of tyrants / From your native land. / Strike the blow to vaccination, / Claim your liberty; / Sound the echo through the nation, / Britons shall be free."[55] Campaigners consistently appealed to the ideal of the freeborn Englishman deployed by radicals from at least the late eighteenth century. They upheld England as the "Land of the Free and the Brave" and argued that Englishmen were born with this love of freedom; it was an innate, natural feeling and their birthright. As such, they would resist "the iron heel of tyranny" at every turn.[56]

Anti-vaccination propaganda contrasted English freedom with the despotism of foreign nations. While they blamed the British state for the coercive vaccination laws, agitators nevertheless associated compulsory vaccination with a foreign element. During the summer of 1881, while a smallpox epidemic raged in the capital, a vaccination scare erupted in the North of England. Rumors quickly spread that foreigners were to be sent to revaccinate all the children attending state schools. In May, the intruders were characterized as "negro doctors"; by June, they had become "American quack-doctors." Parents responded immediately by surrounding the schools and demanding their children. In Derbyshire, a group mainly composed of mothers "smashed the windows and did other damage" to the schools, succeeding in closing them down for the day. In Wednesbury, "alarmed and irate parents" objected to having their children "cut to pieces by *black men, Mr. Gladstone, or anyone.*"[57]

Anti-vaccinators often located this foreign tyranny in Europe or in far-off lands associated with the excesses of the East. In a pamphlet addressed to the secretary of state, the alternative medical practitioner John Fraser suggested sarcastically that the government take the final step toward coercion and send vaccine officials door to door accompanied by policemen to enforce vaccination. He also advised that, "French-like," the vaccinator should ride on the vaccine cow brandishing an "upraised lancet."[58] Although the French did not enforce compulsory vaccination, English anti-vaccinators, in the tradition of popular radicalism, still pointed to their closest neighbors and traditional rivals as the epitome of coercive government. But central European nations also provided a perfect foil for English justice. Gibbs distinguished England from countries such as Austria, "where the number of hens a man may keep in his yard, or the number of bakers, or butchers, in a town, are alike regulated by law, and where the subject may be forcibly seized by the police and carried off and vaccinated."[59] In contrast, they argued, Britons were celebrated for their independence and individuality.

Middle-class agitators were more likely to characterize the East as the antithesis of British democracy. For Wilkinson, the "medical Gladstone Government" was little better than "Egyptian despotism."[60] According to Mary Hume-Rothery, England was not so far removed from a "nation of despised Orientals."[61] The compulsory vaccination laws, these anti-vaccinators suggested, "orientalized" England and led to cultural degeneration. This rhetoric of foreign tyranny took on particular importance as anti-vaccinators staked their claim to citizenship in an imperial context that required them to position themselves in relationship to both the "civilizing mission" and colonial peoples who were also subject to the "parliamentary lancet."

IMPERIAL CITIZENS The anti-vaccination movement reached its peak in the 1880s at a time that saw the passage of a Third Reform Act, which considerably expanded the franchise, the rise of the female suffrage movement, and a heated contest over Home Rule in Ireland. The expansion and consolidation of the British empire in the 1880s and '90s contributed to this fertile climate for debates over British citizenship. Anti-vaccinators seized on the new imperial rhetoric to provide a sense of urgency and scope to their cause. In 1897, William Tebb proclaimed that "anti-vaccinators in England are fighting the battle, not for their own country only, but for the Colonies and the whole of Europe."[62] But the relationship between English anti-vaccinators and colonial subjects was far from straightforward. English anti-vaccinators paid scant attention to their colonial counterparts in India, who from 1880 were also forced to undergo vaccination, and who were engaged in a resistance campaign of their own.[63] Their relationship to Africans was rather more complex. Anti-vaccinators used the suffering of Africans to underscore the tyranny of the state, critiquing the medical component of colonial rule that historians of empire have increasingly characterized as integral to the imperialist project.[64] At the same time, in using African bodies to represent their own, these agitators in fact implied that the privileges of citizenship were to be granted first and foremost to white Englishmen.

Anti-vaccinators routinely criticized both the technologies of imperialism and the excesses of the British imperial state. In the 1880s, they attacked not the need to civilize "darkest Africa," but, rather, the method adopted by missionaries who went forth "with the Bible in one hand and the equally sacred lymph in the other." In 1885, the Countess de Noailles, patron of the anti-vaccination cause, outlined the role of the European civilizing mission. While she commented specifically on the

Belgian Congo, her message was also directed at Britain's African colonies. The "blessings of civilization," she argued, did not lie in the vaccination lancet. The "responsibility" incurred in a "Protectorate over aboriginal races" required colonizers to do them no harm and to "raise them up by the purest common sense of more favoured lands towards the higher levels of health and happiness." This could not be accomplished through "medical experimentation," she maintained, for vaccination would surely spread "the diseases of the old Continents . . . to the veins of poor Africa."[65] While the imperial project itself needed no justification, vaccinators, the countess argued, were bad missionaries.

The *Vaccination Inquirer* reiterated this position but was more critical of the project of "civilizing the natives." In 1887, under the headline "Missionaries as Vaccinators," it described a German cartoon that lampooned the British vaccination of "Caffreland." The *Vaccination Inquirer* critiqued the so-called "civilising" operation, arguing that our "missionary system seems to have unwittingly produced in the national mind an opinion that we are morally justified in introducing, and dutifully bound to enforce, on subject communities every British notion which we may happen to believe to be good for man."[66] In fact, anti-vaccinators maintained, the British penchant for vaccination clearly demonstrated that they were as superstitious and savage as those they intended to convert.

"We are rare promoters of civilisation!" quipped Joseph Towers, an agitator among the working classes in East London. "Among the articles in the treaty of peace with the Zulu chiefs is one which signifies that *no witch-doctors are to be tolerated.* If that be so, the oppressed natives of Zululand are, after all, better off than the be-doctored inhabitants of these northern isles, who are tormented out of their lives by the Compulsory Vaccination Acts. It may be feared, however, that such congratulation will prove but temporary, for the Jennerian boon may yet be conferred on poor Africans if they are sufficiently docile under British rule."[67] Anti-vaccinators were quick to characterize vaccination as "primitive" and implied that Britain itself was devolving into a society that worshipped false idols. Vaccination is a mere "fetish," argued Hadwen, "infinitely more dangerous, than the Medicine Man's charm in Lobengulas' Kraal, or the mystic hieroglyphics of the Wizard of the Arabian Desert."[68] Agitators denounced vaccination as a "foul Jennerian rite" and a "grotesque superstition," more abominable than human sacrifice uncovered "abroad" by missionaries. They frequently compared vaccination to child sacrifice. The compulsory vaccination acts, argued Mary Hume-Rothery, were simply "ACTS FOR THE OFFER-ING UP ANNUALLY OF AN INDEFINITE NUMBER OF HUMAN SACRI-FICES to propitiate an imaginary Devil." Up to 200 children were cer-tified each year as dying from vaccination while "tens of thousands" of other deaths were due indirectly to the operation, argued a sympathizer. What would we say, he added, "of some savage African tribe that every week sacrificed to an idol two children to guard them against small-pox?"[69] By illustrating the parallels between vaccination and so-called superstitious rites, anti-vaccinators suggested that imperial Britain was in fact hardly different from the "primitive" peoples it intended to civilize.

By the 1890s, it had become clear to anti-vaccinators that vaccination was being forced on Africans not just by missionaries but by the impe-rial state, whose arm had grown long enough to reach even far-off colonized peoples. Most anti-vaccinators were at the very least uncom-fortable with the use of vaccination as a way of either incorporating colonial peoples as British subjects or subduing them to be ruled. But in critiquing the technologies of British imperialism, anti-vaccinators were nevertheless more concerned with themselves than with their colonial counterparts. Anti-vaccinators used Africa as a foil for England and invoked the suffering bodies of Africans to make statements about their own domestic condition. Drawing parallels between an oppressed English public and subjected colonial peoples was a powerful political statement. As Antoinette Burton has argued, Victorian feminists used a "variety of colonized bodies" to stake moral claims "on the domestic body politic." They used the "injuries of 'others,' " she maintains, "to (re-)focus the attention of the state on their own desire for inclusion in the body politic."[70] As a group who felt themselves equally margin-alized from the full privileges of English citizenship, anti-vaccinators employed comparable tactics, stressing their solidarity with those who suffered similar bodily violations.

During the 1890s, anti-vaccinators increasingly commented on the parallels between the poor and working classes subjected to compul-sory vaccination in England and their counterparts in the African colo-nies. In the Transvaal, the *Vaccination Inquirer* reported in 1893, the punishment for noncompliance was twenty-five lashes if one were "coloured." "This is about what our own doctors would like to do if they dared," its editor commented.[71] Two years later, *The Graphic*, a middle-class illustrated periodical, depicted the enforced vaccination of "natives" in Natal. "It is useful at least," the anti-vaccination press responded, "to show how the medicos would like to treat the poor of our own land if it were not for the power of the democracy which perforce restrains them."[72] This relationship between domestic and colonial vaccination policy proved politically useful but also troubling for English resisters in that it produced a certain identification with Africans that at the same time they attempted to disavow. In attacking medical imperialism, anti-vaccinators revealed their anxieties over the relationship between their own bodies and those of colonial subjects, critiquing the government for treating its white citizens as it did its colonized others.

The imagined connection between the metropolitan working class and colonized peoples was hardly new. The identification of the poor with colonial subjects and racial others had been established in the early nineteenth century by missionary societies. By the 1870s, the racialization of class difference had become a trope of late-Victorian journalism. The slums of the metropolis were imagined as a dark continent penetrated by urban explorers seeking to uncover the habits and dwellings of savage tribes.[73] This uneasy relationship between a white English working class and racial "others" had also been symptomatic of working-class radicalism since the 1830s. Radicals such as William Cobbett, Richard Oastler, and Bronterre O'Brien all opposed the antislavery movement and attacked the hypocrisy of abolitionists who embraced the liberation of the "negro" while turning a blind eye to the exploitation of the white factory "slave."[74] Indeed, the key phrase in the ten-hours movement was "white slavery," which implied that part of the outrage derived from the fact that the exploited industrial worker was a white Englishman, not a black African. The language of white slavery enabled the working man, largely because of his racial affiliation, to position himself as a citizen entitled to property in his own person and to control over his dependents.[75] Thus, some early Victorian radicals and reformers were torn between rejecting the abolitionist cause and embracing its rhetorical power. They often used the language of slavery to forward workers' claims to social justice while at the same time dismissing the actions of those who prioritized the plight of Africans and African Americans.

In the 1850s, medical dissenters seized on these complex discourses of slavery to stress their position vis-à-vis orthodox medicine.[76] But it was not until the last decades of the century that anti-vaccinators revived the discourse for their own purposes. The language of slavery they mobilized in the 1880s and '90s served as a nostalgic language of suffering for agitators such as William Tebb, who had been active in the American abolitionist campaign before founding the LSACV.[77] No longer a contentious political issue, slavery was used by middle- and working-class anti-vaccinators toward the end of the century as a metaphor for social inequality and coercive governmental tactics. Tebb's most frequent point of reference for vaccination defaulters was to the American fugitive slave. The "hunting of unvaccinated fugitives from parish to parish," he argued, was no different from "slave-hunting in the United States." The treatment of anti-vaccinators in the courts, he proposed, paralleled the infamous Dred Scot case, which established that African Americans did not have the same citizenship rights as whites.[78]

Tebb repeatedly returned to this analogy in the last decades of the century, arguing that English anti-vaccinators, "like the negro race in America during the reign of the Democratic slavocracy, have no rights which magistrates are bound to respect." In 1897, the *Vaccination Inquirer* ran an excerpt from *Uncle Tom's Cabin*, comparing the selling of slave babies to the death of children from vaccination.[79] Correspondence from the United States reinforced and encouraged this relationship, constructing the relationship between parliamentarians and anti-vaccinators as that between abusive master and compliant slave. Writing from Brooklyn in 1884, a subscriber to the *National Anti-Compulsory Vaccination Reporter* compared anti-vaccinators' blind allegiance to political parties (which, he maintained, did little for the cause) to the relationship between "dark-skinned ignorant slaves" and "Ole Mas'r.'" Because "Ole Mas'r'" was a "nice man and allowed them a few sugar-cakes," the correspondent argued, these slaves "forewent their manhood, their liberty, and all their individual rights" and refused to run away.[80]

Anti-vaccinators were quick to draw on the political, emotive, or rhetorical value of the slave, or of the colonized African. They were quicker still to claim that the suffering of white English citizens took precedence over that of the oppressed elsewhere. Tebb declared that he had heard many an escaped slave recount his story, but there were no experiences "more pitiful, cruel, and heart-breaking" than those he had heard "from the lips of English mothers" when detailing the wrongs done to them under the vaccination acts.[81] Anti-vaccinators routinely criticized those who placed the lives and welfare of racial others ahead of suffering English citizens. If the persecution of anti-vaccinators was suffered by "Bulgarians or the Egyptian fellaheen," proposed an agitator, gesturing to Gladstone's concern with the "Bulgarian Horrors," "they might secure at our hands the attention which is withheld from Englishmen."[82] Similarly, Mary Hume-Rothery maintained that it is "English men, women and children themselves who are now the slaves, in stead of poor negroes on distant shores, for whose emancipation, strange to say, it seems to have been far easier to stir up enthusiasm and concentrate effort, than it is on behalf of those whose wrongs and oppression disgrace every town and village in the length and breadth of the land."[83] Hume-Rothery deliberately invoked the "telescopic philanthropy" of Dickens's infamous Mrs. Jellyby, who is so preoccupied with her mission to the natives of Borrioboola-Gha that she neglects her children and her household, which are in a perpetual state of chaos.

Anti-vaccinators employed the familiar discourse of anti-slavery and likened themselves to colonized peoples, then, not because they were highly concerned about the treatment of Africans, but to underscore the perceived irony that those most persecuted by compulsory vaccination were white English citizens and not subjected black Africans. The language of citizenship they deployed was thus an inclusive discourse that allowed a variety of campaigners to participate in the struggle of the people against privilege. But it was also an exclusive language. In appealing to the rights of the freeborn Englishman, anti-vaccinators not only linked their struggle to traditions of popular political protest, they also implicitly asserted that the rights of citizenship were due first and foremost to white Englishmen.

Liberalism and the Middle-Class Campaign

The populist language of citizenship so frequently deployed by anti-vaccinators of all social classes drew on a narrative of popular revolt against privilege and power that served to situate the campaign within a long tradition of popular politics. This was vital to the success of the cross-class alliance, for it united campaigners together and diffused the class tensions evident in the movement. But this attempt to provide common ground for all who resisted compulsory vaccination was complicated by the very real differences between campaigners.

The vaccination laws implicitly targeted the working class. Their implementation, as chapter 4 will discuss, openly discriminated against workers and the poor, for vaccination officials generally did not pursue middle-class defaulters. Middle-class anti-vaccinators thus had little firsthand experience with the vaccination acts. While they attacked the policy of compulsion, they rarely felt the impact of the compulsory clauses on their own bodies. For middle-class campaigners, the issue of the parental rights of English citizens was primarily bound up in larger political debates about the nature of liberalism. Middle-class anti-vaccinators fought to defend the Old Liberal agenda, which privileged individual rights and laissez-faire. But toward the turn of the century, this position was falling out of favor within the Liberal Party. The politics of the middle-class campaign thus centered on the meanings of liberalism and the relationship between the individual and the state. Middle-class anti-vaccinationism was thus more concerned with party politics than body politics.

THE OLD LIBERAL AGENDA   Middle-class anti-vaccinationists' attack on state compulsion and the violation of parental rights was part of a larger critique of the Liberal Party. While these campaigners generally considered themselves liberals, they were highly concerned about the direction of the Liberal Party, which no longer seemed to uphold its principles of individual rights, personal liberty, and laissez-faire capitalism. Mary Hume-Rothery attacked the "Pseudo-Liberal Party," which, although it did not pass the coercive 1867 act, sustained and strengthened it. Appealing to her political roots as the daughter of the Benthamite Joseph Hume, Mary Hume-Rothery claimed that "she also was a politician; she had been born, bred, and cradled in politics, and she held that no man was a Liberal who went in for destroying the liberties of his fellow-men."[84] Her position was shared by Milnes, who was a member of the newly founded National Liberal Club. Milnes maintained that he who did not support the right to refuse vaccination "calls himself a Liberal in vain":

He may be in favour of all the measures in the programme of a Liberal Ministry, but a Liberal he is not. He may get upon one platform and shout for universal suffrage, and upon another and scream for land nationalisation, but a Liberal he is not. He may betake him to the steeple-top and shriek for Christian socialism till he split his throat, still that man is not a Liberal; and calling himself a Liberal, I advise my Liberal friends to tell him that he has misdescribed his party, that he belongs to a party older than Liberalism—a party which was before Liberals were, and a party which unhappily shall be when Tories are no more—he is not a Liberal, he is a liar.[85]

These critiques were leveled implicitly at Gladstone, who had spoken openly about the "great inequality" of the vaccination law but, once in power, did nothing to alter it. By firmly voicing anti-vaccinationism as part of a Liberal agenda, middle-class campaigners attacked not only conservative policies but also emerging interventionist trends in liberalism that had begun to take root within the Liberal Party in the 1870s.

Mid-Victorian liberalism, while associated with the politics and economics of laissez-faire, was never entirely divorced from state intervention. The utilitarianism of the first half of the nineteenth century actually involved a degree of governmental participation in the lives of the British public. In fact, laissez-faire and state intervention were interrelated policies that accompanied the changes wrought by rapid industrialization.[86] Nevertheless, the idea of laissez-faire pervaded liberal discourse throughout the century and became a powerful rhetorical and political tool in the fight against compulsory vaccination. Like the alternative medical practitioners who resisted the disappearance of the medical marketplace, Tebb argued that "there should be free trade in medicine, as in everything else of exchangeable value." The LSACV proposed that there should be "free trade in vaccination; let those buy it who want it, and let those be free who don't want it."[87]

Middle-class campaigners also decried the system of compulsory vaccination because it undermined the idea of equal treatment under the law. The Personal Rights Association, founded in 1871, maintained that it was committed to "the principle of the equality of all citizens before the law, without regard to wealth, birth, sex, culture, race, religious belief, or any other circumstances whatever save the responsibilities which are implied in respect for the rights of others."[88] Compulsory vaccination, one of the Personal Rights Association's leading causes, violated this principle of equal justice at all levels of its administration as it openly discriminated against the working class. It is clear that the vaccination law, argued a widely quoted essay, "was never intended to apply to persons whose station is above that of the lower middle class."[89]

These anti-vaccinators also clung fast to the Old Liberal tenets of individual rights and personal liberty. A true Liberal government, they argued, respected the liberty of the individual above all else. J. H. Levy, professor of logic and economics at Birkbeck College and editor of the *Personal Rights Journal* (later renamed *The Individualist*), maintained that compulsory vaccination was a "gross and cruel invasion of personal liberty," for it interfered with the individual's decision to make choices governing the health and well-being of his or her own person and family.[90] The rights of individuals—in this case, parents—were paramount, middle-class anti-vaccinators argued. The state's purpose was thus to defend and protect personal liberty rather than to impinge on it. This position was central to organized anti-vaccinationism's critique of the Liberal Party, for, as Mary Hume-Rothery argued, a "Liberal was entitled to do his best for his own children, leaving his neighbours to do likewise."[91]

THE CHALLENGE OF NEW LIBERALISM Middle-class anti-vaccinators argued, therefore, that the individual rights and personal liberties of parents were the privilege of all citizens and thus a central concern of liberalism. However, they feared that these principles were being undermined by forces within their own party. "How is it that Liberalism," asked Herbert Spencer in 1884, in "getting more and more into power, has grown more and more coercive in its legislation?"[92] Spencer identified a new breed of Liberals for whom state intervention was not anathema and attacked them for co-opting the paternalistic style of governance that had characterized the Tories.[93] An article in the *Personal Rights Journal* in 1886, titled "The Old Liberalism and the New," articulated this debate within liberalism:

> [T]here [is] a difference between the old school of Liberals and the new. The cry of the old reformers was for political justice. They demanded the reform or the abolition of institutions and laws which imposed a

restriction on the personal rights and freedom of individual Englishmen. . . . [T]he new Liberalism derived its force not so much from the
love of inflexible justice as from a deep pity for the hardships of the
poor, for the misery which remained amongst us, notwithstanding the
growth of national wealth and prosperity.

By the 1880s, this rift between Liberal agendas was firmly entrenched.
While Old Liberals continued to maintain that the government should
"leave us free, and do us no harm," New Liberals began to ask, "How
much can Government do, and do safely, to contribute to the dignity
and greatness of the life of the people?"[94]

Old Liberals such as P. A. Taylor, MP for the anti-vaccinationist
stronghold of Leicester, maintained that "the less the State interferes
with the home management of the various portions of the community,
in regards to their habits, manners, and customs, the better both for the
State and the people."[95] New Liberals, however, argued just as fervently
for state intervention to promote the good of society. A pro-vaccination
pamphlet argued that, just as it provided free education and regulated
the hours and nature of child labor, the state should also contribute to
the health of children through public vaccination.[96] This New Liberal
principle was based largely on T. H. Green's philosophy of positive
freedoms and on the liberal organicist theories of J. A. Hobson and L. T.
Hobhouse, who argued that state intervention, however coercive, was
appropriate where the lives and safety of the entire community were at
stake. These sentiments were already at play in the 1850s in relation to
compulsory vaccination. John Simon argued as early as 1857 that vaccination was to be classed among those conditions "necessary for the
maintenance of life, which a parent should not be entitled to withhold
(any more than food or clothing) from his offspring."[97] This position
had gathered new momentum by the 1880s as New Liberals began to
argue that individual liberty and state intervention were not necessarily
in opposition. Rather, they posited, the state should be a catalyst for the
common good, thus ensuring liberty for the widest number of its citizens.[98] By providing free vaccination, New Liberals insisted, the state
undertook to furnish a basic need and was thus justified in intervening
in private life.

Many middle-class anti-vaccinators vigorously opposed this New Liberal position, which was gaining ground within the Liberal Party toward

the end of the century, as it dramatically reformulated the relationship between the individual and the state. In the wake of the Education Act of 1870, which sought to provide a minimal level of education for all children, William Hume-Rothery contended that the state had no right to compel either vaccination or education, as both were matters of parental choice. Whether it was in the best interests of either the individual or the community was beside the point. Even if vaccination were the greatest blessing, Hume-Rothery proposed, "the State would have no more right to [enforce it] than it would have to enact that every man should bathe himself regularly every morning."[99]

But if Hume-Rothery's position was typical of middle-class anti-vaccinationists, this dogmatic resistance to any and all state intervention did not necessarily characterize all campaigners. Some anti-vaccinators supported compulsory education, and, as we shall see in chapter 6, many in fact demanded that the government step in to deal with the issue of urban sanitation. Elements of New Liberalism thus clearly appealed to those anti-vaccinationists who considered themselves progressive reformers. In the early twentieth century, the idea of equal access to urban amenities became enshrined in the London County Council's political platform of "municipal socialism."[100] In promoting "municipal socialism" in the decades around the turn of the century, many middle-class anti-vaccinators actually supported a limited amount of governmental intervention. Picton, who fought for individual rights in relationship to vaccination, nevertheless served on the London School Board and in the 1880s and '90s became involved with the National Society for the Prevention of Cruelty to Children, an organization that was heavily involved in the policing of parental behavior. Similarly, Russell Rea, who ran for election as a Liberal Party candidate on an anti-vaccination platform in 1900, advocated state-sponsored meals for children and free heat and light a decade later. Conversely, John Stuart Mill, the patron saint of Old Liberalism, was present in the House of Commons when the Vaccination Act of 1867 was passed and did not openly oppose it.[101] Middle-class anti-vaccinators, therefore, were not uniformly committed to the Old Liberal agenda; nor were all Old Liberals anti-vaccinators. Indeed, the vaccination debate reveals the degree to which the meanings of liberalism—in the second half of the nineteenth century, in particular—were pliable and contentious.

Nevertheless, most middle-class anti-vaccinators were Old Liberals and as such were primarily preoccupied with the changing nature of liberalism and the role of the state in daily life. But the middle-class campaign also betrayed underlying anxieties about working-class violence. "It is *dangerous*," cautioned Milnes, "to secure the enmity" of the poor.[102] Josephine Butler warned: "The laws are the real educators of the people, and when they are partial and unjust, class hatred and bitter animosities spread like a poison through the body politic." Compulsory vaccination must be abolished, she said, lest the "violated principles" of democracy "assert themselves in a voice of thunder, in social convulsion and national catastrophe."[103]

This fear of popular revolt, voiced by a variety of contemporary reformers, was as close as middle-class campaigners came to seeing their own bodies as threatened. They often repeated Newman's proclamation: "Against the body of a healthy man Parliament has no right of assault whatever under the pretence of Public Health; nor any the more against the body of a healthy infant."[104] But it was clear that they did not regard their own bodies as vulnerable. Middle-class campaigners were quick to defend the individual rights of working-class parents as part of their commitment to the political principles of Old Liberalism. The language of violation these middle-class reformers mobilized, however, betrayed little concern over the security of their own persons. Thus, while the populist language of rights and citizenship enabled a cross-class alliance to exist, the middle-class campaign rarely engaged with working-class critiques of compulsory vaccination that emphasized the vulnerability of the adult as well as the infant body in the hands of a coercive state. Thus, the middle-class anti-vaccination leadership failed to understand or to address fully the body politics of working-class resistance to compulsory vaccination.

4

The Body Politics of Class Formation

Law should be justice, but mock-justice here

Arrayed in rags of power, to infants dear

Denies the shelter of a mother's love;

Prison and fine the poor man's guerdon prove

For faithful fatherhood—the *rich* can pay

And manage their own babes, in their own way.

Then sweep, oh! sweep this vile class-law away

We humbly ask—we humbly beg and pray!

—W. G. Wood, "The Compulsory Vaccination Law"[1]

The anti-vaccination movement was a cross-class campaign, but this alliance was not unproblematic. While anti-vaccinationists were quick to mobilize the populist discourse typical of both radical protest and liberal reform, the debate devolved as often as not into an issue of class, with an accompanying language of antagonism and divisiveness. When asked by the Royal Commission on Vaccination in the 1890s whether he was opposed to compulsory vaccination, William Kempson, the mayor of Leicester declared: "Yes, I am, decidedly. . . . The feeling is very strong in Leicester; almost enough to set class against class."[2] The cross-class alliance, therefore, was as much a rhetorical strategy as an accurate portrait of the movement.

Anti-vaccinators did come from diverse social groups, but their experiences of compulsory vaccination differed dramatically, as the vaccination administration primarily tracked, fined, and imprisoned working-class defaulters. It was this population that the government deemed most likely to catch and spread disease and accused of being irresponsible parents. The classed nature of the implementation of vaccination policy meant that the values and goals of campaigners were sometimes in conflict. Many working-class campaigners embraced the Old Liberal position and often marshaled the language of individualism and laissez-faire so central to the middle-class campaign. But their resistance to compulsory vaccination was not merely about defending a set of abstract political principles. Rather, it had important bodily implications. Working-class activists easily elided the baby's body with the adult's, implying that compulsory vaccination infringed not only on the rights but on the bodies of adult citizens. They consistently affirmed their bodies as *the* political object at stake in the dispute over compulsory vaccination. Working-class resistance to the vaccination laws thus reveals the centrality of the body to the production of, and the meanings generated around, class in nineteenth- and early-twentieth-century Britain.

Anti-Vaccinationism and Working-Class Politics

Anti-vaccinationism was a national movement, but it found its strongest support in predominantly working-class regions and neighborhoods. Although London was by no means the center of anti-vaccination agitation, working-class districts of East and South London such as Hackney, Shoreditch, Bethnal Green, Mile End, and Southwark were home to various anti-vaccination leagues. The cluster of industrial towns around Manchester, Sheffield, and Liverpool also proved to be a hotbed of anti-vaccinationism, boasting upward of thirty-five anti-vaccination societies.

Grassroots resistance to the vaccination acts was largely mobilized by those who described and identified themselves as workers (although obviously not all workers supported the anti-vaccination position). These resisters were journeyman laborers, artisans, factory operatives, and small shopkeepers. It was primarily this population that was compelled to use the public stations and suffered the indignities of being tracked and punished by local authorities. Local anti-vaccination agitation was generally recognized as a working-class activity by anti- and pro-vaccinators alike. A vaccinator from Lancashire declared that vaccination was "hated amongst the working classes" in his district.[3] In

1905, the *Daily Mail* characterized twenty-six defaulters imprisoned in Derby as "belong[ing] to the working class."[4] Letters to newspapers were often signed "from a working man," while a celebrated parade of women carried banners declaring: "Working Women of South London join us in our appeal to the Legislature!" Anti-vaccinators such as Elijah House, a self-described "working man," positioned and imagined themselves as workers, "clothed in fustian" and a "ragged coat."[5] While it is important to stress that class identities are fluid, not fixed, many anti-vaccinators identified themselves as members of a working class. They expressed a shared experience of the body as violated and coerced and repeatedly voiced their grievances in the political language of class conflict.

Anti-vaccinationism thrived in areas with strong labor movements, for vaccination could impinge on job security. Although they applied only to children, the vaccination acts provoked fears of smallpox that led to the introduction of policies that threatened the lives and livelihoods of adult workers. Some employers demanded that all their employees be vaccinated or else forfeit their jobs. During an outbreak in Sheffield in 1887, thousands were vaccinated and revaccinated in workshops "under the covert threat of dismissal on non-compliance."[6] In Glouces-ter ten years later, a policy of "Vaccination or Starvation" forced "work-ing people" to be vaccinated "or lose their work." Trade unions' involve-ment with this issue confirms the widespread nature of this problem and the successes of solidarity. The Midland Railway Company's em-ployees threatened to strike if forced to undergo vaccination and suc-ceeded in warding off the lancet.[7] Working-class anti-vaccinators thus contended that employers took "advantage of their position and power to force their conscientiously objecting servants to barter their bodies or accept dismissal."[8] Employers must not imagine, argued the *Vaccina-tion Inquirer*, that "wages bought their bodies as well as their labour."[9] Compulsory vaccination thus made workers fear not only for their babies, but also for their own persons.

Anti-vaccinationism quickly established itself as part and parcel of working-class political life. Long before compulsion, William Cobbett, the father of early Victorian radicalism, had opposed vaccination. So did his intellectual descendants, such as members of the Keighley Radical Club, who in 1885 invited "Teetotal, Peace, Antivaccination and Home

Rule Societies" to join them at a political conference.[10] Anti-vaccinationists often allied themselves with these older forms of radical politics that sought the advancement of the working classes. The LSACV advertised in *The Radical*, a short-lived journal devoted to radical politics, while the *National Independent*—committed to "social justice" and the "rights of the working classes"—placed their own ads in the *Vaccination Inquirer*. In 1903, the official organ of the Reading Workers' Electoral League, the *Reading Labour Herald*, published a column of anti-vaccination notes.[11] Some anti-vaccinators considered themselves socialists and belonged to the Independent Labour Party. The London branch of the Marxist International Working Men's Association also supported the cause by publishing anti-vaccination material in its journal, the *International Herald*. The campaign, however, was not readily embraced by all socialist organizations. William Morris's journal *Commonweal* ignored the issue entirely, while Henry Hyndman, the leader of the Social Democratic Federation, was wary of encouraging anti-vaccination support. Instead, he sought to demarcate his serious commitment to Marxist socialism from the type of faddism that many Liberals also resisted. "I do not want the movement to be a depository of odd cranks," Hyndman declared, "humanitarians, vegetarians, anti-vivisectionists and anti-vaccinationists, arty-crafties and all the rest of them."[12] Despite the uneasiness of these emerging socialist organizations to open themselves up to accusations of crankery, resistance to compulsory vaccination was clearly part of a much broader working-class political culture that critiqued the repressive policies of the Victorian state.

Vaccination and the New Poor Law

Resistance to the vaccination laws was part of a widespread working-class distrust of state welfare in general. Compulsory vaccination's relationship to the dreaded New Poor Law ensured that it would be immediately unpopular. "[I]t cannot be refuted," insisted a pamphleteer in 1881, "that much of the defective result of vaccination originated in the operation of the New Poor Law."[13] The laboring classes despised the New Poor Law, for it severely limited their independence, forcing all recipients of government relief into the workhouse, which was notorious for its brutalizing regime. This suspicion of the Poor Law was compounded by the 1832 Anatomy Act, which had given the state unprecedented access to the bodies of the poor. This legislation permitted Poor Law Guardians to distribute the corpses of dead paupers to anatomy schools for dissection. The workhouse thus not only stigmatized the poor but threatened their bodily integrity.[14]

The vaccination services were administered by the Poor Law because the 1853 act had grown out of the 1840 policy of offering free vaccinations to the poor. Although the 1853 act was new, the vaccinators who operated under it often were not. Some had served as public vaccinators for over a decade and continued in these positions, despite the fact that the public requiring their services had changed. In the London district of St. George-in-the-East, many parents refused the services of the public vaccinator, who was also the workhouse surgeon, preferring instead to consult his deputy, who had no parish appointment.[15] A physician at the Manchester Southern Hospital for Diseases of Women and Children declared that, even though Poor Law medical officers had the best supply of lymph, parents refused their services "lest poverty came too near their skirts."[16]

More problematic still, the vaccination officers who tracked down recalcitrant parents often held other Poor Law appointments. Some were relieving officers or rate collectors or held comparable positions with the sanitary authority. In Bromley in 1901, the vaccination officer was also the relieving officer, the registrar of births and deaths, and the school-attendance officer.[17] While the Poor Law Board often refused to sanction the dual appointment of a vaccination officer and relieving officer, this was largely because they felt that relieving officer was a full-time job. The board had no objection to the "Relieving Officer in going his rounds . . . intimat[ing] to the poor persons whom he sees the necessity of having their infant children vaccinated."[18] The vaccination personnel were therefore heavily identified with relief and carried with them the taint of pauperization with its threat of accompanying disenfranchisement.[19]

The vaccination acts were intended to be non-pauperizing, completely divorced from the stigma of relief and the specter of the workhouse. But even pro-vaccinators critiqued the marriage of public vaccination and poor relief. In seeking out the services of a public vaccinator, declared H.

W. Rumsey (who, ironically, was arguably the founder of state medicine),
the laboring classes "are drawn silently and insidiously within the pre-
cincts of pauperism."[20] In proposing the 1853 bill, Lord Lyttleton identified the problem of administering vaccination through the Poor Law but
claimed he could do little to remedy it:

> There now existed a good deal of prejudice among the poor against the
> present arrangement, which they confounded with pauperism, suppos-
> ing that, in taking their children to the public vaccinators, they were
> receiving parish relief. The Poor Law Board, had, indeed, issued an
> order that gratuitous vaccination should in no degree stamp the recip-
> ient with the character of a pauper; but, nevertheless, it was a very
> natural feeling, and if the machinery were separated entirely from that
> of the Poor Law Board, which had not necessarily any particular knowl-
> edge or information of the subject, the system would probably work
> better.[21]

Because this separation was never achieved, vaccination remained
linked to poor relief in the minds of many parents. Even public vaccinators and vaccination officers who operated within the system were confused about the relationship between the vaccination services and the
New Poor Law. Some public vaccinators were unclear as to whether they
were required to vaccinate all persons attendant at their stations regardless of whether they were poor. Others demanded whether the parents
of a child receiving free vaccination were "considered to have received
parochial relief from the fact of having the child vaccinated by the public
vaccinator." Still others requested the ability to withhold relief from
those who refused to comply with the vaccination act.[22] The Poor Law
Board provided the same answer to every query of this nature: Vaccination had no relationship to relief, and all who applied to public vaccinators were to be provided with the service, regardless of their economic
situation and without risk of pauperization. Nevertheless, this position
had to be reiterated time and time again. A headline in the *Manchester
Guardian* as late as 1902 ran: "Free Vaccination Not to Be Classed as
Out Relief."[23]

If the administrative system that linked public vaccination to the
services of the Poor Law challenged working-class ideals of independence and respectability, "a very natural feeling," it also had bodily

implications. Public vaccination was performed at vaccination stations, regarded by many parents as sites of moral and physical pollution. These were not purpose-built buildings but mechanics' institutes, lecture halls, reading rooms, chapel vestries, schoolrooms, inns, pubs, coffeehouses, and, at times, the workhouse infirmary. These stations were often inconveniently located, even for parents living in towns, and posed certain problems. Parents who were forced to take their children to pubs or inns often felt obliged to purchase a drink while waiting. Some may have welcomed this, but for teetotalers or those on a limited budget, this proved uncomfortable.[24] In rural districts, mothers often had to walk miles in both directions and then return again eight days later for an inspection. The process could be both tiring and time-consuming.

At these stations, public vaccinators, who were paid per child, often vaccinated numbers of babies in one day using vaccine matter taken directly from the arm of a previously vaccinated infant. More often than not, as many public vaccinators admitted, they did not fully inspect either the supplier or the recipient for signs of scrofula, syphilis, or other diseases, which many people feared could be transmitted through vaccination. In 1869, *The Anti-Vaccinator* decried the horror of "public-houses where arm from arm vaccination was being carried on according to the Act, and where mothers, too poor to object, were compelled to allow their children to be inoculated with poison from others whose antecedents . . . [could] give no hope of health." The law was most unjust, it maintained, "for the rich man could trace the antecedents of the child, but the poor man had no such power."[25] As the next chapter will discuss in greater detail, the vaccination of children from arm to arm provoked enormous fear of contamination, especially since public vaccination was performed in at least four places. Those who could afford a private doctor could request only one mark and could often have calf lymph or lymph from a healthy child from known parents. Those who could not afford this expense were forced to submit to the matter that was available and to the discretion of the vaccinator, who often had little time for parental concerns. When a mother in Lower Stoke in 1890 requested only two marks, the vaccinator refused, vaccinating each child in three places and hers in four because, he claimed, she "used too much tongue."[26]

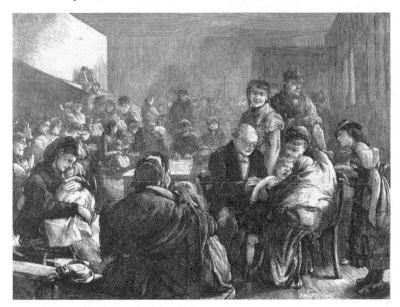

6. "The District Vaccinator," *The Graphic*, 8 April 1871.
By permission of the Wellcome Library, London.

An illustration of an East London vaccination station in *The Graphic*, intended to be an authentic "sketch" of East End life, presented a crowded and unsystematic image of public vaccination to its middle-class audience (see Figure 6). The artist pictured babies, small children, and respectably attired workers huddled together in a single poorly lit room. *The Anti-Vaccinator* condemned these stations as sites of pollution. "Parents are now *compelled* to take their children to the *public stations*," its editor claimed, "where they mix with *paupers*, and are operated on indiscriminately with *paupers*—the operator going from right to left, or *vice versa*, utterly regardless of persons: and thus at the outset we have one great objection to vaccination—it reduces respectable mechanics, &c., to a level with paupers."[27] Public vaccination threatened those who considered themselves members of a respectable working class because it compromised their social status. But it also threw them into direct physical contact with paupers, which produced anxieties over their physical and moral integrity, for the blood of their own "pure" infants was being polluted by that of those with questionable morals and debatable health.

The only thing that recommended the vaccination station over a private practitioner was that it was free, and sometimes even this was not incentive enough to attract a steady stream of babies. In East London at the turn of the century, a Shoreditch vaccination officer resorted to bribing parents with a cup of tea and to offering the baby a sixpence.[28] When Lord Lyttleton was asked whether, if the Local Government Board advised him to send his child, humbly attired, to a public station, he would undertake "such a risk," he skirted the question. "My impression," he declared, "is that the Act does not require anyone to send their children to the public station. I think everyone can get it done in the way he prefers."[29] Obviously, this was not actually the case, as the services of a private physician could be costly. In working-class homes where pennies counted, such an expenditure could not be justified. Thus, by administering vaccinations through the Poor Law Guardians, the government, though insisting that vaccination was to be non-pauperizing, succeeded in stigmatizing those who could not afford the fees of a regular doctor.

Persecution and Prosecution

What working-class anti-vaccinators found most objectionable was the fact that vaccination officers rarely prosecuted middle-class defaulters, unless they were confirmed anti-vaccinators and propagandists. The "word compulsory is a sham," argued the Reverend James Stead. "It means no more than this—those shall be compelled who cannot afford to pay for their freedom from the operation of the Act—a gross injustice. It is one law for the rich and another for the poor."[30] Magistrates, these agitators contended, openly discriminated against the laboring population by fining and imprisoning them while consistently overlooking the delinquencies of offenders "reckoned as being of their own calibre."[31] Testifying before the Royal Commission on Vaccination, Thomas Gordon Collins, a London bookkeeper, declared that he "regarded it as a grievance that clergymen and people of position are not summoned, while workingmen, like myself, are."[32] While not all middle-class defaulters escaped prosecution and imprisonment, even the firmly middle-class Mary Hume-Rothery conceded that it was "*mostly* the poorer and working classes, and the tradesman-class" who were fined and sentenced to jail.[33]

TRACKING AND FINING   Working-class anti-vaccinators accused the
government of discriminating against working people not only by compelling them to use the public stations, but by relentlessly tracking and
fining them. Vaccination officials often understood their vocation as a
form of detective work. In 1863, a public vaccinator complained about
the difficulty of tracing defaulters: "I have one of the largest vaccinations in London, derived from a densely populated neighbourhood, and
which I look closely after; but though I hunt them up like a bloodhound
on the murderer's trail, I am often thrown out."[34] As a result, anti-
vaccinators considered the vaccination officer a "spy" or a "sneak"—an
agent of the state paid to intrude on the privacy and sanctity of family
life. Anti-vaccinators often labeled vaccination officers "Baby Hunter[s]" and "sleuth hounds" and compared them to the "Inquisition."[35]
The vaccination act, wrote one protester, "is the only English law that
encourages spies and informers to hunt down respectable working
men."[36] One defaulter—an advertising contractor, bill poster, and
printer—lapsed into conspiracy theories: "Police Constable 657T and
661T (who I have every reason to believe are also in the pay of the secret
service) . . . tried all they could to entrap me, but thank God they
miserably and lamentably failed in their *grotesque* conspiracy."[37] While
this may be the product of a paranoid personality, vaccination officers in
some districts were paid a fee for each certificate of successful vaccination they obtained, rather than a salary, to encourage them to track
down more noncompliers.[38]

The acts also discriminated economically against working people.
The fine for noncompliance was 20 shillings plus court costs, which
could range anywhere from one penny to over a pound. For the middle
and upper classes, these fines were, if not negligible, certainly afford-
able. For the working class, however, they were more than trifling,
considering that it was not uncommon for a working man to earn
between 15 and 20 shillings a week. The Vaccination Officers' Birth
Books for Enfield in the 1880s and '90s reveal that most defaulters
were factory operatives or journeymen laborers whose salaries could
not have accommodated such a hefty penalty and who could not have
afforded to miss a day of work to appear in court.[39] Even if one could pay
the penalty the first time, the cat-and-mouse nature of the 1867 and

1871 acts, which allowed for repeated prosecution, meant that fines could be levied almost indefinitely for each child, forcing penniless parents into prison. A letter to *The Co-operator* from the wife of an imprisoned defaulter reveals the sad irony of this situation. With her husband in prison, she was left without his wages and feared she would have to enter the workhouse. In the workhouse she knew that her child would be forced to submit to vaccination. Her husband's imprisonment, she lamented, was thus meaningless.[40]

Similarly, defaulters appealed to the LSACV for help. "William Ockwell and I are working men," wrote one resister. "Ockwell has two children, and cannot afford to pay from £3 to £4 as did our neighbour. ... We cannot hold out unless we are assisted either in our defence or in the mitigation of penalties."[41] Fines were often paid by a local anti-vaccination society, many of which had mutual defense leagues attached to them. In 1898, the NAVL, successor to the LSACV, charged subscribers 5 shillings per annum for the first child and 2 shillings 6 pence for each additional child. This entitled the subscriber to have his or her fines and court costs paid by the society, though members of less than six months could claim only half of their expenses.[42] This type of insurance was a typical working-class economic strategy that was similar to burial insurance and boot clubs, savings plans that permitted parents to pay small sums of money on a weekly basis toward the purchase of boots for their children, or to cover the cost of a child's funeral. The defense fund was also common to other radical reform movements that expected their members to be fined or imprisoned.[43]

As a challenge to this perceived economic discrimination, fervent anti-vaccinators sought to accumulate fines in order to become examples of governmental despotism, claiming that as working men they were being milked dry by a law which favored the wealthy and penalized the poor. For working people, compulsory vaccination acted, in the words of one critic, as a "baby-tax" swindled from the poor "in a never-ending stream of cash" reminiscent of the South Sea Bubble scandal.[44] The most famous of these martyrs was Charles Hayward, a mechanic from Ashford who by October 1888 had been fined 53 pounds 12 shillings for the non-vaccination of his two children, much of which was paid for him by the defense fund of the LSACV. The case of Hayward—who the anti-vaccinationist MP (and birth-control advocate) Charles

Bradlaugh characterized as "in a very humble condition of life"—provoked a heated letter-writing campaign by William Young, secretary of the LSACV, to Henry Matthews, secretary of state. In July 1887, Young wrote to Matthews to complain about the "long and malicious prosecution" of Hayward and the "vindictive tyranny exercised towards him" by the magistrates of the Ashford Police Court, who insisted on imposing the maximum fine of 20 shillings, despite the fact that Hayward had already been fined countless times. "I am aware that over the Poor Law Guardians your department has no control," wrote Young, "but I hope that in the interests of our common humanity it is in your power to put some restraints upon the magistrates who disgrace the office they hold by their despicable despotism, and to administer to them a prompt and stern rebuke." The magistrates were so annoyed by the constant reappearance of Hayward before them that, by November, they had refused to continue to listen to him or his defense lawyer and during one hearing left their bench.

This tactic of accumulating fines was intended to demonstrate the folly of the law, which sought to induce vaccination through the threat of penalty: Those who refused to vaccinate, anti-vaccinators maintained, were "conscientious objectors" and would not be deterred by fines. A handbill, most likely issued by the LSACV and titled "VACCINATION LAW TYRANNY. Periodical Persecution and Plunder of a Working Man by the East Ashford Board of Guardians, Aided and Abetted by the Local Magistrates," summed up this position. Giving details of the Hayward case and a list of his fines, the handbill declared: "The purpose of the law, we take it, is to have HAYWARD'S child vaccinated; but inasmuch as the child will not be vaccinated, and cannot be vaccinated without HAYWARD'S consent, what is the use of demonstrating the impotence of the law by the repetition of futile prosecutions?" While the secretary of state's response was a straightforward refusal to take up the case, the tactic seems to have worked, as the case was eventually dropped.[45]

RESPECTABILITY AND THE ANTI-VACCINATION PRISONER   Working-class campaigners objected to vaccination's association with the New Poor Law and to the government's discriminatory practices of tracing and fining only working-class defaulters. They were equally incensed by the state's treatment of anti-vaccination prisoners. The sentence for noncompliance with the vaccination laws was generally two weeks but at times more severe, as in the case of Mrs. Blanchard, who, after serving a sentence of seven days, was sent immediately back to jail for fourteen more.[46] Some resisters chose this option precisely because it provided an opportunity for martyrdom. At the winter meeting of the NAVL in Eastbourne in 1900, the "anti-vaccination martyrs" were presented in prison dress.[47]

Many anti-vaccinationists insisted that imprisonment was the best and only moral response to the vaccination laws, as paying fines was merely caving in to governmental despotism. However, they also argued that, as among the "most-peaceable citizens," they should not be "arraigned, prosecuted, and punished as dangerous criminals" or associated with social outcasts. "I have been a member of a christian church for 17 years, and a Sunday school teacher for about 18 years," declared Richard Vickers, a commercial traveler, "yet by this law I am liable to be treated as a common felon, and handcuffed to a house-breaker, a thief, or a murderer." Similarly, an outraged correspondent to the *Anti-Vaccinator and Public Health Journal* fumed: "A friend of ours, in passing through the streets of Dewsbury, met [Mr. W.] Taylor on his way to Wakefield House of Correction, manacled between two prostitutes!"[48] Anti-vaccinators fervently opposed this type of treatment, not only because they considered arrest and imprisonment a draconian penalty, but also because it allied them to a criminal class from whom they struggled so hard to distinguish themselves. In a notice to the "Working-Men Electors of West Cumberland," the *Vaccination Inquirer* maintained that the vaccination acts were abominable because they turned "worthy men into criminals."[49]

Anti-vaccinators argued that it was not "rogues or vagabonds, not criminals" who were being fined and imprisoned but "honest respectable citizens."[50] Middle-class campaigners attempted to link anti-vaccination resistance to respectability, arguing that "all respectable people, all true men, in every class" should oppose the "tyrannical" vaccination acts. A justice of the peace and a police sergeant both testified in front of the Royal Commission on Vaccination that those who refused to vaccinate were members of a "respectable class" of working men.[51] But working-class anti-vaccinators, like agitators for an expanded male franchise, also relied on the rough-respectable divide. If respectability was a malleable and manipulable concept, it was also integral to working-class identity in the nineteenth century and formed an important part of workers' claims to be incorporated into the polity.[52] For anti-vaccinators, respectability was linked to a Gladstonian discourse of moral responsibility and became a crucial marker of their status as model parents, furthering their claims to be treated not as felons, but as conscience offenders.

In the 1880s, George Russell, a grocer, was charged thirty times for non-vaccination of his children. A letter to the editor of The Echo, a national newspaper sympathetic to the anti-vaccination cause, argued his case by positioning Russell as the epitome of the respectable anti-vaccinationist. "Is George Russell an incorrigibly wicked man from a moral point of view?" the letter inquired rhetorically. "Is he a brutal parent—a bad citizen—a besotted drunkard—a fraudulent tradesman— a lying and dishonourable man?" Russell, the newspaper argued, had "integrity." He was not a "bad citizen," for not only did he lead an admirable domestic life, but he was also an honest tradesman and an altogether moral man. Russell, his defender maintained, was a good father, as opposed to the "demoralised parents, drunkards, and courtesans" who were guilty of "maiming and drowning, and burning their offspring." He was a sober, Christian man, a keeper of the "sacred trust" of parenthood. In short, Russell was a model of the "honest and conscientious parent."[53]

As this defense of Russell makes clear, respectability bridged the worlds of public and private, as it had both a domestic and a public face. What transpired within one's household was an important marker of one's social position within the neighborhood and the larger national community. To be respectable increasingly meant participating in the separation of spheres. Respectability depended on a woman's ability to maintain a domestic haven for her husband.[54] In this sense, anti-vaccinators claimed to be models of domestic respectability. Milnes described them as "Sunday School organizers, friendly society members, building society purchasers their neat, trim, tidy homes, with book-case and harmonium, bear witness to their thrift; their well-shod, well-groomed, well-taught children are living testimony to their love; their lives without are circled with respect, and within are hallowed with affection."[55] Anti-vaccination literature routinely portrayed women as good and thrifty housekeepers who kept their homes "sweet and clean and dainty" and saved their pennies to pay fines for noncompliance. An extended homage to the working-class agitator, printed in *The Anti-Vaccinator* in 1869, described the "cottage" of an "honest mechanic" who was "able and willing to work," as a "scrupulously clean-kept and hard-worked-for home."[56] Even in the early twentieth century, this remained an important and telling marker. In 1905, a pamphleteer argued that anti-vaccinators were working men who saved to have a house "fit for a *man*, and not a house unfit for a pig to live in." They have "good home[s]," he argued, "with bathroom, and hot and cold laid on."[57]

To maintain a respectable Victorian household, a man had to demonstrate his financial independence from the state. For this reason, public vaccination and its associations with the Poor Law system of relief proved troubling to working-class parents. "A British Mother" who wrote to the *Morning Advertiser* in 1866 to complain about vaccination fines enunciated this position. "We are not rich," she argued, but with "constant industry, and care and diligence in business, we are just able to pay our rent and taxes, and support ourselves and two young infants honestly and respectably."[58] Financial independence was intimately bound up with industriousness. The model anti-vaccinator had "the pride of manly independence stamped on his brown face," proclaimed *The Anti-Vaccinator*.[59] Tanned by the sun, his body revealed his status as a steady laborer independent of charity or state relief.

Both inside and outside of the home, anti-vaccinators demonstrated their respectability by observing certain codes of behavior. In contrast to those considered "rough," anti-vaccinators claimed to be sober and religious. In all the years of its existence, and among the thousands of its victims, Milnes argued, the vaccination law had never caught a drunkard yet. Many resisters underscored their temperate or teetotal commitments, claiming to forgo "drinks and smokes" in favor of books, music, and evening classes.[60] Henry Blumberg, a doctor and a magistrate, testified before the Royal Commission on Vaccination that anti-vaccinators were "sober and industrious, good citizens." It was "among the people who never object to vaccination," he maintained, that "you will find the drunken and dissolute classes."[61]

As highly respectable and moral members of society, anti-vaccinators argued that they should not be treated as common felons. Indeed, anti-vaccinationists posed a particular problem for the prison system, as they represented a new type of working-class prisoner who was clearly not a member of the criminal class. This kind of prisoner, which also included members of the Salvation Army, demanded a different type of treatment from that of habitual criminals or the "undeserving classes" and thus eventually helped to reform penal practices.[62] Anti-vaccinationists themselves, however, initially felt they were getting no special treatment. The uniform complaint of those imprisoned was that they were treated not as respectable, law-abiding citizens but were routinely committed to hard labor and suffered just as much bodily and mental strife as the convicted murderer. Until the 1890s, little distinction seems to have been made between these "conscientious objectors" and those penalized for theft, assault, or other criminal offenses.

Vaccination defaulters created a controversy over the classification of criminals. Debates over whether anti-vaccinationists were merely debtors, as they had failed to pay a fine, or criminals, as they had refused to comply with the law, raged in the press and in Parliament. In 1891, in response to political pressure from pro-Irish radicals and to a softening of public opinion, the Penal Servitude Act was passed, which improved penal conditions for "political prisoners."[63] While anti-vaccinationists, unlike militant campaigners for the female franchise, did not explicitly identify with Irish political prisoners, they also insisted on their respectable social status even as they were imprisoned alongside "bad characters."[64]

In 1890, George Bainborough, a grocer at Gainsborough, reported his case to the Royal Commission on Vaccination. Bainborough had been sentenced to fourteen days' hard labor and placed on a treadmill. His sentence was then found to be excessive, and he was compensated 40 pounds.[65] Bainborough's case, and others like it, and the recent shift in policy toward political prisoners exerted pressure on the commission to resolve the issue. In an interim report published in 1892, the commissioners agreed that people imprisoned under the vaccination acts should no longer be subjected to the same treatment as criminals, because in every other respect, anti-vaccinators conducted themselves as "law abiding citizens."[66] This decision meant that anti-vaccinationists—unlike suffragettes, who at the end of the century were often imprisoned as second- or third-division prisoners for their acts of civil disobedience—were regarded as "conscience offenders" and henceforward given the same rights and privileges as Irish political prisoners. This was a small victory for the movement but a victory nonetheless, as it disaggregated working-class prisoners, separating felons from honest citizens who were imprisoned precisely because of their commitment to certain ideals and values.

Vaccination and the Working-Class Body

The imprisonment of working-class anti-vaccinators not only provoked anxieties over their social status. It also threatened their bodily integrity, for it subjected the body to deprivation and discipline. If the vaccination lancet most imperiled the "pure," "healthy," "helpless," bodies of "innocent" babies, the prison regime jeopardized the integrity of adult bodies. Inmates' descriptions of prison life returned repeatedly to narratives of bodily privation—labor, sickness, and pain. Both male and female prisoners accentuated the vulnerability of the respectable working-class body, which was not hardened like that of the criminal. Mrs. Walton, a "Poor Woman," described her brief prison experience as follows:

> I was subject to all the indignity of a felon, ordered by two warders to strip my own clothing, and stand naked as I was born for them to examine what marks were on my body. After this humiliation I would have to be put in a bath. I should then have to have donned the prison clothes, with a number on my shoulder. I would then have to be locked up in a small cell night and day, called solitary confinement. I remained nearly two hours. I was afraid my reason would have given way or I should have died before the 14 days expired. A woman opened the door, and asked me if I wanted anything. I told her I was very faint, and would like a cup of tea. Her answer was, "You will get nothing but bread and water here."

Intimidated by the proposed scrutiny of her naked body, the forced cleansing, the dehumanization of being numbered, and the lack of amenities and nourishment, Mrs. Walton caved in after only two hours.

She contacted a friend to pay the fine and bail her out, for she feared that, had she remained, "it would have either killed me or sent me mad."[67]

Before the 1892 decision, anti-vaccinators, like other criminal prisoners, were subjected to the treadmill, forced to pick oakum, set to sleep on plank beds, shaved and garbed in prison gear, and fed a diet of gruel. J. T. Biggs, a plumber and sanitary engineer, testified to the Royal Commission on Vaccination that an anti-vaccination prisoner had been thrust into a "black hole" and made to suffer "every possible degradation." Ben Turner's celebrated poem "For Conscience Sake" decried the prison regime that provoked his narrator's "troublesome cough" and caused him to "be a consumptive; that, an'not having food enough." "My health is very much injured through my confinement in prison," complained another father. A letter to the *Co-operator and Anti-Vaccinator* in 1871 detailed "the cruel manner" in which Mr. T. Jones was treated at a "House of Correction." The cold cell and poor clothing made his "weak state" even worse. He was unable to eat the food and committed to hard labor, which he could not perform because he was "extremely ill."[68] If anti-vaccinators celebrated the martyred status of the prisoner, they also criticized the harsh penal regime's impact on working-class bodies.

This identification of their bodies as highly vulnerable to state discipline reveals working-class campaigners' concern about the safety and security of not only the infant but the adult. If the middle-class Liberal Alfred Milnes was chiefly concerned that there was "no other law in England which so fundamentally violates the principles of individual liberty," working-class agitators stressed that the vaccination act was "the only law we have interfering with our bodies."[69] Working-class anti-vaccinators echoed their middle-class allies, maintaining that it was the parent's role and responsibility to care for the child and his or her right to make decisions about its well-being. In 1875, a dairyman accused of non-vaccination threw the order to vaccinate at the vaccination officer. He declared that "the children were his own property and not the property of the state."[70] But for workers, the issue of parental rights was not distinct from that of rights to one's own person. Acting as the "Vaccination Inquirer" in Parliament, Thomas Bayley, Liberal MP for Chesterfield, argued that those imprisoned and fined under the vaccination acts believed "that they have control of their own bodies and of their children, and that they should not allow the State or anybody else to tell them what they should do with their bodies or with their children."[71] The adult's body, he suggested, was thus as central to the working-class campaign as the child's.

The vaccination acts of 1853, 1867, and 1871 applied only to infant children. But working-class agitators rarely distinguished between their own bodies and those of their babies. While highlighting the physical purity of the "innocent" child was an effective rhetorical device, an illustration that recurred repeatedly in anti-vaccination propaganda depicted a victim of vaccination as an adult working-class man, one of the many prisoners, soldiers, sailors, policeman, postmen, and government clerks also forced to submit to the procedure under separate government and military initiatives (see Figure 7). For working-class anti-vaccinationists, the adult's body was as much at risk as the child's. "It is not a question of vaccination," argued a correspondent to the *Vaccination Inquirer*. "It is a question of a working man's right to call his body his own."[72] These laws challenged firmly held beliefs that the individual was the best judge of his or her own self. James Burns, the voice of plebeian spiritualism, attacked compulsory vaccination and its quite explicit reliance on the expertise of doctors, defending the individual's right to manage the body. "If nobody wore a body except the doctors," he maintained, "then they would of course have the sole right to discuss the best means of managing such bodies; but it is a palpable fact that all mankind are in the same position respecting bodies, and the health of such bodies, as sailors are in regard to ships."[73] Compulsory vaccination, anti-vaccinationists argued, replaced self-determination with a form of bodily "tyranny." Indeed, anti-vaccinationists compared their movement to the Home Rule campaign. An 1880 pocket pamphlet demanded whether "Englishmen, Scotchmen and Irishmen" were "fit to enjoy Home Rule over their own bodies, and over the bodies of their offspring?"[74] By gesturing to the Irish question, anti-vaccinators contended that their movement was as political as these nationalist claims with a similar goal. Self-governance in this context meant the right to control and manage their own and their children's bodies.

At a distraint sale at Stroud in 1893, an anti-vaccinator expressed these concerns over corporeal autonomy by drawing attention to the

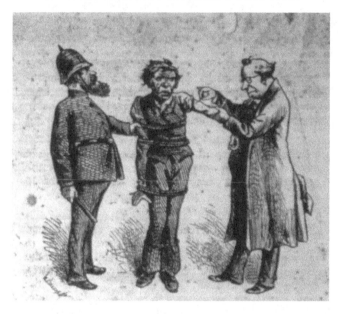

7. Coercive adult vaccination, c. 1882.
By permission of Denis Vandervelde.

vulnerability of his body. The "tedium" of waiting for the auctioneer, reported the *Stroud Journal*, was relieved by the "antics" of a couple of men, "who trotted backwards and forwards under the eyes of the people —the one having on his back an auction bill, and the other fulfilling the role of mock auctioneer. Later in the day the man with the bill appeared with a black face, and carrying in his arms an effigy of a baby, which was supposed to appeal to the compassionate regard of the onlookers. The solicitous parent was rigged up in feminine gear, and occasionally found himself hoisted on the shoulders of some of his compatriots."[75] This anti-vaccinator transformed himself from a white male into a commodity, and then into a black female, stressing the relationship between his own body and those he enacted. His performance with the auction bill underscored a complaint, common among working-class campaigners, that laboring people were treated little better than commercial goods or slave labor to be bought, sold, and bartered, as if they were not "owners of their own persons" but merely "live chattels."[76] As early as 1856, an "intelligent working man" opposed to vaccination argued:

"[T]hey might as well brand us."[77] Branding in this context evoked the marking of cattle, slaves, and criminals, all forms of property. Speaking at the formation of the Kettering Anti-Vaccination League in 1884, Jessie Craigen, working-class suffragist and campaigner against vaccination, vivisection, and the contagious diseases acts, denounced vaccination as a type of branding. The people, she maintained, had become the "doctor's cattle" and the vaccination mark, "his brand." In feudal times, she maintained, serfs were branded "but freemen were unmarked."[78] Since imprisonment was the next stage of the legal process, anti-vaccinationists' bodies were constantly at risk of becoming property to be transferred to the state in lieu of distrained goods. For if there were goods to seize, the government would have them, argued Henry Pitman; if there were none, it would "seize his body."[79]

The use of blackface is significant, as it was also employed at the Leicester demonstration of 1885. Blackface belonged to a tradition of poaching and protest that persisted throughout the nineteenth century in the carnivalesque wakes and fairs, which encouraged disguises, and in the rituals of "mummers."[80] It also appealed to the Victorian working class because, as chapter 3 showed, it allowed them to assert their biological superiority in an imperial hierarchy even as they were being socially denigrated within the British class system.[81] Blackface also directly referenced slavery, a frequent anti-vaccination analogy. In conflating the female, the commodity, and the slave, this anti-vaccinationist revealed his own relationship to these three positions. Though their meanings were multifaceted, they nevertheless all represented a lack of autonomy and suggested the anti-vaccinationist's concern over bodily control and independence. As such, the performance at Stroud echoed the "intelligent working man's" fears of being branded and thus conflated with livestock, slaves, and criminals.

Working class anti-vaccinators thus joined the middle-class leadership of the campaign in critiquing not only the Conservative-implemented acts, but the Liberal Party's perpetuation of compulsory vaccination. They, too, mobilized the language of individual rights and laissez-faire, appealing to the Old Liberal principles their middle-class allies held dear. But for the laboring population, the politics of compulsion transcended debates on the nature of Victorian liberalism and was bound up in a shared personal experience of bodily vulnerability. These anti-vaccinationists deployed the language of class because, regardless of some economic and social differences between them, they maintained that compulsory vaccination nurtured a larger social division: It demarcated those persecuted, surveilled, and compelled to vaccinate from those left to make their own decisions about bodily interventions. This legislation thus helped to reorganize class identities around the site of the vulnerable body, thereby incorporating many individuals into a working class who shared this experience. For, as the next chapter will demonstrate, anti-vaccinationism stemmed not only from a critique of the ideology of compulsion, but also from profound fears about the violating nature of the procedure and the vulnerability of the body to pollution and invasion.

5

Vampires, Vivisectors, and the Victorian Body

> (Pure) lymph, from small-pox'd cow or calf,
>
> From scrof'lous man or child,
>
> Encircled with disease foul,
>
> To which small-pox is mild.
>
> (Pure) lymph, oft fat with redd'ning shame,
>
> With seeds of guilt and crime,
>
> With syphilis inherited,
>
> From wild oats sown in prime.
>
> —Thomas Duxbury, 1884[1]

☞ If an Englishman's house was said to be his castle, anti-vaccinators also imagined his body as an equally sacred fortress—a "little human house"—whose boundaries were not to be transgressed. "The vaccinators not only come into [the Englishman's] house," warned an agitator, "but they get inside of his skin, and invade his veins, so that the blood in his body is not his own."[2] By scarifying the flesh and introducing disease into the system, vaccination threatened strongly held beliefs regarding bodily integrity and blood purity. It also wielded the power, anti-vaccinators maintained, to transform the individual into something "other," a monstrous version of the self. On these grounds, anti-vaccinators attacked vaccination as bodily assault, a violent disruption of the physical integrity of the individual that was harmful both to physical and to spiritual health. In expressing their concerns about the permeability and transformability of the individual body and a trend toward what they considered "violationism,"[3] anti-vaccinators participated in the construction of a gothic body.

The "gothic body" that emerged in the late nineteenth century sub-
stituted a securely bounded human subjectivity with one that was "both
fragmented and permeable." This fin de siècle body was morphic and
constantly in danger of becoming an "other."[4] If the gothic body was
vulnerable to transformation, its boundaries were also constantly
threatened, for it was at risk of violation, penetration, and systematic
disruption. Anti-vaccination propaganda participated in these shared
cultural anxieties and helped to shape these experiences and understandings of bodily vulnerability by maintaining that vaccination violated bodily integrity, polluted the life force, and transformed its victims
into a horrific parody of humanity. Anti-vaccinators' concerns, while
multifaceted, focused on the problems of blood purity and bodily integrity and returned repeatedly to two icons of Victorian gothic culture: the
vampire and the vivisector.

Monstrous Transformations

Anti-vaccinators consistently maintained that vaccination caused inde-
scribable pain and suffering and terribly disfigured the bodies of its
victims. Indeed, nothing was as terrifying to parents as the manner in
which the procedure could physically transform their children into
something monstrous and scarcely human. Vaccination, its opponents
argued, turns the healthy child into "a scrofulous, idiotic ape, a hideous
foul-skinned cripple, a diseased burlesque on mankind."[5] The effect of
these often lurid tales of rotten flesh and scabrous wounds was to
represent vaccination as a horrific nostrum that physically and spir-
itually transformed the innocent victim into a deformed monster in
much the same way that Robert Louis Stevenson's gentleman Jekyll
metamorphosed into the dwarfish and undefinably deformed Hyde.
Propagandists repeatedly deployed a range of fantastic, melodramatic,
and gothic tropes—such as the minotaur, the hydra-headed monster,
the dragon, the incubus, the Chamber of Horrors, and Frankenstein's
creature—to depict vaccination as monstrous. This imagery was a common feature of popular political discourse evident since the early Victorian period.[6] Anti-vaccinators heavily exploited it to capitalize on and
perpetuate parental anxieties. But at the same time, these sensationalist

accounts of vaccination horrors reveal a profound discomfort with the impact of vaccination on the infant's body.

Anti- and pro-vaccinators alike agreed that smallpox was a "monstrous" disease. Medicine, maintained an anonymous pamphleteer, "knows no rival to this monster," which went "licking round its victims," its "clammy grasp" on the "throat of all society." During the previous week, he continued, one in eighteen deaths was due to the "insatiable monster's demands."[7] A pamphlet protesting the erection of a new fever hospital in the fashionable North London neighborhood of Hampstead personified smallpox as a "fiend" that haunted the heath with its diseased minions. But Jenner, maintained a proponent of vaccination, had tamed this "beast of prey" by extracting "the claws and the teeth."[8]

Supporters of vaccination participated in the production of this fantastic and sensationalist imagery. Pro-vaccination propaganda in particular focused on the horrific nature of the disease. The unvaccinated, proponents of vaccination warned, fell "victim" to the "devouring monster" and became loathsome creatures themselves.[9] The "horror and disgust" inspired by the smallpox patient, argued the former vaccinator-general of Trinidad, "the hideous loathsome aspect of the face, the horrid smell, the frightful pits and scars" can be appreciated only by those who have attended during an epidemic. In fact, the patient "attacked with this fell disease becomes a mass of living corruption, so hideous," declared John Shortt, general superintendent of vaccination for Madras, "that the mother sickens at the sight of her child and turns away." If the child escapes with his or her life, "it is so frightfully disfigured as scarcely to be recognized."[10]

Anti-vaccinators inverted this monstrous language, arguing that it was vaccination itself that was responsible for disfiguring their children. Working- and middle-class parents wrote thousands of letters to various newspapers recounting the fate of their children, whom vaccination had transformed from angelic infants with "silvery curls" to terrifying monstrosities.[11] In 1895, Margaret Thompson wrote to the *East London Observer* to complain that shortly after being vaccinated at the Shoreditch public station in East London her child had broken out in a "loathsome eruption." A "bladdery eruption," she recounted, covered the baby's entire body so that there was "hardly a piece of healthy

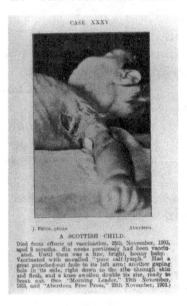

CASE XXXV

J. Pithie, photo   Aberdeen.

A SCOTTISH CHILD.

Died from effects of vaccination, 25th November, 1903,
aged 8 months. Six weeks previously had been vacci-
ated. Until then was a fine, bright, bonny baby.
Vaccinated with so-called "pure calf-lymph." Had a
great punched-out hole in its left arm: another gaping
hole in its side, right down to the ribs through skin
and flesh, and a knee swollen double its size, ready to
break out. (See "Morning Leader," 17th November,
1903, and "Aberdeen Free Press," 28th November, 1903.)

8. "A Scottish Child," in W. J. Furnival, *Professional Opinion
Adverse to Vaccination* (Stone: W. J. Furnival, 1906). *By permission
of the National Library of Medicine, Bethesda, Maryland.*

skin the size of a shilling from head to foot."[12] Parents frequently proclaimed that vaccination had led to the putrefaction of their babies. In
1877, F. Pearse maintained that he had witnessed a child literally rot to
death after vaccination. The arms, feet, hands, face, and head were
rotting away, he lamented, "eaten into the bone" so that the child was
covered in "large holes." The child smelled "like anything rotten"; so
putrid was the odor they could "scarcely bear it."[13] W. J. Furnival's
published collection of photographs of children allegedly contaminated
through vaccination and left permanently disfigured provided anti-
vaccinationists with shocking visual evidence of vaccination's transformative possibilities (see Figure 8).

While most cases of contamination were recounted as stories of dam-
aged children, adults, too, produced narratives of lives and bodies
ruined by vaccination. Among the most well-known testimonials to the
dangers of vaccination came from Ira Connell. Born in the anti-vaccination stronghold of Oldham, Connell claimed that he had been "a suf-

ferer and Victim to Vaccination for the space of Twenty-two Years." In 1869, Connell, with the help of Henry Pitman, published *My Experience of Vaccination*, which recounted the trials he had suffered as a result of vaccination. Connell claimed that he came from "healthy folks" who had no history in either family of any disease. After being vaccinated with "bad lymph" at eighteen months old, Connell maintained, he broke out with wounds on his limbs. He summed up his injuries as follows:

> Soon after Vaccination, my health was seen to decline; and, directly after, large wounds broke out in different places about my person, which have caused the left arm and hand to be quite useless, and also my left foot. I have had as many as from 14 to 15 wounds at once upon them—all these to be re-dressed every night of my life. . . . There is not even one limb that has escaped the malady. I have a wound that covers the whole of the back of the left hand, which along with the elbow, is quite stiff and useless. There are three large wounds on the left foot, and three on the right foot. The right foot is almost the size of two feet. The pain I suffer from these wounds is of an indescribable character.[14]

Connell was apparently reduced to spending his days moving around on his knees like an animal, having lost the use of his legs. In 1884, Mr. Cunningham, a thirty-one-year-old sufferer, told a similar story. Attempting to seek treatment for his condition, Cunningham visited "scores" of doctors (both orthodox and heterodox) and at least three institutions, to no avail. He tried a host of patent medicines and was visited by "a large number of doctors and medical students" while in the Manchester Infirmary, but nothing helped. Cursed with a "lump of raw beef" in place of a foot, he smelled so disagreeable that disinfectants had to be applied to the bed to keep down the odor. With their useless and rotting limbs, Connell and Cunningham resembled the "abhuman" objects that run rampant through late–Victorian gothic fiction.[15]

If vaccination could physically deform the body, its monstrous nature also derived from its ability to pervert the spirit. Nonconformist antivaccinators, who objected to vaccination on religious grounds, proposed that physical health and spiritual health were intimately related. The magnetic and botanic practitioner D. Younger maintained that one should try to make the physical body a "fit dwelling-place for a pure, happy, uncontaminated, and well-developed spiritual body."[16] Vaccination, its opponents argued, introduced "demons" and "ghouls" into the "glorious tabernacle" of the body, the "inside of which they should never see."[17] Indeed, anti-vaccinators played up the sinister implications of the late-night session of Parliament at which the first Compulsory Vaccination Act (1853) was passed. They likened Parliament to a black sabbath: "[I]n a dark midnight hour, when evil spirits were abroad, when nearly all slept save a few doctors, who were rather awake, whose dictum or nostrum carried the night, this Act was passed, this deed was done. It was a deed worthy of the night, dark as the night. No light shone on it, the blackness of darkness hovered around it. It was a deed that can but lie in the night; light is fatal to its being."[18] According to this version, doctors convened in Parliament under the cover of night as if they were a coven, to prepare their "nostrum," which one critique denounced as a brew no better than the "poison of adders, the blood, entrails and excretions of rats, bats, toads and sucking whelps," all ingredients familiar to the witches' cauldron.[19] Vaccination was a potion or a curse, these anti-vaccinators implied, and the vaccination acts a dark deed. Similarly, campaigners cast vaccination as a supernatural and decidedly "unChristian" rite, a type of "devil-worship" that could transform an angelic child into an "anti-Christ."[20] Vaccination appeared, then, as a satanic perversion of Christian sacraments, which were supposed to secure the safety of, if not the body, then certainly the soul.

The relationship between bodily and spiritual purity was particularly important, anti-vaccinators implied, in relation to the child. By the Victorian period, the Romantic notion of the child as innocent, as opposed to the Calvinist conception of the child as tainted by original sin, had come to dominate the discourse of childhood. Evangelical writing highlighted both the fragility of the child and its redemptive power. For this reason, the child served Victorians as an important symbol of purity and grace.[21] Anti-vaccinators believed that interference with the child's body was doubly transgressive, as it defiled the individual in its purest state and threatened the soul, forestalling the child's redemptive possibilities.

Religious anti-vaccinators interpreted vaccination as sacrilege precisely because it interfered with the body of the child "just after God has given it you." In 1877, Mr. G. J. Pratt of Brighton refused to vaccinate his child because, he claimed, the child was "as God gave it him."[22] It was unnatural and irreligious to tamper with the body that, formed by God, was perfectly constructed, particularly when it was fresh from its Maker and in its purest state. Vaccination, maintained a book by "a Christian" titled *Jenner or Christ?* is the "most outrageous blasphemy against God, [and] against Nature."[23] Anti-vaccinators condemned public vaccinators as "baby-defilers" who were responsible for the moral corruption of the infant souls on which the entire nation depended. In resisting the "defilement" of babies' bodies, trumpeted William Hume-Rothery, we are striving to "uphold the souls of their parents, and the faith of our nation."[24]

To underscore the grave dangers of vaccination, anti-vaccinators drew on millenarian language and the rhetorical power of the Book of Revelations. They cautioned that compulsory vaccination fulfilled an apocalyptic prophesy, for Revelations 16:2 warned that "foul and evil sores came upon the men who bore the mark of the beast." "Whatever the spiritual interpretation may be of this prophecy," maintained Mary Hume-Rothery, "it is clear that it has received a most singular realistic fulfillment in modern Christendom."[25] Condemning vaccination scars as the mark of the beast, a symbol of the damned and a sign of the apocalypse, was the stock-in-trade of anti-vaccinators. In the 1860s, Thomas Orton, secretary to the Sheffield Anti-Compulsory Vaccination Society, issued a handbill titled, "Compulsory Vaccination the Mark of the Beast." Similarly, in 1894 "A Worcestershire Parent" released a pamphlet titled, "The Parliamentary 'Mark of the Beast.' "[26] This apocalyptic language of spiritual perversion served to enhance the widespread discourse of monstrous physical transformation, both of which had roots in profound anxieties about bodily violation and blood purity.

Bodily Violation and Blood Purity

In wounding the skin, vaccination violated the biblical proscription "Ye shall not make any cuttings in your flesh . . . nor print any marks upon you."[27] But it also threatened what many considered the inviolate boundaries of the individual body. Vaccination was dangerous and disruptive, its opponents insisted, because it "violate[d]" the "physical integrity" of the human body by puncturing the skin.[28] In an 1873 call to mothers to resist vaccination, the ACVMPS insisted that vaccination means "cutting and wounding" the infant's "tender flesh."[29] Anti-vaccinators consistently claimed that the body was a "fortress" to be protected from invasion and that no government had any right "under any pretence to violate the bodies of its subjects." Our bodies, argued the health reformer John Fraser, are governed by "sacred" physical laws. But vaccination, he maintained, "trampl[es] down the defensive battlements" of the body, leaving it exposed to invading forces of disease. Should Englishmen not also declare "My skin is my castle"? trumpeted P. A. Siljeström, a widely quoted Swedish campaigner.[30] Anti-vaccinators feared this wounding of the skin because it allowed access to the internal body and, hence, the blood, the body's life force. Vaccination "violates the body," argued J. J. Garth Wilkinson, "by an actual wound into the blood."[31] The vaccinator's lancet "puncture[s]" the "skin-tissues, designed by nature to guard the blood from contact with all foreign and injurious matter," warned Mary Hume-Rothery, just like "the thorns and spines of poisonous plants, the stings of noxious insects and the fangs of reptiles."[32]

This fear of bodily violation was intimately bound up with concerns over the purity of the blood and the proper functioning of the circulatory system. Throughout the nineteenth century, both professional and popular opinion imagined good blood as the key to a healthy constitution. "The blood is the life," maintained a pamphlet on smallpox, "and *pure* blood is *healthy* life." Each drop of blood, it continued, "is conveyed over the entire human frame once in less than five minutes, carefully leaving in proper *situ*, like a skillful builder, such concrete, foundation, bricks, mortar, flooring, roof, scantling, plaster, wood, and metal-work, iron, bell-handles, chimney-tops, windows, drainage, kitchen-range, and wash-house, as an erection for modern occupancy requires to pass the survey of the lynx-eyed inspectors of a building society, or fire insurance board."[33] Blood was thus imagined as the building blocks of life, ensuring a healthy physical foundation for this "little human house." Anti-vaccinators took seriously the biblical tenet, "[T]he blood is the all in all—the individual himself—in short, the very life," and maintained that pure blood was vital to health.[34] Anti-vaccinators who came from alternative medical circles had long articulated the importance of the proper circulation of good blood. The hygiest John Morison argued, "[A]ll diseases arise from an impurity of the blood." Health, as a general principle, maintained Fraser, "depends upon the purity of the blood," for the blood is the "forming agent of the body."[35] But even for those anti-vaccinators who did not actively practice some form of alternative medicine, the blood commanded an important place in their understandings of bodily economy. The best guard against smallpox, maintained a Midland anti-vaccinator, is to keep "the blood pure," the bowels regular, and the skin clean.[36] Anti-vaccinators regularly asserted that obeying the laws of hygiene, getting plenty of fresh air and exercise, and eating nourishing food was nature's way of keeping the blood pure and free of disease.

Based on a fluid reading of bodily economy, this focus on the blood as the root of disease and the seat of health was widespread in popular medical culture. It stimulated the production of a plethora of cure-all patent medicines that were marketed to the public as blood purifiers. Clarke's World Famous Blood Mixture maintained that, no matter what the symptoms, the "real cause" of most diseases was "bad blood." "Keep your blood pure," Clarke's advertised in the *Family Doctor and People's Medical Adviser*, "and the health of the system will follow." Similarly, Swift's Specific Vegetable Blood Purifier portrayed itself as a noble soldier, protecting a classical maiden from the enemy—"blood poison"—and from the demon-like inefficacy of "other mixtures." Even non-medicinal products championed their effects on healthy blood. An 1898 advertisement for Van Houten's Chocolate titled, "The Little Soldiers in Your Blood," maintained that the product helped to fortify the corpuscles in pure blood—"our soldier friends" who fight disease germs.[37]

Anti-vaccinators argued that vaccination polluted the blood by introducing foreign material into the healthy human system. Regardless of the nature of vaccine matter, adding something to the blood was adulteration of the body's most important substance, they insisted. Archdeacon Colley of Durban, South Africa, whose pamphlet was widely quoted in England, warned of the dangers of blood contamination by arguing that one knew very little of the blood's "supreme powers, marvellous qualities, and inner sanctities." It would be a grave mistake, he

argued, to commingle things "not by Heaven's will originally com-
pacted."[38] Similarly, a banner at the Leicester Demonstration in 1885
demanded, "Pure blood and no adulteration."[39] Since healthy blood
was vital to a healthy constitution, any interference with it put the
individual at risk for any number of diseases, resisters argued. As F. W.
Newman insisted, "Tampering with the blood is an abomination." Anti-
vaccinators attacked compulsory vaccination as "State blood poisoning"
or, worse still, "blood assassination." Vaccination is "pollution of our
veins," maintained Newman in 1882. In fact, argued an Earlestown
father, his child was so poisoned by vaccination that for months the
baby had not a "drop of pure blood in its body."[40]

Blood purity for many anti-vaccinationists was part of a larger concern with "physical Puritanism," a preoccupation with physical and
moral purity that often dovetailed with ideas of individual independence. Physical puritanism also had a decidedly feminist dimension
that articulated the vulnerability of women to bodily pollution and violation at the hands of state medicine.[41] Anti-vaccinationism thus found
allies in the temperance and anti-tobacco campaigns, which also attracted a female following. A correspondent to *The Anti-Vaccinator* declared, "If there is anything that I detest more than others, they are
vaccination, alcohol, and tobacco."[42] Temperance Halls were frequently
home to anti-vaccination lectures and meetings, and many campaigners against compulsory vaccination considered themselves teetotalers.
In addressing the British Temperance League Conference on the subject of anti-vaccination in 1869, Pitman illustrated the ties between the
movements. "We may rejoice at being life-abstainers, and that we come
of a pure teetotal stock," he maintained, "but our rejoicing must be with
trembling, so long as our children may be (and are) by law poisoned
with the blood of the drunkard." Like seeks like, Pitman argued; thus,
children contaminated with the blood of those who drank alcohol also
craved it.[43]

In its quest for physical purity, the anti-vaccination campaign also
became closely aligned with vegetarianism, a movement that arose in
Britain in the 1840s and had a decidedly populist and, later, feminist
tone. The ties between vegetarianism and anti-vaccinationism were
strong: Richard Butler Gibbs, founder of the organized anti-vaccination
campaign, was a noted devotee of vegetarianism. Newman, a promi-

nent anti-vaccination and anti–contagious diseases acts campaigner, was president of the Vegetarian Society of Great Britain from 1873 to 1884, and William Tebb, founding member of the LSACV, launched his social-reform career as a paid organizer for the vegetarian movement. Vegetarians maintained that all animal products polluted the natural purity of the body and resisted incorporating animal matter in any form. A piece of anti-vaccination comic relief made these links explicit: A doctor seeking to vaccinate a child, reported the *Vaccination Inquirer*, reassured the mother by insisting that he would use "the purest calf-lymph." "Then sir," replied the woman, "that settles it, for we are vegetarians!"[44]

As campaigners for food reform in general, anti-vaccinators and vegetarians maintained that vaccination had the same, if not worse, deleterious effects on the body as did the adulteration of food. Vaccination, argued Pitman, is "national adulteration" not just of the people's food, "but of their life's blood."[45] There was a limit to what the people would stoop to eat, anti-vaccinators suggested, and if some animal products were not fit to eat, then they were not fit to be inserted into the body in any manner: "What is not fit for a child's bread and butter is not fit for its blood," argued Furnival.[46] In 1890, the *Vaccination Inquirer* reported on cab horses sold for sausage meat and beef tea. Cab horses with "greasy legs" were always rejected, it claimed. But although "the greasy heels are too horrible to be allowed to approach a sausage, they are," it continued sarcastically, "just the thing to exude 'pure lymph' for insertion in little children."[47] Adulterated food and vaccination were directly related issues in the case of "vaccinated veal"—meat sold for human consumption that derived from the carcasses of cows used in the production of vaccine matter. According to John Burns, president of the Local Government Board, during 1905 and 1906, 600 calves used in the production of lymph were slaughtered and sold for food at Smithfield Market.[48] Temperance, vegetarianism, food reform, and anti-vaccinationism were thus related movements that encouraged abstention from drink and flesh to purify the blood and ward off disease. Proclaimed the hydropath T. L. Nichols: "[T]emperance men and vegetarians need never fear small-pox, however produced. Make the blood pure and it offers no foothold."[49]

Contaminated, Deteriorated, and Despoiled

If anti-vaccinators imagined that the health of the body depended on the proper circulation of pure blood, vaccination represented the ultimate disruption of the body's economy and its contamination by impure sources. As an animal product, anti-vaccinators argued, vaccine was already a corrupted substance that became even more polluted and polluting when passed through a multitude of children.[50] The arm-to-arm method practiced at public stations, parents maintained, threatened to contaminate their respectable working-class infants with the blood of animals, paupers, syphilitics, and degenerates.

ANIMALS   Although anti-vaccinators were ostensibly concerned with good blood, what was actually being transferred in the vaccination process was lymph—a mucus-like substance that contained the essential element of vaccinia. Vaccination was performed by inserting lymph cultivated from a calf, or a human vaccine vesicle, into the arm. However, one could never be certain that lymph did not also contain blood. In testifying before the Royal Commission on Vaccination, the medical officer of health for Harrogate expressed his concerns over calf lymph. "The first specimen of calf lymph I got [from the Local Government Board] frightened me when I got it. . . . [T]here was so much blood mixed into it that I hesitated to use it."[51] In practice, then, blood and lymph could never be considered discrete substances, as they were intermingled bodily fluids.

Part of the objection to vaccine lymph was that it derived from animals. Lymph was the product of a cow, for cowpox produced an immunity to smallpox without being communicable within a human population. In the late eighteenth and early nineteenth centuries, cartoonists satirized popular fears surrounding cowpox inoculation. In James Gillray's 1802 etching "The Cow-Pock—The Wonderful Effects of the New Inoculation," the vaccinated sprout horns from their heads and fully formed cow carbuncles from their noses, cheeks, and buttocks. These associations continued well into the 1890s as the bovine nature of lymph shaped an understanding of its effects on the human body. At a meeting of the British Medical Association in 1890, a speaker on vaccination rashes produced a child who the *Vaccination Inquirer* reported was "covered with little horn-like excrescenses, which had resulted from vaccination."[52] Some parents feared that vaccinated children might adopt cow-like tendencies. A report on the Gloucester epidemic of 1895–96 maintained that parents had been unwilling for "a beast [to] be put into their children," as they had imagined that they might come "to low and to browse in the fields like oxen." Similarly, a father summoned to the Woolwich Police Court in 1891 asserted that he resisted the vaccination of his child for fear of a nineteenth-century version of mad cow disease: "[I]t is well known that the bulls go mad every seven years, and that the cows make them mad"; when these same cows are used for vaccinating children, he reasoned, the children go mad. "The madhouses are full of vaccinated children."[53]

Anti-vaccinators were anxious that calf lymph could also transmit animal diseases. In her memoir, Amy Frances Gomm remembered that her parents, caretakers of a landed estate, had resisted vaccination in the 1890s. "The cow came into it," she recounted, "and people in villages knew about cows. 'The most cancerous and consumptive animal there is.' I can hear Dad saying it now."[54] Anti-vaccinators repeatedly characterized vaccine matter as a "loathsome virus derived from the blood of a brute," which could harbor animal diseases as yet unknown to humans. In a report submitted to the Royal Commission on Vaccination in the 1890s, J. T. Biggs, a plumber and sanitary engineer, claimed that a child had caught what the parents maintained was "a sort of foot-and-mouth disease" from calf-lymph vaccination.[55]

It was bad enough that the "disease of a *beast*" be forcibly communicated to the "tender bodies" of "*human* children," anti-vaccinators maintained, but worse still that one could not be sure of the beast that emitted it.[56] While vaccine was supposed to be the product of the cow, it was often produced by injecting different forms of animal poxes or human smallpox into the cow. Anti-vaccinationists insisted that one could never be certain how many different animal diseases were communicated through vaccination. The original vaccine virus was said to be derived from the horse grease, which was as objectionable as the cowpox. Vaccine virus, claimed a pamphleteer, derives from the "stinking heels of an emaciated horse in the later stages of phthisis."[57] In 1902, Walter Hadwen insisted that the latest batch of vaccine matter supplied by the National Vaccine Establishment had been produced by inoculating smallpox into a monkey and then monkey pox into a calf.[58] Anti-vaccinators reasoned that repealing the compulsory clauses would allow "the deluded ones" to "humanize, bovinize, equinate, assinate, or assassinate, to their hearts' content with any lymph they please" while protecting those who did not want their bodies contaminated with a menagerie of polluted fluids.[59] To anti-vaccinators, then, "pure lymph" was an oxymoron, for lymph was by definition an impure substance of questionable origin. How could one have "Clean dirt, and healthy cow-disease!"[60]

Those who objected to vaccination were also uneasy about the moral and mental effects of incorporating an animal product. "True the physical horns and hoofs do not show themselves," warned a pamphleteer, "yet the mental horns and cloven hoofs too frequently shoot out."[61] Anti-vaccinators feared that vaccination could "stimulate their animal propensities" and thus "brutify" and "lower" human nature. By infusing the human system with the "passions of the beast," argued Archdeacon Colley, the person is "dehumanized" to the degree in which "the animal has been implanted."[62] These concerns over physical and moral bestialization occasionally manifested themselves in anxieties about devolution, a specter raised by Darwinian theory. Even if we are "ascended from gorillas," Wilkinson argued, we nevertheless refuse to have our "natures mixed again with the disease of beasts."[63] Diluting or replacing human blood with that of the beast could reverse the process of evolution, these campaigners implied, returning man to an ape-like state.

PAUPERS While animal lymph posed serious concerns for anti-vaccinators, human lymph was equally, if not more, problematic. Until the 1898 Vaccination Act mandated the use of calf lymph supplied by the National Vaccine Establishment, public vaccination was generally performed from arm to arm. In London in 1893, there were only two public vaccination stations that claimed to use calf lymph. While some vaccinators clearly preferred to use preserved calf lymph, many claimed that human lymph was purer and less liable to contamination. However, there was no clear consensus within the medical community as to which substance was safer.[64] The arm-to-arm method was widespread because it was preferred by the government. Since this was the cheapest way to ensure a continuous supply of vaccine matter, it was "humanized" lymph that was most commonly used in public vaccination.

All vaccinated infants were required to be brought back to the vaccinator eight days after the procedure to check whether the vaccination had "taken." These children with fully developed vesicles were used at public stations as the vaccinifier, or "stock-baby," from which matter would be taken for use in other operations. This ensured that a supply of fresh lymph was always maintained in the community. Refusal to supply lymph for use in public vaccination could result in a hefty 20 shilling fine. In 1891, Lydia Cook, the wife of a railway laborer who earned 19 shillings a week, was fined 1 shilling plus 25 shillings 6 pence costs and threatened with fourteen days in prison for refusing to allow lymph to be taken from her child. Her family had a history of consumption, she claimed, and she did not want to contaminate other children.[65]

The Cook case, an anti-vaccination cause célèbre, exemplified the recurrent complaint that public vaccinators were not discriminating enough about the lymph they employed. Since blood was regularly transferred with lymph, vaccination exposed children to a variety of diseases that, campaigners maintained, could be transmitted through the blood. Vaccination, its opponents argued, could spread scrofula, cancer, leprosy, idiocy, consumption, epilepsy, erysipelas, syphilis, deafness, blindness, and a variety of other hereditary and contagious diseases (see Figure 9).[66] A poem that appeared in 1881 in *Fun*, a periodical with primarily a lower-middle-class readership, made light of what was clearly a source of concern for those who used the public stations:

> So submit to legislation,
> And apply for vaccination
> To condemn to extirpation one particular complaint;
> And instead of one affection
> You can have a whole selection;
> So you'll kindly choose your favorite hereditary taint.[67]

What the poem satirized was working-class parents' lack of control over which lymph was used to vaccinate their infants. Unlike the private doctors employed by the middle classes, who often used calf lymph

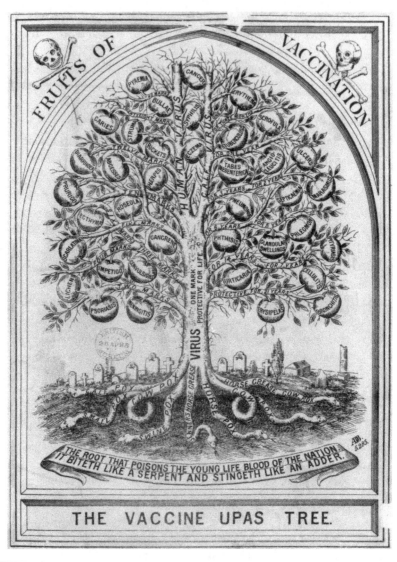

9. "Fruits of Vaccination," c. 1885.
By permission of the British Library, shelfmark 1881.c.16(40).

because they considered it safer, the public vaccinator was not being paid by those he vaccinated. The laboring classes who were forced to use his services therefore had no choice in the lymph. The public vaccinator, claimed the feminist Ursula Bright, vaccinates with "*what lymph he likes*," for the transaction existed outside any real medical marketplace.[68]

If anti-vaccinators held fast to beliefs about blood purity and the integrity of the body, pro-vaccinators produced their own bodily imaginary. Public vaccinators were instructed to select children of dark complexion, with brown eyes and thick, smooth, clear skin, as vaccinifiers. Fair children with blue eyes, they feared, might be scrofulous. In addition, they were encouraged to choose legitimate children from parents personally known to them "whose family history is good" and to avoid the first born to weed out hereditary conditions. They were routinely cautioned not to draw blood when pricking to collect lymph.[69] How carefully public vaccinators followed these recommendations was another matter entirely.

Working-class anti-vaccinators were highly concerned that at public vaccination stations, lymph was taken from children without inspecting them or their parents for signs of contagious or hereditary disease. In public stations, *The Anti-Vaccinator* maintained, there was not the "slightest discrimination exercised as to the purity of the source whence the matter was derived." The lymph at vaccination stations, argued Tebb, was positively "reeking" with scrofulous and syphilitic contaminations.[70] Even doctors conceded that the collection of lymph for public vaccination was not always carefully performed. In a lecture delivered at the Richmond Athenaeum, the senior surgeon for Richmond Hospital in the 1880s maintained that when he was a medical student, lymph was taken from "crowds of squalid, unhealthy, scrofulous-looking children. No questions were asked. Neither mothers nor children were examined as to whether they were fit persons to vaccinate from."[71] Something must be done to secure the quality of lymph, he declared. Anti-vaccinators asserted that little had been done to ensure the purity of lymph because its victims were the poor. Once the "reckless severities of the public stations" are imported into the private drawing rooms of "Grosvenor-place," a higher standard of vaccination will surely be mandated, the *Vaccination Inquirer* argued.[72]

For respectable working-class people, the public stations thus posed the risk of having lymph from an unknown and potentially contaminated source infused into their children. Lymph from paupers, *The Anti-Vaccinator* insisted, could "give no hope of health."[73] However, it could be equally alarming to be vaccinated from someone one knew. Faith Dorothy Osgerby, born in 1890 to a stonemason turned cattle dealer, remembered that she was used as the vaccinifier for six of her schoolmates. As she looked back at the age of seventy, the process seemed "horrifying" to her.[74] Similarly, Gomm recalled that since "everybody knew everybody else," one would know that "so-and-so's baby had more than a fifty/fifty chance of growing up mentally defective. All the family were."[75] Since not all babies were equally desirable as vaccinifiers, parents regularly attempted to control the origin of the lymph to prevent contamination from diseased or morally questionable families. The vaccinator was assailed with questions: "Is the matter good?" "Where did you get it?" The cautious parent stated, " 'I would not have it from that child; he has bad blood," or "I would not like it from the other, his parents have ugly disorders."[76] But even careful vaccinators could not guarantee the quality of lymph, for hereditary taints were not always written on the body. Scrofula, argued the hydropath Mary Nichols, "often lurks in the veins of the most beautiful, fair, and apparently robust and healthy infant." Even a "neighbour's healthy-looking child," anti-vaccinators cautioned, could communicate foul diseases, whether handpicked or not.[77]

Since the poor, unlike the middle and upper classes who used private physicians, could not readily select the vaccinifier, and since even seemingly healthy children could harbor disease, public vaccination multiplied the amount of disease in any given community, its opponents suggested. The poor, claimed Wilkinson, are all "imbrued in each other's taints"; vaccination "mingles in a communism of blood the taints of the community." Since blood was transmitted through "hundreds of thousands of beings" by way of arm-to-arm vaccination, every "hereditary sewer opens up into every nursery; nay, into each infant's very heart," Wilkinson warned.[78] The sewer, which carried the waste of society and which had connotations of sexual pollution, was infecting the child, who was supposed to be pure and innocent, untainted by physical and moral corruption. Since vaccination had passed blood from arm to arm to arm, no matter how healthy a child seemed, each vaccinated infant was a repository for the diseases of the entire community. Each person's blood was no longer his own, Wilkinson suggested, for each individual shared in the diseases with which the "residuum" infected the social body. Vaccination, its critics maintained, was thus a dangerous form of "body-mixing."[79]

The mingling of blood and other bodily matter also raised important, if difficult to articulate, moral questions. Some anti-vaccinators suggested that vaccination not only could pass physical disease between bodies but also had moral consequences. Vaccination, argued a draper from Evesham, exercised an injurious effect on the *"moral nature."* Mary Hume-Rothery argued that, while "corrupting" the physical body, vaccination also "debased the *moral* life-blood" of all who submitted to it.[80] What these two critics implied, the *Eclectic Journal and Medical Free Press* made explicit: It denounced the system that obliged "respectable" working-class parents to have their children vaccinated from paupers, who, it suggested, communicated their debased moral conditions along with the lymph.[81] If the blood of individuals "inherited from their ancestors" was now to be mixed with "the blood of the entire people in an adulterous union," what was to become of class distinctions and family bloodlines? According to William Hume-Rothery, vaccination was a form of "adultery," as it combined the blood of one family with that of another. Blood mixing not only raised concerns regarding the physical body. It also blurred social distinctions, which threatened to degrade the laboring classes whose morality was already heavily scrutinized.[82]

SYPHILITICS The relationship between physical and moral taints became inextricably linked in debates over the transmission of syphilis via vaccination. Since the 1860s, anti-vaccinators had insisted that vaccination was directly responsible for an increase in syphilis morbidity. Between 1872 and 1874 in London alone, argued William Young, 1,074 children under the age of five had died of syphilis; the rates, he claimed, had doubled since the introduction of compulsory vaccination.[83] Charles Creighton, an expert on epidemics, concurred, maintaining that cowpox itself was really a venereal disease. The vaccine virus "in its original or primitive form," argued a pamphlet from the Mile End branch of the NAVL, "is syphilitic virus."[84] Most, however, argued that in the process of transferring the lymph from arm to arm, blood tainted with congenital or hereditary syphilis could also be passed along. The compulsory vaccination laws are nothing less than the "deliberate incorporation of national syphilis by Parliament," a pamphlet on invaccinated syphilis warned. Popular conceptions of syphilis as blood poisoning only served to strengthen the perceived ties among vaccination, syphilis, and bad blood.[85]

Syphilis was particularly problematic because, unlike scrofula and erysipelas, it had a moral dimension and carried a social stigma. Until the 1880s, both scientific experts and the lay public understood syphilis to be a sexually transmitted disease contracted from prostitutes and through other "impure" sexual relations. Indeed, syphilis carried such a loaded moral charge that it was the quintessentially "nameless" Victorian disease.[86] But in the last decades of the nineteenth century, the medical profession also began to focus on what it termed "congenital" and "hereditary" forms of the disease.[87] If the problem of how "innocent" children acquired venereal diseases stimulated heated debate among late-Victorian medical professionals, invaccinated syphilis raised even more troubling questions. Doctors were largely resistant to accepting the possibility that syphilis could be spread via vaccination, for it implicated the medical profession itself in the transmission of this particularly pernicious disease. Some pro-vaccinators did concede that syphilis could be passed from congenital or hereditary cases by careless vaccination. In 1886, Jonathan Hutchinson—the leading British expert on syphilis—reported that in studies of fourteen children vaccinated from a carefully selected vaccinifier, eleven had become infected with syphilis.[88] In an ironic twist of fate, the most convincing evidence for invaccinated syphilis was supplied by Dr. Robert Cory, head of the Local Government Board's animal vaccine station, who infected himself in the course of an experiment intended to demonstrate the impossibility of transmitting venereal disease via vaccination.[89]

Despite a new scientific focus on the nonsexual transmission of venereal diseases, anti-vaccination literature did not sever syphilis from its explicitly sexual connotations. Vaccine matter, argued Archdeacon Colley, is a "fungoid, yeasty, abominable mixture of corruption, the lees of human vice, and dregs of venial appetites, that in after life may foam upon the spirit, and develop hell within, and overwhelm the soul." Drawing on the medical language of fermentation, Colley insisted that vaccine was always tainted by syphilitic conditions that could literally engulf the soul. Because the soul was housed in the body, he implied, it was constantly at risk of physical contamination. Even if invaccinated syphilis was not physically apparent, its dangers were ever present, for it might manifest "morally" and lead its victims forth "by the ways of impurity, and nameless filthy sins, addicting the victims to habits of intemperance, and vices too hideous to name."[90] Although he could not bring himself to name the disease, William Hume-Rothery also warned that syphilis caused "moral degradation" that could itself become hereditary.[91]

Those who contracted syphilis from vaccination were eager to deny any responsibility for the disease whatsoever. In 1885, a Camberwell child developed a case of what one doctor identified as "hereditary syphilis" and died. The father "indignantly repudiated the heredity, both for himself and his wife." The doctor subsequently admitted that the disease had probably been transmitted during vaccination. However, he registered the primary cause of the baby's death as meningitis, as he was reluctant to admit to having infected the baby. The outraged father insisted that the death certificate should read "invaccinated syphilis," but the doctor refused, offering instead to add syphilis as a cause of death. The father balked at the suggestion, maintaining that he did not want it to be construed as a "reflection upon the parents." Printed in the *Vaccination Inquirer*, this story served as a cautionary tale: Young men and women entering wedlock, it warned, should consider the vaccination question carefully, for they ran a terrible risk of living their lives "under the cruel suspicion of having corrupted their offspring by the results of their own vice."[92] If a child contracted a venereal taint from vaccination, the humanitarian Joseph Collinson argued, the blame would fall on the parent whose moral standing was compromised.[93] Vaccinal syphilis brought "misery and domestic unhappiness," argued *Disease by Law*, for "happy homes" were wrecked by "unfounded marital suspicions."[94] Vaccinating one's child left one's own and one's family's sexual practices open to scrutiny, campaigners suggested, for the risk of contracting syphilis from vaccination was considerable.

DEGENERATES   In late-Victorian culture, the syphilitic functioned as a paradigm of degeneracy that threatened not only the individual's health but also that of the nation. National health became an important topic of public debate in the late nineteenth century as Britain attempted both to manage an expanding empire and to deal with waves of eastern European immigration to a metropolis that was already struggling with the problems of rapid and increasing urbanization. Darwinian and Lamarckian fears of devolution; eugenic concerns over social hygiene; and a developing science of criminology with roots in physiognomy, phrenology, and anthropology provided theoretical support for popular concerns over class conflict, miscegenation, and national decline.[95]

Anti-vaccinators participated in and helped to shape a widespread discourse of national efficiency, physical deterioration, and degeneration that escalated toward the end of the century. As early as 1856, *The Hygiest*, a health-reform magazine popular among alternative practitioners, warned that vaccination led to "degeneration of the human race."[96] Many anti-vaccinators used the term *race* as a synonym for humankind. Vaccination, argued *The Anti-Vaccinator* in 1869, threatens to undermine the health and strength of the "entire human race."[97] Campaigners against compulsory vaccination continued into the twentieth century to attack vaccination in these broad terms. The vaccination laws, argued a speaker at the 1907 NAVL annual meeting, strike "at the physical stamina of the race."[98] But some anti-vaccinators not only critiqued the general effects of vaccination on the human population but specifically lamented its impact on the British nation.

Vaccination, its opponents argued, weakened Britain's future citizens and threatened the nation's health. In 1883, Jessie Craigen accused vaccinators of "stamping out the energy of the nation."[99] As good citizens, anti-vaccinators maintained that compulsory vaccination compromised national efficiency and the state apparatus. "Does the State need strong and healthy citizens," demanded Mary Hume-Rothery, "or puny and diseased ones?"[100] Long before the panic precipitated by the Boer War, anti-vaccinators warned that Britons were deteriorating in stature. The standards for recruits were significantly lower than in the early part of the century, according to a correspondent to the *Anti-Vaccinator and Public Health Journal* in 1872; this "deterioration and dwarfing," he feared, was jeopardizing national security.[101] By the early twentieth century, the government became increasingly concerned with the quality of men volunteering for military service and launched an investigation into physical deterioration. Anti-vaccinators attempted to make vaccination a priority for the Physical Deterioration Committee of 1904, suggesting to committee members that they investigate vaccination as the root cause of this widespread physical decline. The committee acknowledged that it was a worthy subject of inquiry but declined to take up the issue. Parliament had expended enough time and money on the Royal Commission on Vaccination, they argued, and was not inclined to undertake another investigation.[102]

Fears for the British nation were intimately bound up in concerns for the white English race. If the people continue to be "contaminated, deteriorated, and despoiled" by vaccination, argued a campaigner in 1870, then the "Anglo-Saxon race—once the finest race of people—will sink into effeminacy, disease, and premature death."[103] It was the "people of Europe," insisted George Gibbs, whose "physical stamina" was depleted by vaccination.[104] In an article printed in the *British Medical Journal* in 1903, these fears of race—and thus, blood—purity were carefully articulated. The purity of the bloodstream of the human race is of such importance, argued Dr. Josiah Oldfield, secretary of the Vegetarian Federal Union, that to pollute it with animal lymph would be as "desecrating" as to "marry the daughter of a royal line of kings to a negro husband."[105] Blood purity, suggested Oldfield, was as much about keeping the races distinct as it was about separating the classes or the human from the animal. Indeed, pro- and anti-vaccinators alike warned that skin color—an important marker of race—could be transmitted via vaccination. Dr. Bakewell of Trinidad reported that a white child had become "piebald" shortly after being vaccinated from a "negro" child. After the healing of the pustules, reported the *National Anti-Compulsory Vaccination League Occasional Circular*, the child became "spotted over the whole of the body with black hairy marks . . . as in the negro."[106]

In a guide for British mothers in India, Mrs. Howard Kingscote, a popular novelist and the wife of a commanding officer in the Indian Army, attempted to dispel some of these clearly widespread fears. It was perfectly safe to vaccinate from a native child, she insisted, whose physiology was no different from that of a white child. While Kingscote attacked this "misconception and prejudice," she nevertheless recommended using a European vaccinifier if at all possible, for no other reason than the implicit assumption that it was preferable that the races remain separate in this as in all other things, for the empire rested on a colonial hierarchy that depended on a "symbolics of blood." As Ann Stoler has argued, late-nineteenth- and early-twentieth-century discourses on miscegenation "combined notions of tainted, flawed, and pure blood with those of degeneration and racial purity in countless ways."[107] Vaccination, in its mingling of the blood, posed the threat of miscegenation and thus degeneration, which many argued would ultimately lead to the collapse of the Anglo-Saxon race and the downfall of Imperial Britain.

Toward the end of the century, these fears of syphilization, degeneration, and miscegenation also found expression in the eugenic movement, which had roots in a type of social Darwinism. However, there was no single, fixed relationship between vaccination and eugenics. Compulsory vaccination could be construed as a eugenic tool that protected against national decline by ensuring a population free of smallpox. *Punch* denounced the 1898 conscience clause, fearing it would lead to a decline in vaccination, as the "TRIUMPH OF DE-JENNER-ATION" (see Figure 10). Alternatively, in 1896 a correspondent to the *British Medical Journal* using the pseudonym "Political Economist" argued that compulsory vaccination undermined the eugenic program, as it gave "an unfair advantage" to those who otherwise would not be vaccinated. The correspondent declared that the wise are vaccinated and the unwise are not, ensuring the "survival of the fittest" and the death of the "residuum." "Scientifically speaking," he continued, it would be better to let well enough alone and let nature take its course.[108]

Although he did not share the eugenic goal of an eradication of the "residuum," a politically loaded term, the anti-vaccinationist and whole-meal–bread manufacturer Thomas Richard Allinson nevertheless envisioned anti-vaccination as a part of a larger social-hygiene program. In 1887, Allinson described what he considered an ideal "physical millennium," in which none but the healthy could marry and then only after attaining certificates of health. "If this were the case now," he maintained, "we should have a finer race and stronger children, with fewer infantine deaths. As it is, cripples, delicate, or diseased persons may marry, and no one can stop them. This may result in delicate or deformed children or children with not enough vitality in them to last many years. These consume our food, increase our death rate, and are no benefit to society at large." He continued, "We take greater care of

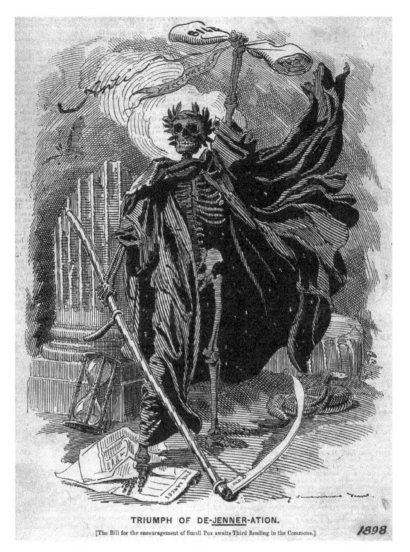

TRIUMPH OF DE-JENNER-ATION.

[The Bill for the encouragement of Small Pox awaits Third Reading in the Commons.]

1898

10. "Triumph of De-Jenner-Ation," *Punch*, 30 July 1898.
By permission of the Wellcome Library, London.

our animals than we do of our own kind, we let our animals come to maturity before we breed from them, and then we choose the best sires we can get." But among human beings, Allinson concluded, everything is left to "chance or fortune." Allinson, who was explicitly concerned with good breeding, thus denounced vaccination as a threat to the "health of the race."[109]

The Gothic Body

The language of violation, contamination, and degeneration was central to the anti-vaccination campaign. But this discourse was not merely sensationalist propaganda. Anti-vaccinators articulated their bodily anxieties through the horrific genre. Like feminist campaigners against state medicine in general, they drew on "gothic sensibilities" and a "rich symbolic network" of tainted blood to express their fears about personal and national health and security.[110] Indeed, anti-vaccinators consistently returned to two telling icons of Victorian gothic culture: the vampire and the vivisector.

THE VACCINATION VAMPIRE   In *The Vaccination Vampire*, an 1881 handbill, Wilkinson drew on a number of related metaphors to construct vaccination as vampiric. Compulsory vaccination, he maintained, is the "bloodhound" of the childbearing woman. The bloodhound, an image deployed in the 1860s by a public vaccinator forced to "hunt" down noncompliers, served as the symbol of detection. The state tracked anti-vaccinators, pursuing them like criminals through the use of a creature that, like the vampire, was specifically trained to track the smell of the blood. Vaccination, Wilkinson further argued, was like a raven perched on "parturient" sheep, waiting to pluck out and devour the eyes of the newborn lambs. It "hover[ed]" over the pregnant woman who waited in the "shadow of its wings," primed and ready to attack the infant. Winged and hovering, vaccination here figures as both a bird of prey and a vampire haunting the laboring mother. The vampire's concern is with the blood, but, according to Wilkinson, vaccination disrupted the entire fluid economy of the body. The "Vaccination Vampire" polluted the "pure babe" precisely at the point of its "suckling," the handbill warned,

for the mother's milk was "blighted" by fear of the "poisoned lancet'";
thus, the "Vaccination Vampire" was a source of "universal pollution"
and degeneration, for it led to "degradation and extinction." The "cradle
is born to an immediate medical hell," Wilkinson warned, for the "Vaccination Vampire" "befouls" and "demonizes" and is the "Supreme
Quack and grand Apollyon or Destroyer of the Human Race."[111] Wilkinson's "Vaccination Vampire" thus epitomized what anti-vaccinators considered an invasive and violating operation.

Published in 1881, *The Vaccination Vampire* deployed a literary trope that
was not yet a century old, for the vampire was a distinctly nineteenth-
century phenomenon. While the word *vampire* made its debut in English writing in the 1730s, John Polidori's "The Vampyre," a short story
published in 1819 and originally attributed to Byron, was the first of a
series of Regency and Victorian vampire tales and plays that culminated
in 1897 in the immensely popular *Dracula*.[112] By the 1850s, the vampire
had become a stock character, popularized and commercialized for a
mass-market audience in Britain largely by James Malcolm Rymer's
Varney the Vampire. Serialized with illustrations in 109 penny install-
ments between 1840 and 1842, *Varney*, a pot-boiling "penny dreadful"
was a smash success. It was reprinted in 1847 and then again in 1853, the
same year compulsory vaccination was enacted.[113] The vaccinator and
the vampire were thus products of the same historical moment. Indeed,
according to anti-vaccinators, they had much in common.

Although its metaphorical value was multivalent, from midcentury
the vampire came to symbolize the bloodthirsty doctor. Orthodox medicine was seen to be vampiric because of the Galenic tradition of bloodletting. In 1850, the medical botanist Albert Isaiah Coffin declared that,
since the doctor asserts that disease is in the blood, he "attacks your
veins like a vampire."[114] In 1885, Wilkinson claimed that medicine was
dead "but stirs and rises from its grave as a vampyre; and is the night-
haunting demon of the end of the Nineteenth Century."[115] In language
that was apocalyptic as well as gothic, Wilkinson both dismissed orthodox medicine as dead and yet feared its reanimated return, for vaccination, he implied, had breathed new life into the medical profession.

The linkages among medicine, vampirism, and reanimation to which
Wilkinson alluded were also bound up in the early-nineteenth-century
discourse of blood transfusion. The obstetrical patient, weak from loss

of blood, was the prime candidate for this experimental practice in the 1820s. The Romantic imagery of the swooning, bloodless mother found in accounts of blood transfusion had much in common with contemporary tales of victims of vampirism. In this context—and, indeed, in *Dracula*—the medical practice of blood transfusion appears as the antidote to the wasting sickness caused by the vampire's bloodsucking.[116] But the transfusing doctor was not always the Romantic hero who reanimated the dead. In 1896, a year before the publication of *Dracula*, Mary Elizabeth Braddon's story "The Good Lady Ducayne" appeared in the *Strand Magazine*, an illustrated monthly featuring popular fiction. In this story, the heroine discovers mysterious bites on her arm, only to find that she is regularly being lanced by a foreign doctor to infuse her blood into the aging Lady Ducayne. The doctor both saps and infuses the veins, just as the vampire sucks blood but leaves a transformative material behind to turn his victims into monsters themselves. Although it is not actually a vampire story, for the doctor is a mere mortal, "The Good Lady Ducayne" nevertheless points to the cultural intersection of medicine, blood tampering, parasitism, and, interestingly, a wounded arm.[117] With its medical associations already established, then, the vampire served anti-vaccinators as the perfect foil for the vaccinator who "invad[es]" the blood, inserts "a foul enemy," and leaves his victim monstrously disfigured or dead.[118]

The vampire's relationship to the doctor was also bound up in medicine's social position as an aristocratic profession. The vampire evolved out of a gothic genre that was a "late product of the controversy generated in Britain by the French Revolution."[119] The vampire operated in many ways as a symbol of the ancien régime that lingered and haunted Britain's own stately homes. The aristocracy's power in the nineteenth century derived from its being both dead and in fact not dead. The vampire's preoccupation with blood has thus been read as an aristocratic concern for the perpetuation of hereditary bloodlines.[120] Polidori's vampire Lord Ruthven was brought to life at the same moment as Frankenstein's monster, both creations of a now legendary 1816 meeting of the Shelleys, Byron, and Polidori on the shores of Lake Leman. It was Lord Ruthven, a clearly Byronic character, who established the literary relationship between the vampire and the aristocracy that was perpetuated by Rymer's Sir Francis Varney and Bram Stoker's Count Dracula. Thus, when anti-vaccinators drew on this metaphor, they were gesturing to medicine's established aristocratic associations. Although by midcentury most orthodox medical practitioners were decidedly middle-class, anti-vaccinators generally attacked doctors as aristocratic tricksters. In this they were not unlike other medical reformers who proclaimed physic to be a "genteel profession" and physicians no better than empirics clothed in "gilded and gorgeous trappings."[121] Indeed, when Josephine Butler campaigned against the compulsory medical inspection of prostitutes under the contagious diseases acts, she identified those "terrible aristocratic doctors" as the root of medical corruption.[122]

Anti-vaccinators considered medicine to be an aristocratic profession and, like the vampire, linked to "Old Corruption." But both medicine and the monster would take on middle-class associations over the course of the nineteenth century. Rymer's vampire, Sir Francis Varney, claimed a title and in many ways served as a symbol of the bloated and parasitical aristocrat. However, Varney had been a highway robber; once transformed into a baronet, he sought not blood but money. The vampires that were to follow him also prioritized the accumulation of wealth. Mr. Vholes, the lawyer in *Bleak House*, drains away his clients' money with such alacrity that Dickens notes he has "something of the Vampire in him."[123] Dracula, too, hoards his bounty in the back passages of his decrepit castle and "bleeds" a stream of gold coins when attacked. The relationship between the vampire and the accumulation of capital thus positioned the monster as a member of the bourgeoisie. No invocation of the vampire makes this association more explicit than Karl Marx's famous epigram, "Capital is dead labour, that, vampire-like, only lives by sucking living labour, and lives the more, the more labour it sucks."[124] It was Marx's 1867 *Capital*, Nina Auerbach argues, that "sealed the vampire's class descent from mobile aristocrat to exploitative employer."[125] *Sealed* may be too strong a term, for anti-vaccinators used the vampire as a complex symbol of both an aristocratic profession and the bourgeois capitalist state. These institutions were linked by the figure of the public vaccinator who was both a "qualified" medical practitioner and a state employee.

Public vaccinators, according to Lieutenant-General A. Phelps, president of the NAVL from 1897, were "grasping vampires" who operated on the sick and healthy indiscriminately in search of "blood money" to sustain them.[126] But the public vaccinator was not the only target of vampiric accusations. Anti-vaccinators combined both the medical and the political meanings of the vampire that circulated in popular and political culture to attack a range of state officials who, they claimed, were motivated by a corrupt lust for blood and for money. Anti-vaccinators accused the government of being a "State vampire." They inverted the notion that parasites such as paupers preyed on the state and proposed instead that the state fed off its citizens. Similarly, anti-vaccinators accused vaccination officials of "thirsting for blood." Vaccination officers, maintained Mary Hume-Rothery, were "parasites of tyranny . . . taught to live as blood-suckers upon the oppression of their fellows."[127] Anti-vaccinators regularly denounced the spies and informants who forced noncompliers to bribe them as "vampire[s]" who must be silenced, although the victim risked being "bled again and again."[128] Vaccination officials were literally vampiric, anti-vaccination propaganda suggested, as they pierced the skin and drew blood. They were also economically vampiric as parasites who profited from what vaccination's opponents considered a corrupt compulsory system that taxed the people to pay a legion of officials out of the public rates. In sum, the "Vaccination Vampire" represented a host of demonic state agents who literally and symbolically bled the people dry.[129] In using the vampire as a metaphor for vaccination, anti-vaccinators critiqued the marriage of old and new forms of corruption that state medicine in general, and public vaccination in particular, had come to represent.

By the time Dracula, the most famous vampire of all, made his entrance, anti-vaccination propaganda had already heavily exploited the symbolic value of the vampire. *Dracula* appeared in 1897 just after the Royal Commission on Vaccination had reached its conclusions and at a high point in the anti-vaccination campaign. Stoker's vampire was not a metaphor for vaccination (although Stoker himself was surely aware of this relationship),[130] and anti-vaccinators never referred directly to the novel. However, *Dracula* perpetuated many of the anti-vaccination campaign's anxieties. It cemented the relationship between the vampire and the vaccinator in horrific ways by consolidating the affinities among bodily violation, blood, degeneration, sexual pollution, and miscegenation.[131] Stoker's novel, David Punter argues, demands to know: "[T]o what extent can one be 'infected' and still remain British?"[132]

If *Dracula*'s meanings supported the anti-vaccination campaign's metaphorical use of the vampire, it also elaborated these associations. Stoker's novel, in its concern with multivalent, dangerous, penetrative sexualities, explicitly eroticized bodily violation in ways at which the anti-vaccination campaign only hinted. It also extended the racialization of fin de siècle fears of degeneration and blood pollution in important ways by preying on anxieties about Jewish immigration.[133] Although the "Vaccination Vampire" was not an anti-Semitic apparition, anti-vaccinationism did express a profound fear of pollution from contaminated Others. Thus, while *Dracula* contributed to and enriched fears around the permeability and transformability of the body, its popular success was nevertheless due in part to its mobilization of a shared cultural symbolism already articulated by anti-vaccination propaganda.

THE INFANT VIVISECTOR   If anti-vaccinators capitalized on the Victorian vampire's symbolic purchase, they also expressed the uneasy relationship between the doctor-scientist and his often working-class patient through that other Victorian gothic figure: the vivisector. Like the vampire, the vivisector had by the Victorian period come to be "indelibly associated" in the popular mind "above all, with blood."[134] In the last decades of the nineteenth century, anti-vivisection propaganda shaped an image of the vivisector—a physician or scientist who experimented on live animals—as a cross between a mad scientist, a butcher, and a mass murderer. It deployed a religious language of shedding light on "dark practices" that was also a gothic language of dark deeds, arcane practices, and monstrous attacks on the body. Physiology, proclaimed the animal-rights campaigner Louise Lind af Hageby, is a "bird of prey" that carries "the mutilated bodies" of weak creatures in its "murderous fangs"—rhetoric reminiscent of Wilkinson's critique of compulsory vaccination as a ravenous raven.[135]

The anti-vaccination and anti-vivisection movements, as I have noted, were intimately related. They shared personnel, an interest in vegetarianism, and a concern for animals used in the production of vaccine.[136] Vaccine matter was harvested from calves, which members of both movements claimed were treated in an abominable manner. "The luckless calves," the *Vaccination Inquirer* maintained in 1895, "must no longer be strapped and fixed and shaved and scarified and poisoned, and fastened in their stalls with fourscore aging sores on their bellies, and their tails tied over their backs, lest in seeking allevia-tion of their miseries for themselves they rupture their vesicles and ruin the stock-in-trade of the virus-mongers."[137] Since vaccination and vivi-section were "twin monsters," the anti-vaccination movement is a "nec-essary part" of the anti-vivisection movement, a member of both cam-paigns claimed.[138] These two agitations shared a rhetoric that both reflected and perpetuated anxieties about bodily violation, anatomiza-tion, and human experimentation well into the twentieth century.

Anti-vaccinators and anti-vivisectionists decried the violence of medi-cal science in general. Vivisection, its opponents claimed, was merely the butchering of helpless animals in the name of medical progress. Frances Power Cobbe, founder of the British Union for the Abolition of Vivisection, proclaimed that vivisection was no less than the "cutting up alive, the flaying, starving, baking, boiling, stewing alive" of sensitive creatures.[139] Anti-vaccinators deployed a similar language of savagery and violation. Because the instrument used for vaccination was a type of lancet (a surgical tool), the technique of vaccination provoked anti-vaccinators to condemn doctors as butchers who "cut and puncture with knives and lancets, till the blood gushes out."[140] They regularly denounced scientific medicine's "cuttings, stabbings, rippings, slash-ings, vivisections, roughnesses, [and] brutality" and rejected the notion that these "druggings . . . cuttings and maimings" could be for the public good.[141]

If animals could be exposed to these trials, anti-vivisectionists feared that it would not be long before "our idiots, lunatics, [and] babes" were subjected to the same treatment.[142] Campaigners against vaccination argued that science, in its zeal for slicing and dicing, had already pro-gressed from animals to babies. They attacked public vaccinators as "Baby Cutters," "baby-slashers," "baby-sticker[s]," and "butchers" guilty of "puncturing babies." Anti-vaccinators drew explicit parallels between vaccination and vivisection. These "cutters and carvers" were also "blood poisoners and vivisectors," declared Mary Hume-Rothery. Vaccination, agitators insisted, was actually "vivisection of the arm."[143]

As I argued in chapter 1, these anxieties over the violation and pen-etration of the flesh were part of (often working-class) fears of heroic medicine evident from at least the 1850s and perpetuated well into the twentieth century. The English working class was in general highly suspicious of medical technologies and regarded not only vaccination but also thermometers, surgery, and hospitalization as "unnatural and dangerous assaults on bodily integrity."[144] Vaccination, agitators insisted, was merely a new form of medical torture, similar to vivisection. In a vision of vivisection, Anna Kingsford, a vegetarian, anti-vivisectionist, and Christian esotericist, described her dream about an underground vivisector's laboratory as a "torture-chamber" where men were hard at work "lacerating, dissecting and burning the living flesh of their victims," both animal and human.[145] Anti-vaccinators concurred. "Some of the vaccinators use real instruments of torture," argued a Cheltenham doctor. "Ivory points are driven into the flesh, and wounds ensue." Lancets, anti-vaccinators claimed, are "bodily weapons" that "lacerate the skin" and cut holes into the flesh of a "little healthy babe's arm."[146] A cabman prosecuted for non-vaccination in 1865 defied the law precisely because he would not allow his child to be "tormented by a lancet."[147] An 1884 LSACV pamphlet characterized compulsory vaccination as a "system of tyranny and torture" comparable to the "Inquisition."[148] Opponents considered vaccination particularly pernicious because the torture was enacted on the bodies of "helpless" children. In 1886, Tebb had tried unsuccessfully to attract the interest of the Society for the Prevention of Cruelty to Children, claiming that it was neglecting the "cruelties of vaccinators."[149]

The rhetoric of the "baby-slasher" envisioned vaccinal vivisection as butchery and torture. Anti-vaccination literature also linked the vivisector—and hence, the vaccinator—to the emerging cultural figure of the mass murderer. Anti-vaccinators regularly denounced vaccination as "child-murder." The vaccination station, argued the *Anti-Vaccinator and Public Health Journal*, was a "Murder shop." In a torchlight procession that paraded through the streets of Bath during February 1888, an anti-vaccinator carried a banner bearing a cartoon of a "man (presumably a doctor) standing over the body of a child, a knife in his hand, and surrounded by the dead bodies of several little children." Just a few months later, Jack the Ripper took London by storm, leaving in his wake the mutilated bodies of the prostitutes he had murdered. In the heat of the investigation, Frances Power Cobbe suggested that the Ripper might very well be a "physiologist delirious with cruelty."[150] This cartoon also appeared three years after the Maiden Tribute scandal, which advertised that the virginity of a young girl could be purchased for a mere 5 pounds by lust-driven "minotaurs." The image of the minotaur was also employed by anti-vaccinators who warned that vaccination's "giant paws" entrapped the "innocent child-life" of the country.[151] Feminists regularly linked medical and sexual violation; thus, in this context, the banner's image suggested the vaccinator's almost pornographic delight in the slaughter of young children. At is most extreme, anti-vaccination propaganda depicted vaccination as a "diabolical rape" or as "Murder and Mutilation"—sensationalist and lurid discourses also to be taken up in the accounts of the Whitechapel murders.[152]

It was not merely that the vivisector violated and mutilated the body physically, and possibly sexually. He also threatened to turn those most helpless into experimental fodder. The vivisector represented a type of "mad doctor," an archetype that had long circulated in Victorian culture. H. G. Wells's 1896 novel *The Island of Doctor Moreau* consolidated an image of the vivisector as a Faustian mad scientist driven by a lust for experimental material.[153] In the novel, Moreau, exiled from Britain after a vivisection scandal, vivisects the animals on his island to transform them into humans. The result is the construction of a race of monstrous beast men, one of whom is the agent of Moreau's own demise. Wells made the links between the vivisector and the vaccinator patent. In explaining his experiments to the protagonist and narrator, Moreau maintains that he can transform not only the outward form of an animal but also its physiology. The "chemical rhythm of the creature," he proposes, can also be made to undergo a modification, "of which vaccination and other methods of inoculation with living or dead matter are examples that will, no doubt, be familiar to you." A similar operation, Moreau suggests, "is the transfusion of the blood."[154] Wells thus perpetuated and reinforced a perceived relationship among blood tampering, vaccination, and vivisection.

Like Moreau's exotic hybrids and the dogs, horses, and other "non-human[s]" that animal-rights campaigners struggled to save from "murderous experimentation,"[155] anti-vaccinators regularly insisted that their children had become unwilling subjects in a medical experiment. They looked forward to the day when, in the words of Tebb, "the pretended duty of experimenting upon our neighbour's children will cease to supersede the real duty of protecting our own."[156] Anti-vaccinators objected to the manner in which the laboring classes were used to train vaccinators. "We cannot see," argued the *Eclectic Journal and Medical Free Press* in 1869, "why the young pupils of surgeons should be allowed to go from house to house trying, as we have heard them say, 'experiments on the poor.'"[157] At the turn of the century, they also attacked the state for using "the children of the working classes" as guinea pigs to test new vaccines. Is it justifiable, argued the *Vaccination Inquirer* in 1900, to enforce the use of glycerinated lymph, a new form of purified vaccine matter, "by way of experiment upon the children of the poor?"[158] S. Monckton Copeman, a bacteriologist and medical inspector to the Local Government Board, was vilified in 1902 for performing vaccine trials on unwitting infants: "Dr. Copeman says 'every batch of lymph should be tried on children before being distributed, as effects on the calf were not an infallible criterion.' That is to say, some child is to serve as the *corpus vile* for testing some new pox on before it can be regarded as safe for general circulation. We should like to know whether the parents of this 'experimental child' are to be warned of the empirical and vicarious purpose their infant is to subserve for the good repute of the National Vaccine Establishment."[159] It was outrageous to assume that any child, whatever his or her social class, could be used as experimental material, the *Vaccination Inquirer* opined. In 1904, the *Vaccination Inquirer* attacked Copeman again for performing "gruesome and audacious experiments" on children using "corpse lymph"— smallpox crusts cultivated from dead bodies.[160]

In an 1884 letter to the *Preston Chronicle*, Mr. Cunningham (whose rotting foot we met earlier) drew explicit connections between the vaccinated and the vivisected. Cunningham complained about his treatment after suffering numerous injuries following vaccination. After consulting a number of doctors he was admitted to the Manchester Infirmary. There they "not only took my portrait," he stated, "but they seated me in a chair upon the dissecting table, while references were made to my particular case, and examinations made by those who were present."[161] What Cunningham objected to was his positioning as an object of scientific study. Not only was he examined by all and sundry, but he was displayed on the dissecting table as if he were already dead, an anatomized or autopsied corpse, or about to be vivisected like an anaesthetized dog.

This fear of becoming merely experimental material dates back at least to the early eighteenth century and is particularly evident in a variety of anti-medical literature from the 1830s through the early twentieth century.[162] As early as 1833, John Morison, purveyor of Morison's vegetable universal medicines, insisted that there had been no end to doctors' "fruitless tortures, trials, and experiments on the human body."[163] In 1854, Wilkinson maintained that "poor people" avoided hospitals precisely because they felt that "within those walls" they were held captive by doctors who "may try experiments with them."[164] A medical student at the London Hospital in Whitechapel in the 1880s recalled that "quack doctors" often attempted to cash in on the "popular horror" of the hospital: "Don't go in there," they would shout to the patients, "they'll cut you up alive."[165] In 1903, the Personal Rights Association denounced legislation for the compulsory notification of infectious disease, maintaining that once within the hospital, the "medical inquisitor" might "choose to make experiment *in corpore vili.*"[166] In her 1928 memoir, Kathleen Woodward underscored these anxieties. She remembered that as a child of the Victorian slums, she believed, "for it was repeatedly said, that the hospital existed to 'do things with knives.' "[167] Thus, the Battersea Anti-Vivisection Hospital explicitly advertised not only that it refused to employ vivisectors, but that it conducted no experiments on its patients.[168]

While anti-vivisectionists proved important allies, anti-vaccinators often undermined animal-rights campaigns to enhance their own position. Anti-vaccinators were quick to note a primary difference between the two campaigns: the lives and bodies that anti-vaccinators defended were "helpless human children," not "dumb animals." Even the worst "monstrosities" of vivisection, the *National Anti-Compulsory Vaccination Reporter* argued, could not compare to the "anguish and suffering" inflicted on babies by "Infant Vivisectors." We have often wondered, it claimed in 1883, "why no society for the Prevention of Cruelty to Infants should exist" while that for the protection of cruelty to animals was so active.[169] In the last years of the campaign, anti-vaccinators attacked anti-vivisectionists who appeared to attract more funding than themselves. One would have thought, declared Charles Gane, honorary secretary of the NAVL, that "to save children from the tortures of vaccination was, in its way, more laudable than to save animals from the pains of vivisection." He continued: "I presume [that] the reason is that the wealthy classes are much more closely concerned with the welfare of their horses, dogs, and cats, and vivisection is brought more closely home to them. Thus they contribute large sums of money to protect their pets from torture. The Anti-Vaccination movement, on the other hand, is mostly concerned with the poor." Anti-vaccinators resented legislation passed in regard to cruelty against animals while compulsory vaccination was stringently enforced. "Infants will soon be the only creatures not protected by law against vivisectional cruelties," lamented the *Vaccination Inquirer* in 1894.[170]

By drawing explicit connections between the vaccination of children and the vivisection of animals, anti-vaccinators capitalized on and contributed to an already pervasive discourse of scientific cruelty. While they supported their animal-rights allies, anti-vaccinators also manipulated the discourse of suffering creatures to underscore vaccination atrocities, which they considered more tyrannical precisely because the victims were human children. The vivisector functioned as a horrific figure that, like the vampire, inspired dread among many Victorian parents who sought to protect their children from the murderous and mutilating lancet. These gothic discourses were not only an emotive language. They pointedly reveal widespread anxieties over the transgression of a number of boundaries that compromised anti-vaccinators' spiritual and physical health, their morality and sexuality, their racial identity, and even their humanity. As David Glover has argued, in *Dracula*, as in Victorian culture at large, "it is matter out of place that matters, the contamination and dissolution of the pure and sacred that counts, the transgression of boundaries and borders that is the ultimate horror."[171] As we shall see in the next chapter, these boundaries and borders not only applied to the individual's body, which vaccination made all the more vulnerable, but also to the social body, which was constantly threatened by contaminating forces.

6

Germs, Dirt, and the Constitution

Oh! sweet and precious is the thought

Foul germs to find wherever sought!

Fresh fields for ever bless our view

Of cultured filth, and *Pasteur*'s new!

—"Civis Brittanicus," 1882[1]

☞ Vaccination posed a problem for the integrity of the individual body and the purity of the blood. But as a preventive strategy for a contagious disease, it was also part of a larger debate regarding the health of the social body. Proponents of vaccination and its detractors relied on a language of contagion drawn from a number of medical theories that by the 1880s included the germ theory of disease. Nineteenth- and early-twentieth-century theories of disease transmission, however, were adaptable and could be shaped to accommodate a variety of social, political, and medical exigencies. Thus, although bacteriology provided pro-vaccinators with a widely agreed on scientific theory to bolster their empirical claims, it did not entirely reconfigure the terms of the debate. In fact, germ theory also furnished anti-vaccinators with a new, authoritative medical language to articulate what they continued to identify as smallpox's material and social cause: dirty environments and compromised constitutions.

There was little doubt throughout the second half of the nineteenth century that smallpox was contagious, that it could be passed from person to person or through contact with infected items such as money, clothing, letters, or books. But exactly what *contagious* meant was never self-evident. In the early Victorian period, in particular, medical discourse focused on the "predisposing" and "exciting" causes of disease. Predisposing causes related to the general state of the victim's constitution. Exciting causes were specific events, often environmentally driven, that set a disease off. Predisposing causes were not limited to hereditary conditions, however; they were also thought to be the result of environmental influence. Thus, "vitiated air" and overwork—because of their long-term effects on the human constitution—could also be understood as predisposing causes that, in a popular Lamarckian model of evolution, could then be passed down to future generations.[2]

In 1871, Henry Pitman emphasized the relationship between constitution and environment. The "constitutionally strong, who live in a pure atmosphere" suffered little smallpox, he argued.[3] A decade later, William Tebb continued to deploy this model of disease causation. Smallpox is found, he maintained, "amongst the poor, ill-fed, uncleanly, intemperate, over-worked populations of Hackney, St. Giles's, Bethnal-green, Poplar, Shadwell, Bermondsey, and Southwark, amongst those who live in the courts and alleys, in old and decayed habitations, and in the miasmatic atmosphere in which the neglected residuum of this immense city are reduced to dwell."[4] Smallpox was caused both by "ill-fed," "overworked," and thus depleted constitutions (the predisposing cause), he maintained, and by the "decayed" and "miasmatic atmosphere" of certain poverty-stricken urban sectors (the exciting cause). Those who fell victim to the disease were both constitutionally weak due to poor nourishment, lack of hygiene, drunkenness, and overwork, and constantly exposed to dirty environments whose effluvia could themselves spark disease. Whether one caught smallpox was thus entirely dependent on the relationship between the state of one's constitutional predisposition and the presence of the disease, understood in this case as the miasmatic product of rotting matter.

With the development of various germ theories in the 1870s, the mechanisms and meanings of contagious disease were changing as new theories built on these established understandings of disease processes. The vaccination debate provides an important context for mapping the shifts and continuities in these disease theories. But the debate over the mechanism of smallpox contagion was also intimately bound up with larger social questions. While engaging with medical theory, anti-vaccinators consistently tried to shift the debate over disease causation from a strictly scientific framework to a discussion of underlying social problems, which they believed were being left behind in the wake of bacteriological advances.

The Problem of Dirt

The passage of the first Compulsory Vaccination Act in the 1850s was premised on a widespread understanding of smallpox as an infectious disease that generally originated with the poor who then spread it to their social betters. The nidus of smallpox in Charles Dickens's *Bleak House* (serialized 1852–53) was Tom-All-Alone's, a slum home to "a villainous street, undrained, unventilated, deep in black mud and corrupt water . . . and reeking with . . . smells." From these streets that propelled one "every moment deeper down, into the infernal gulf" the disease spread quickly from the "corrupted blood" of the poor to work "its retribution, through every order of society, up to the proudest of the proud, and to the highest of the high."[5] The morbid products of unhealthy blood circulated not only through the individual body, Dickens suggested, but also through the social body, oblivious to class distinctions.

Dickens's portrayal of smallpox and its mode of infection reveals how complex understandings of contagion were at midcentury. The depiction of Tom-All-Alone's as a contaminated, ill-ventilated, and marshy environment which propagated disease was firmly rooted in a miasmatic interpretation of smallpox etiology. Miasmatic theory proposed that disease was caused by nonspecific gaseous material given off by decomposing organic matter.[6] Bad smells could indicate the presence of disease; hence, the importance of proper ventilation. Miasmatic theory proved a dramatic language in which to evoke the dangers of dirt and fumes. In *Bleak House*, however, the protagonist Esther Summerson contracts smallpox not through a wafting miasma but, rather, through social contact with her maid Charley, who has carried the disease with her from the pestilential slum after nursing a dying child. This zymotic theory, popular from midcentury, held that disease was caused by the introduction of specific animal poisons into the bloodstream. Zymotic diseases were those conditions characterized by a spreading internal rot that derived from an external rot and could be communicated to others.[7] Zymotic diseases were specifically those diseases passed from person to person. However, the terms *zymotic* and *miasmatic* were often employed interchangeably in both popular and professional circles through the 1860s. They were both used to signify diseases caused by dirt, for zymes were not disease entities but catalysts that in the right environmental conditions could spark disease processes.[8] Smallpox, Mary Hume-Rothery argued, "like other zymotic disease, is eminently a filth-disease."[9] Through the 1860s, then, contagious diseases were not necessarily distinguished from those with environmental origins. Smallpox, though transmissible from person to person, it was widely believed, could in the right environment spontaneously generate.

The miasmatic and zymotic theories thus linked dirt and disease. This explanation for smallpox appealed to anti-vaccinators who stressed the urban nature of the disease and its roots in filthy environments. When he analyzed the victims of the 1870–72 epidemic, John Pickering, editor of the *Anti-Vaccinator and Public Health Journal*, found them among "the very lowest classes of society." They were "children that were filthy, neglected, and ill fed, others living in houses that were overcrowded, destitute of proper ventilation, and in courts and alleys where sanitation is a term unknown."[10] Indeed, pro- and anti-vaccinators alike feared that contagious diseases emanated from the poorest sectors of urban centers. "The slums," argued J. J. Garth Wilkinson, "are the causes of Small-pox." A correspondent to the *Vaccination Inquirer* echoed this sentiment, maintaining that he had never heard of an outbreak of smallpox having its rise in the fashionable haunts of "Belgravia or South Kensington"; rather, it invariably breaks out in the "dirty parts of the metropolis."[11]

Dirt for anti-vaccinators was inseparable from poverty. "Bad air, foul water, bad food, bodily fatigue, exposure, anxiety, [and] sorrow"—in short, the emotional and physical strains of poverty—argued "Medicus," generally predispose the body to contagious disease.[12] Thus it was not the poor per se, anti-vaccinators suggested, but the squalid conditions in which they were forced to live that were to blame for smallpox. The poor, argued Wilkinson in 1881, were "the rotten sheep of health." Reworking the biblical reference to the sorting of individuals on Judgment Day, Wilkinson insisted that smallpox deaths should not be sorted into vaccinated and unvaccinated; instead, they should be classified by levels of poverty. A thousand other factors "which cannot be causal would, as *sorters*, produce the same effect as non-vaccination," he continued. "Thus, the people who wear best black and employ fashionable tailors, die of small-pox at a vastly less rate than those who wear fustian; and these again, than those who are in rags. The drinkers of the best port die less in the case than the drinkers of the cheapest beer."[13] The poor contracted smallpox at a much higher rate, he reasoned, because their poverty both forced them into polluted environments that harbored disease and perpetuated the conditions that made them vulnerable in the first place.

Although, as we shall see, an exclusively environmental explanation for smallpox emphasizing spontaneous generation had fallen out of favor in medical circles by the 1880s, throughout the nineteenth and early twentieth centuries anti-vaccinators continued to identify contagious disease in general, and smallpox in particular, as primarily a problem of dirt. "Small-pox," argued Walter Hadwen in 1894, "is essentially a dirt disease. Get rid of the dirt, and you get rid of the disease."[14] Vaccination could not address the issue of dirt, its opponents argued, for even if it succeeded in reducing smallpox mortality, the perpetuation of insanitary conditions would merely give rise to other contagious diseases whose root cause was poverty.[15]

Anti-vaccinators emphasized that only sanitary measures could prevent the spread of contagious diseases. Since the physician's job is to cure disease already manifest, argued William Young, it was not to medicine, "which can prevent nothing," that one should turn but to "civil engineers, sanitary inspectors, and an efficient staff of scavengers." Vaccination, claimed W. J. Collins, a medical doctor and Progressive MP for St. Pancras, was "inoperative in the absence of sanitation and superfluous in its presence." Indeed, anti-vaccinators regularly pitted sanitation against vaccination as two separate schools of thought. "Sanitation *not* Vaccination," advertised a banner at the 1885 Leicester Demonstration. Vaccination was opposed to sanitation, the *Vaccination Inquirer* proposed, because it distracts one from "the higher and truer cult of cleanliness." More significantly, vaccination conflicted with the principles of sanitation as it makes "a treaty with the powers of dirt" and attempts to domesticate rather then eradicate it. How can one "combat dirt with dirt?" anti-vaccinators demanded.[16]

Some historians have cast anti-vaccinators' consistent and continued focus on dirty environments and thus sanitary solutions to smallpox as a preoccupation with an increasingly outdated Chadwickian "sanitary idea," and have thus dismissed their preventive strategies as "anti-scientific."[17] While their attention to dirt shared with the sanitarianism of the early nineteenth century a focus on nonmedical approaches to public health, anti-vaccinators were far from disciples of Chadwick. Anti-vaccinators lobbied for a continuous supply of pure water, an effective system of drainage, the prevention of overcrowding, the erection of well-ventilated urban housing, and the creation of more public baths, parks, and open spaces—demands that far exceeded the water and sewers that characterized Chadwick's public-health scheme.

Indeed, for anti-vaccinators public health was highly politicized. "We need pure air, pure food, pure blood; equity, equality, and the opportunity to be healthy," insisted a correspondent to the *East London Observer* in 1907.[18] "Society can only escape from disease by removing the causes," argued Joseph Collinson, a member of the Humanitarian League, the "drunkenness, impurity, slums, dirt, [and] injustice that makes men work for starvation wages."[19] Rather than embracing Chadwick's program, then, anti-vaccinators attacked these government public-health schemes for failing to address the larger problems of industrialization and urbanization, such as low wages and inadequate food, that preoccupied anti-vaccinators in particular, and the working class more generally.[20]

Roy MacLeod has nevertheless argued that the vaccination debate "crystallised" the argument between germ theorists and sanitary reformers, who, MacLeod implies, eventually lost out. In the same vein, Dorothy Porter and Roy Porter maintain that from the 1890s, preventive medicine grasped the "bacteriological baton," leaving "the 'dirt' theories of the Chadwickian era behind."[21] These historians position the rise of the bacteriological germ theory of disease as a watershed that marked the advent of a new and thoroughly modern medicine. However, recent studies have challenged this assumption by focusing on the local contexts and "communities of discourse" that informed debates over germ theory.[22] Germ theory did provide pro-vaccinators with a scientific explanation for the success of vaccination and, in hindsight, laid the foundation for the immunological "body system" that was to play a dominant role in twentieth-century medicine.[23] But it also furnished anti-vaccinators with a new medical language to conceptualize and articulate the problem of dirt. For as Michael Worboys has recently argued, nineteenth-century germ theories were "additive and adaptive" in that they built on and reworked older concepts of contagious disease to suit a new language and new ideas. The rise of germ theory should not be seen as "a series of conflicts between competing, incommensurable paradigms," he insists.[24] Rather than clarifying divisions between dirt theories and germ theory, the vaccination debate provided a contentious context for negotiations over the meanings and implications of germs at a time when dirt remained an important, culturally loaded, and not yet "anti-scientific" category.

Germ Theory and the Vaccination Question

From the late 1860s through the 1870s, the idea that diseases were caused by nonspecific microscopic living organisms present in the air— or panspermism—began to challenge the predominant miasmatic or zymotic theory. What was significant about panspermism was that it theorized that diseases did not spontaneously generate but were "ancestral," that they always had roots in other living disease entities and thus could not emerge *de novo* merely from environmental conditions. This theory was widely debated and heavily criticized by sanitary reformers such as Florence Nightingale, who in 1869 proclaimed this "Disease Germ-Fetish" to be merely a "superstition." Disease was not caused by separate entities that existed independently, as did cats and dogs, she asserted; diseases were conditions. Smallpox could grow independently in a closed room or overcrowded ward, without being imported by any outside source. Indeed, a disease could grow and "pass into" another. "Now, dogs do not pass into cats," Nightingale argued; thus, diseases could not possibly be discrete organisms.[25] A handful of anti-vaccinators concurred with Nightingale. They considered germ theory "too absurd for serious criticism."[26] William Hume-Rothery dismissed germs as mere "chimeras," for, he proclaimed, disease is a "condition," not "an organised and living entity." If this panspermism were true, he argued, "these germs would eat up the human race, as maggots eat up a dead rat."[27]

While the Hume-Rotherys consistently attacked the germ theories of disease that were being formulated and debated in the 1870s and '80s, pro-vaccinationists and anti-vaccinationists cannot be neatly categorized into those who espoused germ theory, on the one hand, and those who rejected it, on the other, as some historians have implied.[28] Middle-class campaigners in particular, some of whom were doctors and scientists themselves, kept abreast of the developments in medical research and participated in scientific debates over the meanings of germ theories at a moment that saw considerable discussion of their implications. Many, if not most, anti-vaccinators incorporated the discourse of germs into their own understandings of disease transmission. This did not mean that they abandoned other scientific explanations for the spread of disease. Rather, anti-vaccinators manipulated new and older disease theories to fit their agenda. Some of these anti-vaccinationists were in fact well-regarded medical professionals, among them the bacteriologist Edgar Crookshank, who favored isolation over vaccination, and Charles Creighton, renowned for his work on the history of epidemics who was converted to the anti-vaccinationist position in 1888 while writing the *Encyclopedia Britannica* entry for "Vaccination."[29] They were dismissed by their medical colleagues as cranks, not because they lacked the appropriate credentials, but because they refused to endorse the scientific community's pro-vaccinationist position and thus, in general, to further medicine's sole authority to deal with the problems of contagious disease.[30]

The discourse around early germ theories focused on the presence of contagions in the air and thus could be interpreted by both professional and lay communities as a renewed call for sanitation as germs and filth became interchangeable concepts. Indeed, panspermists from Joseph Lister on stressed the importance of a clean environment. Alfred Carpenter, the medical officer of health for Croydon, used germ theory to support sanitarianism in the 1870s. A member of the Royal College of Surgeons insisted in the 1880s that insanitary conditions "predispose strongly to epidemics of variola by providing a germ-laden atmosphere." The idea that dirty environments nurtured the growth of germs was in fact perpetuated by some medical professionals into the twentieth century. A pro-vaccinationist Torquay physician proposed in 1901 that "[p]athogenic or disease-producing germs" are harmless when subjected to "sunlight and fresh air"; they become virulent only under favorable conditions in which to breed: bad ventilation, darkness, and filth.[31] The *Journal of State Medicine*, the official publication of the Royal Institute of Health, reported in 1900 on the environmental conditions that offered a breeding ground for "microorganic contagions."[32] Germ theory, then, in its initial formulation and for many decades hence emphasized the relationship between disease organisms and their environmental conditions. This understanding of the nature of contagion allowed anti-vaccinators to use the discourse of germs while remaining committed both to environmental and to constitutional explanations for disease, even in the age of bacteriology.

BACTERIOMANIA   Through the 1870s, doctors, scientists, and government administrators regularly correlated the steady decline of smallpox over the course of the century with the rise of widespread vaccination. In addition, they proclaimed that empirical and anecdotal evidence proved that the vaccinated rarely contracted smallpox, and those who did had a much lower mortality rate than the unvaccinated.[33] However, pro-vaccinators offered no widely agreed on theory for how or why this was the case. Indeed, while vaccination has come to represent the triumph of germ theory, it predates it by almost a century and as a practice was based entirely on empirical evidence rather than on scientific theory or controlled experimental practices. Because no verifiable explanation for its success could be found, it appeared, charged an anti-vaccinator in 1876, that vaccination worked by "some mysterious cause."[34]

In the 1880s, however, in response to new developments in bacteriological research and to the challenges presented by anti-vaccinators, pro-vaccinators began to advance microbiological explanations for the functioning of vaccination. The bacterial theories of the 1880s, unlike the panspermism of the previous decade, theorized germs as organisms that were specific to certain diseases. Thus, tuberculosis could be contracted only through the absorption of the specific *Tubercle bacillus* into the body, and not merely from exposure to generalized disease germs present in impure air. The implication of bacteriology was that inclusive approaches to disease prevention, such as sanitation, were ineffective and inefficient. Instead, preventive medicine should focus on identifying specific germs, containing their spread, and, when possible, inoculating against them.

The rise of laboratory science across western Europe in the late nineteenth century led to the isolation of anthrax in 1876, typhoid in 1880, tuberculosis in 1882, and a string of other agents soon after.[35] This fueled the search for the micro-organisms specific to dangerous contagious diseases and, significantly, led to the identification of a number of bacteria that would later be debunked.[36] These developments within scientific medicine were rapidly absorbed into popular culture. By the 1880s, germs were everywhere. In 1884, the *New York Times* sarcastically observed that "every few months" Louis Pasteur announces "the discovery of a new germ." There were microbes of sport responsible for "the sporting mania," satirized the *Daily News*, and microbes of old age that were the direct cause of growing old.[37] Patent-medicine dealers exploited "bacteriomania," appropriating the microbe to sell a range of products. In the 1890s, Leo's Microbe Pills advertised that they could promptly eradicate "Bacteria" from the human system. These pills combated the "Microbes of Rheumatism, Gout, Lumbago, Consumption, Nervous Debility, Indigestion, Bronchitis" and countless other disorders, including "piles" and "sciatica." Radam's Microbe Killer, a cure-all patent medicine, also capitalized on the currency of germ theory. William Radam invited his customers to his offices on Oxford Street to see "Micro-Photos" of the microbes of "Cancer, Consumption, Cholera, La Grippe, Diphtheria, Malignant Oedema," and others.[38]

Pro-vaccinationists were quick to jump on the bacteriological bandwagon. Theorizing that smallpox and cowpox were little different from typhoid or tuberculosis, they began to search, unsuccessfully, for what they termed the bacillus, virus, or specific germ of the disease. Finding the germ was not crucial to diagnosing, treating, or preventing smallpox; indeed, all of these had been possible for 100 years. In fact, throughout this period bacteriology actually did little to advance scientific knowledge of smallpox. Pro-vaccinationists turned to bacteriology more for political than for medical reasons. They used the growing authority of germ theory to strengthen their argument for the power and necessity of vaccination at a time that saw a general decline in smallpox morbidity. This strategy mirrored that of medical and public-health practitioners in general who seized on a single germ theory of disease as a means of advancing their own professional authority, even though multiple and sometimes conflicting germ theories remained constantly in play.[39]

Anti-vaccinators understood the professional stakes involved in the promotion of bacteriology and critiqued this popular fascination with microbes as a fad engineered by medical practitioners to keep the public in their thrall. "This *infection-scare* is a SHAM," complained Mary Hume-Rothery, "fostered, if not got up originally, by doctors, as a means of raising their own importance and tightening their grasp on the throat of the nation's common sense which has lain so long paralysed and inert in their clutches."[40] Germs were not just the latest harmless enthusiasm, remarked some anti-vaccinators: "[T]his miserable craze of microbe-mongering" was creating widespread hysteria over infectious disease.[41] While anti-vaccinators participated in a sensationalist scare campaign of their own, as chapter 5 noted, they accused their opponents of fear-mongering to encourage the practice of vaccination and to ensure that only scientific medicine could control disease prevention. In 1885, Thomas Baker, a lawyer and ardent vegetarian and anti-vaccinationist, maintained that medical officers of health were being paid by the government to keep "the people in a perpetual state of disease panic; frightening the entire community over 'contagious germs.'" Twenty years later, the complaint was the same: "We are being frightened to death by microbes. It is germs, germs, germs everywhere," lamented Walter Hadwen. Must one give up shaking hands, kissing, eating, and drinking? With all the germs ever-present, he smirked, "it is a wonder that any of us are alive at all."[42]

Anti-vaccinators consistently challenged the practices and theories of the new germ theory. Some resisted bacteriology because of its associations with animal experimentation. As we have seen, many anti-vaccinators opposed what they considered the inhumane practices of vivisection. Since the emerging science of bacteriology was based largely on animal trials, anti-vaccinators regularly linked germ theory to vivisection. But more often they stressed the fact that, despite new advances in bacteriology, no one was yet able to identify or to cultivate the germ of variola (smallpox) or vaccinia (cowpox). Throughout the 1880s, a number of different scientists claimed to have isolated "cocci" and "microbes" within vaccine lymph, but the leading British microbiologists S. Monckton Copeman and E. E. Klein dismissed these claims. In 1900, the *Transactions and Annual Report of the Manchester Microscopical Society* maintained that "although bacteria are invariably present in vaccine lymph, and a large number of different micro-organisms have been identified no specific bacillus peculiar to vaccinia or variola has yet been positively discovered." *Public Health*, the journal of the society of medical officers of health, confirmed this observation the following year.[43] Thus, anti-vaccinators rejected the government's claims that medical science could make vaccine matter safer.

Because the disease-causing agent itself could not be identified, anti-vaccinators dismissed outright attempts to purify lymph with glycerine to destroy any other organisms that could be transmitted along with the vaccine. In 1891, Copeman, the newly appointed medical inspector to the Local Government Board, declared that the glycerination of lymph removed any "extraneous" organisms that might interfere with the action of the "essential" organism of vaccination.[44] Largely on Copeman's recommendation, the glycerination of lymph became mandatory under the 1898 Vaccination Act, when the government switched from arm-to-arm methods to the use of preserved calf lymph. Fear that syphilis and other diseases could be passed through lymph during vaccination, as I argued in chapter 5, had provoked considerable resistance to the procedure. The government thus endeavored to curb agitation by removing this threat. By using vaccine matter produced, purified, and distributed by the National Vaccine Establishment, public vaccinators could ensure the quality of the lymph and reduce the possibility of transmitting diseases from one child to the next. However, anti-vaccinators deeply resented the state's reversal of its position on contaminated lymph. The introduction of so-called pure lymph suggested what the government had consistently denied: that many thousands of children had already been contaminated by a substandard product. They argued that despite government reassurances, this "pure lymph business" was in fact an "impossibility," for if the microbe for either cowpox or smallpox could not be identified, how could glycerine "preserve and separate" it? Glycerine, a correspondent to the *Personal Rights Journal* main-

tained, cannot possibly possess the "weird power of selecting and kill-
ing all noxious germs, while sparing and fostering all others."[45]

Other anti-vaccinators claimed that the fact that the specific bacteria
could not be found proved that it did not exist. In 1891, the *Vaccination
Inquirer* maintained not that microbes did not exist, but that vaccine
matter is a "non-specific thing" related to all microbes and thus having
no specific protections against any of them. In an article titled, "The
Microbe Craze," Tebb maintained that the "same microbe" was found
in puerperal fever, diphtheria, foot-and-mouth disease, and scarlet fever
and in diseases resulting in blood poisoning.[46] Hadwen argued in 1905
that the science of bacteriology had a valuable place, but he insisted that
it promised more than it delivered. Scientists, he maintained, have
theorized that "all the acute specific diseases owe their origin to a specific microbe, and yet an undoubted specific microbe has never yet been
discovered as the unerring cause of a single one of them."[47] Hadwen
misrepresented the actual achievements of bacteriology, which continued to garner authority toward the turn of the century. Nevertheless,
he expressed a widespread frustration among anti-vaccinators with the
shortcomings of bacteriology in relationship to smallpox. After more
than two decades of a concerted search for the specific disease agent,
scientists had emerged empty-handed. They had assumed that smallpox was caused by a virus (an organism much smaller than a bacterium), but it was not until the late 1930s, with the invention of the
electron microscope, that the smallpox virus could actually be seen and
identified.[48]

GERMS AND THE ENVIRONMENT   This focus on the nonspecificity
of disease germs allowed anti-vaccinators to retain a panspermist theory, with its focus on contaminated air, and to adopt germs as a new way
of articulating the problem of dirt. Since medical professionals themselves continued into the 1880s and '90s to draw a connection between
germs and dirty environments, it should come as no surprise that anti-
vaccinators seized on this discourse and regularly used germs and filth
as interchangeable concepts. Bacteriology may have transformed medical theory and practice in the twentieth century, but in the late nineteenth century germ theory emerged as "a new way of coding 'cleanliness.' "[49]

Whether they believed in the specificity of germs or not, from the 1870s well into the bacteriological era many anti-vaccinators incorporated some form of germ theory into their etiology precisely to use it to forward their own sanitary agenda. Smallpox, explained "Abdiel" in an 1882 anti-vaccination pamphlet, is caused by "living organisms" that enter the human system either through "contaminated air" or "vitiated, creature-tainted food or drink."[50] Germs, anti-vaccinators argued, were the direct result of unsanitary environments and used dirty media as their mode of conveyance. Smallpox, argued Alfred Russel Wallace, the co-founder of the theory of evolution and a committed anti-vaccinator, is a zymotic disease caused by a "minute organism." The conditions that favored this type of disease were "foul air and water, decaying organic matter, overcrowding, and other unwholesome surroundings."[51]

Anti-vaccinators mobilized germ theory to critique, rather than support, the practice of vaccination itself. Since cleanliness prevented the presence of "organisms" that could "infect" the body, the solution anti-vaccinators offered to the presence of germs was sanitation. Mary Hume-Rothery, who did not believe in germs, nevertheless summed up the anti-vaccinationist position:

> Supposing the new theories as to microbes, bacilli, bacteria, &c., &c., as cause of disease to be founded in fact, the Anti-vaccinating school would meet the danger by *destroying* these parasites by sound hygienic means; by pure air, . . . cleanliness, disinfectants, and especially by cultivating that *health* of the system which is impervious to their attacks; while the Vaccinating school proposes by cultivating and "attenuating" the viruses which contain them and inoculating these into every human and animal body, to render these insusceptible of the mischief from them![52]

Keeping the body and its environment both clean and healthy, Hume-Rothery insisted, would naturally eradicate the microbes and prevent them from finding a habitat conducive to their cultivation. This was clearly a widespread popular belief, for Arnold's Soap advertised in the 1890s that disease could be prevented and removed by "washing its germs out of the body."[53]

What anti-vaccinators explicitly opposed was the tendency within professional medicine to deploy the bacterial theory of specificity to

promote vaccination and other exclusive preventive methods that
closed down their efforts at sanitation. Those anti-vaccinators who opposed germ theory were in fact primarily critiquing bacteriology's implications for the practice of municipal and personal sanitation. Germ
theory, maintained Mary Hume-Rothery, distracted from the principles
of cleanliness, ventilation, and pure food and drink.[54] The germ "hy-
pothesis," argued Sir J. Clarke Jervoise, MP, magistrate, and a correspondent of Florence Nightingale, is directly at variance with sanitary
experience. To accept it would be to negate all public-health measures.[55]
Correspondents to the *Vaccination Inquirer* regularly reiterated this
position. In 1893, Lieutenant-General A. Phelps, future president of the
NAVL, inquired rhetorically whether "infection [by germs was] merely a
theoretical bogey, worked to frighten laymen, and diverting attention
from the real enemy of the human race, dirt?"[56]

In the dissenting report of the Royal Commission on Vaccination,
J. A. Picton and W. J. Collins, the two lone anti-vaccinators left on the
commission after the death of Charles Bradlaugh, used bacteriology to
argue that vaccination was unnecessary. They concluded that the sim-
plest and most effective ways to prevent the spread of smallpox were to
separate the diseased from the healthy and to disinfect infected persons, places, and things.[57] This system of isolation and notification was
based on a bacteriological understanding of disease, for it maintained
that microbes could be eliminated through a process of containment,
which prevented them from moving on to a new host. Since the 1870s,
the city of Leicester had provided a model for an efficient system of
notification and isolation. In Leicester, the medical officer of health was
notified in all cases of smallpox. Infectious people were then isolated in
the town's Fever and Smallpox Hospital, and all contacts were quarantined. Those subjected to quarantine were, however, financially compensated for loss of wages. The patients' premises were then thoroughly disinfected. With a vaccination rate of about 2 percent and with
consistently low rates of smallpox mortality, Leicester exemplified the
success of "the stamping out system."[58] While isolation was rejected by
many anti-vaccinators as another form of tyrannical state intervention,
for others it was part and parcel of a sanitarian approach that favored
using a variety of methods of prevention and containment that would
make vaccination totally unnecessary. Indeed, proper sanitation, ar-

gued the *Vaccination Inquirer* in 1903, would make even isolation obsolete.[59]

GERMS AND THE CONSTITUTION   Instead of rejecting bacteriology
outright, most anti-vaccinators seized on the language of germs, which
in the late nineteenth century was itself imprecise, to further their own
agenda. According to T. R. Allinson: "Small-pox is a germ disease, it
breeds amongst filth, thrives best in dirty slums and overcrowded
streets, and only attacks those whose systems are in a bad hygienic
condition."[60] Here Allinson, like other anti-vaccinators, moves easily
between the idea of the germ, the dirty environment, and the compromised constitution. Indeed, anti-vaccinators used germ theory as a way
to promote their enduring commitment not only to improving the environmental conditions that nurtured disease, but also to resisting inoculating the body with a dirty substance that, they insisted, would only
compromise the constitution. Thus, to anti-vaccinators, germ theory
provided a new way of conceptualizing both the predisposing and exciting causes of disease that continued to dominate their conception of
smallpox.

Developments in bacteriology from the mid-1880s provided those
who promoted vaccination with a scientific theory to support a practice
that was almost a century old. However, it also enabled anti-vaccinators
to make new claims for an even older focus on the importance of a
healthy constitution. In the 1880s, pro-vaccinators proposed that germs
required proper nutrients to live. They settled in the human body and
fed off its "soil."[61] As cowpox and smallpox were almost identical diseases, scientists maintained that they required the same type of suste-
nance. Thus, inoculating the body with cowpox prevented any subsequent smallpox germs from surviving. Just as an attack of smallpox
"eats up and devours—neutralizes, or sterilizes" the smallpox microbe's soil, narrated a popular tract, introducing vaccine matter into
the body allowed the cowpox germs to eat all the available nutrients,
thus providing no appropriate soil for the smallpox germ to take root in
and feed off.[62] As the scientist John Dougall explained in 1886, the "first
harvest" of vaccine "cells" "exhausts" some special ingredient or "pabu-
lum in the soil" so that it is unable to "feed" another crop of the same
cells or "virus" for several years.[63] An 1884 article in *The People*, a cheap

weekly newspaper with a mixed-class readership, compared this process to the Australian rabbit infestation: Vaccine destroys the smallpox germ's habitat just as, in Australia, "the rabbits, though the smaller animal, are beforehand in devouring the grass, and leave nothing for the sheep to eat."[64]

Anti-vaccinators debated the logic of this theory and used it not to dismiss germ theory but, rather, to underscore the importance of a healthy constitution, whether or not germs were specific to the disease or more generally harmful. Testifying before the Royal Commission on Vaccination in the 1890s, George Newman, secretary to the Gloucester Anti-Vaccination League, declared that he did not believe in contagion from smallpox patients unless the person catching the disease was "in a fit state to have it." He explained: "If I throw wheat down on the ground it will not grow, but if there were earth and water and warmth it will grow, but it will not grow without it."[65] This explained why some members of a family or community escaped disease while others suffered its ravages.[66] For anti-vaccinators, a healthy constitution, as I argued in chapter 5, depended largely on the state of the blood. Animal—and, in particular, human—blood seemed to be germs' "favourite pasture," argued a magnetic and botanic practitioner. These micro-organisms, anti-vaccinators agreed, required a suitable soil in which to grow or appropriate nutrients to eat. Since these did not exist in perfectly healthy blood, to combat germs one must only cultivate good blood, they generally maintained—hence, their concern with maintaining pure blood unpolluted by animal diseases. The real safety from smallpox, maintained an anonymous pamphleteer, was to "live a pure and healthy life. . . . Germs will not live unless they find appropriate nutriment."[67]

This idea of good blood, so significant to anti-vaccinators throughout the campaign, took on new importance on the brink of the twentieth century. By the mid-1890s, bacteriology had begun to redefine public health. The trend toward preventive medicine already present in the 1850s had consolidated by the end of the century as new vaccines became available for a number of different diseases. But bacteriology was also beginning to contribute to curative medicine, as antitoxins for diseases such as diphtheria appeared in the physician's pharmacoepia. Anti-vaccinators denounced this medical trend on the same grounds as vaccination: that it polluted the bloodstream with contaminated animal material. In 1897, Hadwen lamented that, with the rise of serum therapy, the "inoculation of every kind of filth" had become the "vogue of the up-to-date physician."[68] Serum theory, Hadwen proposed, was a ridiculous remedy precisely because it introduced a dirty substance into the body and in the process compromised the constitution. "No germ can live in healthy blood"; when a child's blood is already "inflamed" by the "morbid products" of disease, why pollute the "life-stream" still further "with the poisoned blood serum of horse?" he argued.[69] Both vaccines and sera, as quintessentially dirty substances, should be withheld from healthy blood, which was the body's own natural defense against harmful microbes, anti-vaccinators argued. Immunity due to vaccination, maintained Collins, could equally be conferred by health. If antidote theory is true, he reasoned in a marginal notation to Klein's essay on micro-organisms, then "immunity due to Vaccination is of the same kind as the immunity due to health i.e. the elaboration of an inimical chemical substance."[70] Serum therapies and preventive vaccines, anti-vaccinators consistently argued, discounted the importance of maintaining a healthy body that could then resist disease itself.

As medical researchers began to theorize the process of producing immunity, so the constitutional basis for disease began to assume even greater importance to anti-vaccinators. By 1901, the *Saturday Review* was able to offer its readers a complicated theory of immunity: Immunity, it reported, is a "complex problem involving the delicate interplay of the activities of life, the attractions and repulsions of contending cells, the production and warfare of toxins and anti-toxins, the nature of microbes and microbial poisons."[71] This, however, was a problem for the bacteriologist, not the layman, the reporter declared. From the 1890s, this research into the science of immunity was used to explain vaccination by reasoning that the body produced cells that ate invading microbes. In an 1891 report on the discoveries of Elie Metchnikoff, a Russian microbiologist and pathologist who won the Nobel Prize in 1908 for his immunological studies, the *Newcastle Daily Chronicle* described the actions of "amoeboid cells" for a popular audience. Cells, the report explained, "eat up the attacking microbes." Vaccination alerts the cells and puts them on the offensive, endowing them with a "specific power of resistance" to bacteria. The immunity produced by vaccination, it continued, is an "acquired tolerance" of the cells of our body to the "specific poison of the special bacterium" of the disease against which an individual is vaccinated.[72] These devouring cells were called "white corpuscles," "leucocytes," or "phagocytes."

Hadwen dismissed Metchnikoff's claims, likening phagocytes to a "Thames policeman" who supposedly went "rollicking round, gobbling up the disease germs and thus extinguishing the imaginary source of disease."[73] This theory, he suggested, implied that the body was a disorderly state that needed constant policing rather than an organic self-regulatory system that relied primarily on proper circulation. But Alfred Russel Wallace mobilized this theory to explain the importance of both sanitation and a healthy constitution. He argued that as long as we live in "tolerably healthy conditions," our "leucocytes or phagocytes" are able to deal with "disease-germs" that gain entry to the system. But when we live in "impure air," drink impure water, or eat unwholesome food, the system becomes enfeebled, and "our guardian leucocytes are unable to destroy the disease-germs."[74] While the language used to describe the process of infection was adopted from the discourse of a nascent immunology, the real cause of disease, Wallace insisted, remained the insanitary conditions and poor nutrition that compromised the constitution, the body's best defense.

Germ theory therefore became a key discourse in which to frame the importance of constitutional predisposition to disease and thus the need for blood purity. As we have seen, it was an equally powerful language with which to focus attention on environmental conditions and could thus be used effectively to champion sanitation. For germ theory, however transformative, did not entirely replace older models or languages of disease causation.[75] Instead, germ theory was layered on earlier conceptions of disease processes so that, like a palimpsest, the older theories were still evident in the new. Anti-vaccinators thus engaged with germ theory but nonetheless critiqued both scientists and government officials for using it to perpetuate and encourage the practice of vaccination rather than as further proof of the value of sanitation and healthy blood. The emphasis on preventive methods that focused on individual bodies rather than on environmental conditions, these anti-vaccinators feared, undermined efforts to achieve large-scale sanitary improvements that they claimed were the only way to address the problem of urban poverty, the root of epidemic disease.

While anti-vaccinators had championed cleanliness since the begin-ning of their campaign, by the turn of the century sanitation had be-come intensely politicized. Focusing on sewers and dirt was not merely an outdated way to imagine disease processes. Instead, it was a rejec-tion of limited and targeted solutions to disease that ignored larger issues of social inequality. Smallpox could not be stopped by vaccinat-ing the poor, anti-vaccinators argued, for vaccine matter was no better than dirt and compromised those who were already most vulnerable to disease. Ending epidemic disease, they proposed, required a much larger commitment to bettering the living conditions of the urban poor. Indeed, Frank Goss recalled that his mother's resistance to vaccination came from a "deep, sincere and abiding conviction that medical science was a professional racket bolstered up by the State to mask its own deficiencies in not providing decent feeding, housing and living stan-dards for its people."[76] Ironically, what anti-vaccinators lobbied for may indeed have been a much more intensive and interventionist system of policing and regulating the public's health.[77] But however much sanita-tion and isolation interfered with personal liberties, unlike vaccination, these strategies for dealing with disease did not impinge directly on the body and thus had vastly different meanings and resonances, particu-larly for working-class activists.

Rather than entirely reconfiguring the debate, then, some advances in bacteriology were absorbed into anti-vaccinationists' theories of con-tagion. Many campaigners readily adopted germ theory and partici-pated in debates over its meanings and ramifications at a time when bacteriology, particularly in relationship to smallpox, was still in the process of establishing its authority. Understanding anti-vaccinators as adherents to an older model of disease causation that inevitably was to become outdated and thus "unscientific" de-historicizes both germ the-ory and sanitary practices. Instead of serving as a great divide that radically reformulated popular and scientific ideas about contagion, the germ theory of disease has a much more complicated and uneven history of its own. Vaccination and the eradication of smallpox have come to represent the triumph of germ theory. But it was not until well into the twentieth century that the virus could be identified and, thus, the success of the procedure could be adequately accounted for. At the end of the nineteenth century, it was not yet certain that germ theory would triumph and what exactly it might mean. The vaccination debate was therefore a particularly important place in which the social implications of germ theory were being worked out. Ironically, it was just as germ theory ventured a scientific and theoretical, rather than purely empirical, explanation for vaccination that the compulsory policy gave way to a more permissive system that vindicated the anti-vaccinationist position.

7

Class, Gender, and the Conscientious Objector

You can vaccinate a magistrate

Against smallpox for ever,

Against his being something great,

Against his being clever;

But there is no vaccine can be bought

For bags of shiney tanners,

To keep bad ways from being taught,

Or guard him 'gainst bad manners.

—"Pick-Me-Up," 1900[1]

☞ In 1898, the British government attempted to resolve the vaccination issue by introducing a conscience clause. This allowed anti-vaccinators to claim certificates of conscientious objection by applying to a magistrate for an exemption. While the conscience clause proved a contentious issue for pro- and anti-vaccinators alike, it gave the working and lower middle classes a measure of relief from repeated fines, each of which could amount to 20 shillings plus court costs, and from the threat of imprisonment. By the end of 1898, 203,413 certificates of conscientious objection had been issued. Many of these were granted in anti-vaccination strongholds where the conscientious-objection rate accounted for a majority of all births. In 1904–05, the Registrar General reported that in Loughborough, Northampton, Banbury, and Keighley, approximately half of the births were granted certificates of exemption.[2]

The registers of conscientious objectors for Enfield and Hammersmith, which were not known as a centers of anti-vaccination agitation, document that most certificates were issued to the working and lower middle classes—specifically, to a mixture of semiskilled factory operatives, journeyman laborers, and, to a lesser extent, master artisans, policemen, postal workers, porters, and small tradesmen.[3] Conscientious objection was so popular among the working classes at Higham Ferrars, Northamptonshire, that in December 1898 several factories had to close down as all their "hands" had left work to apply for certificates before the 12 December deadline.[4] The first widely acknowledged conscientious objectors, therefore, were not the pacifist or socialist "conchies" identified with World War I but, rather, working- and lower middle-class anti-vaccinationists.

The vaccination conscience clauses were controversial. As most of the applicants who applied for these exemption certificates came from the working classes, and many were women, these acts generated a national debate over the classed and gendered nature of the conscience and the meanings of conscientious objection. The years between 1898 and 1907 thus mark a significant moment in the making of the modern subject and citizen. As the debate over conscientious objection to vaccination reveals, who exactly was entitled to make a claim to possess a conscience, with its concomitant rights, was itself a contested issue.

The Conscientious Objector to Vaccination

The conscientious objector to vaccination eventually became a legal category because politicians acceded to an already pervasive popular discourse that claimed conscientious beliefs as the property of all citizens, whether male or female, rich or poor, educated or uneducated. From their very earliest resistance to compulsory vaccination, agitators insisted that their objections were "conscientious." In 1854, both the hydropath John Gibbs and the medical botanist John Skelton pointed to compulsory vaccination's attack on the "conscientious convictions" of parents. As early as 1858, George Ridley of Bury St. Edmunds, a vaccination defaulter, used the term *conscientious objection* to plead his case in court. By 1870, anti-vaccinationists were regularly mobilizing this defense—significantly, long before a conscience clause was in place. Indeed, these were anti-vaccinationists' own terms. Between 1853 and

1907, anti-vaccinationists repeatedly argued that they had "consciences" and were acting on them. They often described themselves as "conscientious" parents, and declared that they struggled for the "liberty of conscience."[5] In fact, they suggested that anyone with a conscience would naturally oppose compulsory vaccination. In a mock advertisement for the services of a "Baby Hunter"—a vaccination officer paid to trace noncompliers—an anti-vaccinationist cautioned, "No Person with a Conscience Need Apply."[6]

What it meant to have a conscience was not easily definable, and few tried to delineate its meanings. The conscience was generally imagined, like the spirit, to be incorporeal, intangible, and indefinable. It was certainly allied to "opinions," "moral feelings," and "religious principles" in the mind of the hygiest John Fraser; Mary Hume-Rothery argued that it had some relationship to the soul. Significantly, although some linked the conscience to religious sensibilities, anti-vaccinators generally used the term within a secular context, proposing that the rights of "conscience are not confined simply to theological questions." The *Vaccination Inquirer* reasoned in 1884 that "conscience" means "the feeling a man has that his actions are right or wrong."[7] However vague this definition seemed to be, it nevertheless came very close to the Oxford English Dictionary's own definition and underscored the widely applicable nature of the conscience to a whole range of moral dilemmas.[8]

What resisters could agree on was that the conscience was not something to be evaluated, but "as a conscience it is entitled to respect," whatever its character.[9] In reference to the proposed conscience clause, the NAVL, formed in 1896 to consolidate the agitation, contended that it was an "insulting mockery" to suggest that the "validity of the parents' conscientious objection [was] to be determined by any justice, guardian, or other official."[10] The conscience, they argued, could never be assessed by anyone but the individual, for there was simply no way of adjudicating another's personal convictions and moral values. Argued A. T. Guttery: "My conscience is the grandest thing I possess, and when you take that away from me you take everything from me that is worth possessing."[11]

The vaccination question thrust the conscientious objector into the forefront of public debate in the late-Victorian period. The 1909 Oxford

English Dictionary's earliest reference to the "conscientious objector" was to an 1899 text regarding the 1898 Vaccination Act. However, the precedent for conscientious objection in Britain had been established both by the laws relating to oaths and those concerning compulsory education. The Toleration Act of 1689 established the right of Protestant dissenters to object to taking a religious oath on grounds of conscience and allowed them instead the legal right to affirmation. This principle was extended in the Oaths Act of 1888, which allowed any person who objected to swearing an oath because it was contrary to his or her religious belief, or because he or she had no religious belief, to affirm rather than swear in any legal proceeding.[12] Similarly, the Militia Acts of 1757 exempted Quakers from paying rates and supplying property for military use, as this contradicted their religious beliefs.

In accordance with these principles of religious freedom, when the Education Act of 1870 was formulated, it included within it a conscience clause. This enabled parents to exempt their children from religious prayer or teaching within the public school system, thereby anticipating and eradicating any potential objection to the religious content of compulsory education.[13] The issue of the conscience and education was raised again in 1902 when denominational schools were integrated into the public school system and supported by taxes. Passive Resisters—nonconformists who refused to pay school taxes, as most of this money supported Anglican schools whose religious teachings they did not condone, also considered themselves conscientious objectors. In the early twentieth century, anti-vaccinators tried to recruit Passive Resisters to the Education Acts to their cause, for they insisted that both groups were victims of "coercion of conscience."[14]

Pro- and anti-vaccinators alike appealed to these precedents, arguing that vaccination was also an issue of conscience. In an assessment of how to treat vaccination prisoners, prison and Home Office officials aligned anti-vaccinationists with education defaulters and members of the Salvation Army as "conscientious offenders."[15] Anti-vaccinators used these already familiar forms of conscientious objection to argue for their own entitlement to similar legal exemptions. An anti-vaccination pamphlet demanded whether the state had any more right "to enforce a medical belief, than it once had to enforce a religious one." It is today, echoed the Health and Liberty League, considered intolerable that anyone should suffer for their "theological convictions," and yet similar persecutions are carried out in the name of vaccination. If there are religious conscientious objectors, reasoned the *Hydropathic Record*, why can there not be medical?[16]

The idea of the medical conscientious objector had already been established by some religious sects—most notably, the Peculiar People, who resisted all forms of orthodox medical treatment, opting instead for the practices of faith healing. These people were never given a legal status, for the state insisted that neglecting one's child—which included withholding medical aid—was a criminal offense.[17] Most anti-vaccinators (though some did belong to similar religious sects) turned away from this model of conscientious objection and attempted to establish a secular moral position. They emphasized instead the intelligence, convictions, and devotion of the conscientious parent. In *The Conscientious Objector: Who He Is!* W. J. Furnival proposed that the conscientious objector was a

> parent residing in England, who, by reason of certain mild or bitter experiences of his own, by observing what has occurred in other families, by studying the special investigations of gifted scientific men, and by personal "bed-rock" inquiry into the real nature of vaccine itself, has become so firmly convinced of the futility, repulsiveness, and dangers of the operation of vaccination, that he cannot, as a devoted and intelligent parent, conscientiously consent, to subject the beloved children of whom he is natural protector to such a rite.[18]

The conscientious objector, Furnival argued, was "prepared to suffer" for his "honest belief." According to Furnival, the conscientious objector was not someone who merely reasoned that vaccination was wrong, or one who rejected it because it was incompatible with religious beliefs. The conscientious objector had thoroughly investigated the issue and was neither irrational nor negligent. The conscientious objector, he maintained, was "intelligent," loving, and "devoted" to protecting his children.

Despite the fact that anti-vaccinationists had mobilized this rhetoric of conscience and conscientious objection, they did not lobby for a conscience clause. Anti-vaccinationists worthy of the name, declared John Bonner, a paid lecturer for the NAVL, do not want and will not have thrust on them "tickets-of-leave to keep their children healthy, no matter how inexpensive and easily obtainable."[19] The "ticket-of-leave" was conferred on criminals who were released from prison before serving their entire sentence. By comparing their own treatment to that meted out to criminals, anti-vaccinationists proposed that certificates of exemption "insult the objector by converting him into a licensed lawbreaker," a "position of odium to which no self-respecting citizen can willingly submit."[20] The ticket-of-leave rendered one a marginal figure, still under state surveillance and not fully incorporated back into society. Certificates of conscientious objection, anti-vaccinationists suggested, would serve as a stigma, branding objectors as exempt from what was otherwise mandated as a civic and social duty and thus challenging their status as British citizens. Anti-vaccinationists maintained that since vaccination was a matter of conscience, the procedure—and, in fact, all medical interventions—should be entirely voluntary, not something that one was forced to "opt out" of. Their clamorings backfired. The government seized on the anti-vaccinationists' own language of conscientious objection to introduce not total repeal of the acts but exemption certificates.

The 1898 Conscience Clause

The introduction of exemption certificates became possible in 1898 for several reasons. First, smallpox was on the decline. While there were local outbreaks in the 1880s and '90s, the last major epidemic had occurred in 1871. The decline was due in part, but not solely, to vaccination. A number of factors played a role, including variations in the virulence of the virus strain; the expansion of other preventive methods, such as isolation and notification; and the development of port sanitary authorities to prevent the importation of foreign disease.[21] Further, the resilience of the anti-vaccination movement had demonstrated that it was not a passing fad, that objectors were committed and sincere. Finally, after deliberating for seven years, in 1896 the Royal Commission on Vaccination recommended the introduction of a conscience clause.

THE POLITICS OF THE CONSCIENCE   The Royal Commission on Vaccination was appointed in 1889 in response to anti-vaccination pressure.
Its mandate was to investigate the administration of the vaccination acts
and to draft recommendations for improvements in the efficiency and
safety of vaccination. Stacked with eminent medical practitioners who
almost unanimously supported vaccination, the Royal Commission was a
protracted affair. It sat for seven years before publishing its final report.
During this period, many districts declined to enforce the vaccination acts.
In 122 of 620 reporting districts, Boards of Guardians responded to
pressure from anti-vaccinationists who argued that it was unjust to prosecute while vaccination remained under investigation by temporarily halt-
ing all prosecutions for default. In 1896, the medical officer of health for
the working-class district of Mile End in East London reported a vaccination rate of only 43 percent due to "pronounced" opposition and the
refusal of the Board of Guardians to prosecute. In Coventry in 1895, the
medical officer of health declared the vaccination acts a "dead letter" while
the commission continued to deliberate.[22]

The Royal Commission released its final report in 1896. It concluded
that vaccination should remain compulsory so that children would not
go unvaccinated through the neglect or indifference of their parents.
However, it cautioned that parents who were "honestly opposed" to the
procedure should be exempt from prosecution. To encourage vaccination while at the same time allowing for conscientious objection, the
report proposed that the number of fines an individual could accrue
should be limited to two and that a conscience clause should be added.
While the commission was vague about how to separate legitimate
objectors from the negligent, it proposed either that the parent appear
before a magistrate to "satisfy" him that his or her objections were
conscientious, or that the individual make a statutory declaration to that
effect, though the former solution received only scant support. The
commission made no attempt, however, to define what constituted a
legitimate conscientious objection.

In response to the report, Henry Chaplin, president of the Local
Government Board from 1895 to 1900—and, according to anti-vaccinators, "the Toryest of Tories"[23]—introduced a bill to amend the vaccination acts in March 1898. The bill extended the period within which to

procure vaccination from three to twelve months of birth. It replaced public vaccination stations with domiciliary visits and, hence, the arm-to-arm method with lymph preserved in glycerine. It also limited penalties for default to one fine under Section 29 of the 1867 act and another fine under Section 31. It said nothing of a conscience clause. Anti-vaccinationists were outraged. This is a "dishonest Bill and a reckless Bill, and nobody likes it," argued the *Vaccination Inquirer*. "It is neither fish, flesh, fowl, nor good red herring," denounced *Reynold's Newspaper*. "How large is the world governed by asses!"[24]

By April, the need for a conscience clause was under discussion in the House of Commons, as many members believed that limiting the number of fines would serve neither to promote vaccination nor to curb the active resistance of those who objected wholeheartedly to the procedure. While they debated the terms of the clause, parliamentarians of all sorts agreed that the conscience was largely indefinable. They consistently used the terms *honest, genuine, serious,* and *convictions* in an attempt to clarify what was meant by conscientious beliefs, but they generally defined the conscientious objector only in relation to his opposite, the "lazy," "indolent," "indifferent," or "negligent" parent. A few members of both houses maintained that vaccination was not a matter of conscience at all, as conscience in their definition was tied to religious beliefs. However, the question of religion was scarcely raised at all. What was established again and again was that the objection need not be well founded, or "right," as long as it was sincere. It had to be based on a belief that the procedure would injure the child.

At stake in debates over the introduction of a conscience clause was largely how one tested the conscientiousness of an individual's objection and thus who could legitimately claim a conscience in the first place. In July, Sir Walter Foster, the Liberal MP for the anti-vaccination stronghold of Derby, introduced an amendment allowing for a statutory declaration. The model for this, he maintained, came from the union of Barton Regis, where the Board of Guardians had taken it upon themselves to circulate instructions to the parents of newborn babies. On signing a declaration witnessed by a magistrate, the circular explained, those with "conscientious convictions" could exempt themselves from compulsory vaccination. Only those with honest, conscientious convictions—"as honest in their convictions as ourselves," Foster maintained

—would take such a serious step.[25] This was the best means of establishing conscientious objection, supporters of the amendment maintained, because, as Henry Labouchere argued, "when you get on to conscientious objections you get on to very difficult ground." Indeed, former Home Secretary H. H. Asquith asked: How can one "get beyond a man's statement, 'I do conscientiously object to vaccination,'" in the absence of any definition of conscientious objection? It was also in line with the precedent set by the Oaths Act of 1888, Asquith proposed, whereby a person's statement in court was sufficient without the need for evaluation by any external arbiter.[26]

As the conscience clause was being debated in the Houses of Parliament, the death of C. T. Murdoch, Conservative MP for Reading, forced a by-election. At recent elections for the Reading Board of Guardians, anti-vaccinationist candidates had won a sweeping victory, revealing the town to be an important center of agitation. The NAVL had in fact convened in Reading earlier in the year for its second annual meeting. The by-election put anti-vaccinationists on the offensive. They sought to throw their support behind any candidate willing to run on an anti-vaccination platform, regardless of party affiliation. They polled the two candidates on their position and received the resounding support of the Liberal candidate, G. W. Palmer, a biscuit manufacturer who had little other backing from any but an Irish bloc and a small group of campaigners for women's rights.[27] The local Anti-Vaccination Society immediately moved to give its support "irrespective of political creed" to the Liberal candidate who had denounced compulsory vaccination and presumably the proposed conscience clause, for the NAVL still pressured for total repeal of the vaccination acts.[28]

The events in Reading alarmed the Conservative government and immediately raised the stakes considerably. It was in the midst of the Reading election campaign, just a few days before the votes were to be cast, that A. J. Balfour, the Conservative Lord of the Treasury, introduced an amendment that he repeatedly hailed and promoted as a "compromise." This would allow for exemptions but would require all applicants to satisfy a magistrate that his objections were indeed conscientious. Public opinion and political expedience had forced the Conservative government to act, for the anti-vaccinationist lobby had proved itself a formidable political force. The election on 25 July confirmed the

Tories' worst fears. Even Conservative anti-vaccinationists supported Palmer, who won by a majority of 694, the largest ever in the borough.[29] Palmer's victory revealed the extent of anti-vaccinationists' political influence and put pressure on the government to act.

With a general agreement that the law had to be passed by the end of the session, as it was already long overdue, and with the anti-vaccinationist victory in Reading fresh in the minds of Liberals and Conservatives alike, Balfour's amendment was pushed through both Houses of Parliament, despite the fact that it was a bad compromise and proved satisfactory to none of the interests involved. The Vaccination Act of 1898 mandated domiciliary vaccination with glycerinated lymph, limited fines for default, and allowed conscientious-objection status for any parent or guardian who "satisfied" two justices in petty sessions or a stipendiary police magistrate within four months of the child's birth that he "conscientiously believe[d] that vaccination would be prejudicial to the health of the child." By legislating that the magistrates had to be "satisfied" of the conscientiousness of the objection, the 1898 act disregarded the recommendation of the majority of Royal Commissioners. It also deliberately ignored the historical precedents provided by the Education Act of 1870 and the Oaths Acts of 1888, whereby all who claimed a conscientious objection were entitled to this right without requiring the approval of any outside authority.[30] Nevertheless, it was hoped that the act would serve as a "truce and an armistice" to mollify resisters while still retaining state control over the process of granting exemptions.[31] Far from reducing martyrdom and curbing resistance, the 1898 act actually created new controversies. As the Liberal MPs who opposed this process of "cross-examination" had predicted, the implementation of the first conscience clause only aggravated the already difficult relationship between working-class anti-vaccinationists and unsympathetic magistrates.

CLASS AND THE CONSCIENCE   Before the bill was passed, the *Vaccination Inquirer* stood firm, arguing that the NAVL would have none of the idea of a conscience clause. It campaigned for total repeal of the compulsory clauses and considered the conscience clause "a concession not to be tolerated at any price."[32] The formation of the NAVL to consolidate resistance in the wake of the Royal Commission's report itself revealed that the anti-vaccinators' battle was not yet complete. Obtaining conscientious-objector status would cost time and money, the anti-vaccination leaders reasoned; thus, their goal remained the complete repeal of the vaccination acts. Once the bill became law, the NAVL nevertheless claimed at least a partial victory, although it maintained that the struggle for repeal continued.[33]

Reactions to the Vaccination Act of 1898 were varied. The Oldham Anti-Vaccination Society decided against applying for certificates of exemption, arguing that it was a "retrograde and humiliating step to seek by purchase of certificate exemption from an oppression we have already cast off."[34] The Kettering league agreed, but the NAVL wavered. In September 1898, it claimed a "notable victory" with the conscience clause but insisted that the fight continued.[35] In a letter to *The Times*, William Tebb declared that the people had now been "liberated from the most cruel features of an odious and long-standing tyranny."[36] Scarcely a month later, the NAVL was plunged into doubt and disagreement. Its policy, the October issue of the *Vaccination Inquirer* declared, was not to apply for certificates. Every man who stays at home and "lies low and sez nuffin'," it proposed, "is a source of doubt and perplexity to the foe." Applying for certificates would merely be delivering oneself into the "power of a bullying magistrate." There is a danger, it warned, "lest a crowd of certificate-hunters at the door of the court be taken as *pro tanto* testimony that we are satisfied with this Act as a compromise."[37] At the NAVL's annual national conference in 1898, the conscience clause was a source of much debate and disagreement. All that could be agreed on was that the league would not interfere with certificate seekers but would maintain the necessity for further united action. The NAVL realized that, for working people, the conscience clause could provide some measure of security against financially crippling prosecutions.[38]

The vagueness of what it meant to have a conscientious objection was the central problematic of implementing the 1898 Vaccination Act. "There is no definition of a 'conscientious objection,'" argued the medical officer of health for Paddington, "and it is difficult to understand what that term implies."[39] The act was so vague as to what it meant to "satisfy" a magistrate that magistrates immediately became wary of hearing applications. The *St. James' Gazette* reported that the first applicant for conscientious-objector status was met with confusion. "I don't know, I am sure, what I am to do," proclaimed the magistrate. "The act of Parliament says I am to be satisfied you have a conscientious objection. I don't know whether you are simply to come here and say so, and then go away, or what you are to do. You might never satisfy me. I don't know I am sure. I don't understand the Act. I have seen you, and you have told me you have a conscientious objection; I don't know whether that is enough. To satisfy myself I might want to have the doctor and all sorts of people called in."[40] Similarly, a "respectable looking working man" who applied to the Highgate Police Court for an exemption certificate soon after the act had come into effect was sent away again. "We don't understand the Act yet," according to the *Vaccination Inquirer*, was all the clerk could offer.[41] In an attempt to deal with this confusion, a special meeting of the metropolitan magistrates was immediately convened to discuss how best to deal with the new act. It was resolved that London magistrates would hear applications and would not require applicants to be sworn; if they were satisfied by the verbal statement of conscientious objection, they would issue a certificate at the cost of 1 shilling.[42] This hardly clarified anything but the cost of exemption. What it meant to be satisfied was still open to debate.

Since the conscience was intangible, it was impossible to evaluate unless it could be rendered visible or measurable. As Victorians grew increasingly reliant on new scientific technologies that rendered the unseen visible to the naked eye, the very intangibility of the conscience made its existence both suspect and highly problematic.[43] Lamented a magistrate at Bromley: "We have no Roentgen rays with which to examine your conscience, so I suppose we must accept your assertion."[44] This meant that application hearings often devolved into a yes-I-do, no-you-don't circular argument. At the Thames Police Court, Mr. Mead, a notoriously unsympathetic magistrate, told an applicant that he needed to be satisfied that he had a conscientious belief. The applicant replied, "I have," and Mead responded, "No, you have not."[45] This invariably went nowhere, prompting some officials to refuse outright to hear applications.

Depending on where one lived, satisfying a magistrate could prove to be a daunting task, for police-court magistrates enjoyed a "great latitude" in dealing with those who sought out their services.[46] Applicants who declared that they had a medical objection, or that vaccination had killed or injured another child, were often ridiculed and denied a certificate. Those who could not claim to have had another child die from the procedure were equally likely to be denied in some courtrooms.[47] When a "young man" applied for an exemption at Westminster, declaring that his other child had caught diphtheria after vaccination, the magistrate denied his claim. One might as well say, the magistrate replied, that they got diphtheria (a disease for which the germ had recently been identified) "after cutting their toe nails." Another who claimed that vaccination would be bad for the child's health was told that his objection was not "conscientious" and sent away. A father was refused at Castle Eden because the magistrate would grant a certificate only if the child was not in a fit state to be vaccinated.[48] This was common enough, though an absolute misreading of the act, for there had always been exemptions for sickly children.

Since magistrates set their own standards of evaluation, reasons for rejection were often based on the whims of the official presiding. If a magistrate "is pleased to say that he is *not* satisfied," complained the *Vaccination Inquirer*, "no power on earth can prove that he *is*."[49] When a man at Marylebone Police Court refused to respond to the magistrate's query about how far he would go for a certificate—and whether prison was far enough—he was denied an exemption. Other magistrates refused to grant certificates to those who applied at the last minute. Parents who were vague about their objections, claiming that vaccination was "no good" or that they did not "hold" with it, were also routinely denied, as were those who had previously been fined for noncompliance. Some officials felt that vaccination was not a matter for the conscience at all. An applicant at Cheshire was denied a certificate and pleaded, "That means that you say my conscience is nothing?" "Well," replied the magistrate, "not in vaccination."[50] This position was echoed by the conservative press. In 1901, the *Saturday Review*, the voice of Tory regulationism, maintained that since vaccination was a matter of public health, it was not about the individual conscience at all; rather, it was about the safety of the community. "Let us be as conscientious as we please for ourselves," the newspaper argued. "[I]f we must, let us burn ourselves. . . . [B]ut let us see that we do it in such a fashion that our funeral pyre or the fumes of it do not offend our neighbours." To make a conscience clause work, the article continued, the unvaccinated conscientious objector must not be allowed in public except "ringing a bell and clad in a warning garb" like the leper.[51]

While Jennifer Davis has argued that magistrates—at least, at mid-century—attempted to remain morally neutral, much of the animosity generated by the conscience clause stemmed from the inability of many magistrates to overlook their own judgment and values. Magistrates, argued John Brown, president of the Mile End Anti-Vaccination League, often "made their consciences rather than the conscientious belief of the parent the point on which the Act turned." Some are reported to have said that they had a "conscientious objection" to giving out certificates of exemption.[52] This meant that magistrates regularly asserted and attempted to enforce their own value system on anti-vaccinators. Magistrates often "bully and terrorise" applicants, claimed one anti-vaccinationist, turning what was meant to be a "measure of relief" into a new "weapon of persecution."[53] In Stratford in 1902, a magistrate refused to grant a certificate and added insult to injury by declaring that he hoped the applicant would be sent to prison. Some magistrates who did grant certificates nevertheless verbally abused the applicants, claiming that they were not the ethical people they claimed to be. At Chelmsford in 1901, a conscientious objector was given a certificate but not before the magistrate had questioned his moral standing. "I should be very sorry to do what you are doing," maintained the magistrate. "I should consider I was doing a wicked, cruel thing." Another declared an objector "an enemy of the human race."[54] Many anti-vaccinationists refused to appear before a magistrate because they did not want to submit themselves to the indignity of being "heckled" and "bullied for their conscience sake."[55]

Magistrates who refused to grant certificates, and who instead acted according to their own consciences, often did so precisely because they felt that working people could not possibly make conscientious choices themselves. Magistrates often made assumptions about a person's claims to conscience based on his or her class position. As in prosecutions for noncompliance, working people felt that they were unfairly treated by the new conscience clause and dismissed as genuinely conscientious precisely because of their social status. Millicent Garrett Fawcett reported that the working man is "roughly handled by the magistrates, held up for ridicule," and discharged without a certificate. A barrister who followed one such incident remarked, "If you think you are going to bully me as you have bullied that working-man you are mistaken," she reported. "I have a conscientious objection. . . . I claim a certificate." He was duly awarded one. But when Mr. Hodgson, former editor of the *Northern Light*, a cheap weekly paper, applied for conscientious-objector status, he was sent away and told to return in two weeks. The magistrates, reported the *Holloway Press*, had declared that they "found it difficult to discover whether a person had a conscience at all!" To the best of his knowledge, retorted Mr. Hodgson, "he did possess a conscience" and was prepared to take his affidavit, or what he called his "Alfred David."[56]

A poem printed in the *Blackburn Standard* ridiculed the working man's conscience. The working-class father depicted in the poem knew neither his child's sex nor its name. All he knew, the poem asserted, was that he claimed to be a conscientious objector.

> I conscientiously objeck
> To vaccinatin' of my kid;
> In vaccination as a check
> I don't berlieve, an' never did.
> I do berlieve it's bin imposed
> The workin' classes to annoy;
> And that is w'y I ain't disposed
> To try it on my girl—or boy.
>
> I says my boy or girl becos
> I don't know if it's he or she,
> But my old woman 'ere is poz
> That it's a girl—so let it be.
> But wot she's called I couldn't say;
> I know my wife is called the same,
> I think it's Rose, or Kate, or May,
> Or Poll, or Sue, or some such name.
>
> I ain't quite certain w'er we live,
> W'en she was born I couldn't tell;
> I didn't come up 'ere to give

'Er blooming pedigree as well.
If you want facks you'll 'ave ter go
And arst my missus, I expeck,
But for meself, I only know,
I conscientiously objeck.[57]

The author of the poem mocked the working-class father as a figure who lacked both the intelligence and the moral fibre associated with conscientiousness. This father, like all working-class fathers, knows nothing of his family or domestic life, the poem implies; hence, he is not in a position to make medical or ethical choices on their behalf. He protests vaccination, but his opposition bears no relationship to conscientious convictions. Critiquing the policy of vaccinating all workhouse infants, George Gibbs attacked precisely these kinds of generalizations and assumptions about the poorer classes. "[O]ur humane laws," he argued, "recognize no right of conscience in a *pauper* parent."[58]

Anti-vaccinators contested this inconsistent and condescending treatment by the courts in three ways: by seeking out officials sympathetic to the anti-vaccination cause; by attempting to use the letter of the law to their advantage; and by lobbying the Home Office. If some magistrates and justices were excessively stringent in their measures and denied almost all applicants their certificates, others overcompensated. By granting certificates without even the pretense of considering whether or not the objection might be sincere, and by encouraging swarms of people to apply at once, sympathetic officials in anti-vaccination strongholds turned the process into what the prominent medical journals called a "farce" or a "Gilbert and Sullivan comic opera."[59] In Oldham, an important center of anti-vaccination agitation, the mayor and a magistrate agreed to hear applications each evening at six o'clock and each Saturday at three o'clock to accommodate working men's schedules. Night after night, the *Oldham Chronicle* reported, large crowds of people converged on the town hall to apply for certificates of exemption. By the middle of December 1898, the Oldham magistrates were rumored to have granted between 34,000 and 40,000 certificates.[60] Other sympathetic justices, such as the Yorkshire trade unionist Ben Turner, allowed conscientious objectors to approach them day and night, signing certificates in passing on the street. It was said that at Keighley, anyone could apply, merely nod his or her head, and say "yes" in reply to the magistrate's question and be granted an exemption that instant. Eight hundred certificate seekers applied on one day.[61] The reputation of some magistrates prompted desperate anti-vaccinationists to journey into other districts to obtain their certificates. A man from Chesham traveled to Southwark to obtain an exemption; another traveled 280 miles to Heywood on hearing of a sympathetic magistrate.[62] In districts such as these, vaccination was said to have decreased from 95 percent to 2 percent of all births by the end of 1898.[63]

When faced with magistrates who were not as supportive of conscientious objectors, anti-vaccinators used the precise wording of the act to argue that any who claimed his or her objections were conscientious should be granted a certificate. In effect, the anti-vaccination leadership attempted to school the public in the basics of legal rhetorical performance to help conscientious objectors manage the unequal power dynamic within the courtroom. London leagues placarded Battersea with exact directions as to how to obtain exemptions; they also stationed a volunteer outside the Thames Police Court to provide applicants with information on how to go about making a statement of conscientious objection.[64] The NAVL published two pamphlets in 1898 explaining that applicants should apply at the nearest police court, stating that they "conscientiously believe that vaccination would be prejudicial to the health of the child. . . . [C]onfine yourself to this form of words, and decline to be drawn into an argument with the Magistrates." Anti-vaccinationists were particular about these points. "Stick tight to the words of the Act," they cautioned. *The Star*, which was sympathetic to the campaign and well aware of the abuse often heaped on conscientious objectors, warned parents to answer only certain questions. All others were to be met with the firm statement, "THAT IS NOT IN THE ACT."[65]

Magistrates often objected to these tactics. One applicant was turned away from a police court, a magistrate claimed, precisely because he had been coached by the newspapers. If one is told exactly what to say, the magistrate implied, then the honesty and sincerity of the declaration is open to question. Since magistrates often denied the conscientiousness of personal statements made by those unused to speaking before the court, applicants for exemption certificates often fell back on the advice of the anti-vaccination press and made uniform declarations. Either way, it was a gamble, for some magistrates were put off by those who parroted the act, and others by long-winded personal stories.

The behavior of magistrates toward predominantly working-class applicants prompted many conscientious objectors to petition the Home Office, complaining of unfair treatment. By 1904, the Home Office had received about 500 complaints against justices and magistrates who refused to grant certificates to those claiming to be conscientious objectors. Concerned with promoting equality under the law, the Home Office issued memoranda in 1904 and 1906 in an attempt to encourage greater uniformity among magistrates in the evaluation of conscientious objectors. The issue at stake, the Home Office maintained, was whether the applicant had an "honest conscientious belief" that vaccination would, as the act stated, be "prejudicial to the health of the child," whether or not this position was "reasonably founded."[66] Conscientious objectors, the Home Office insisted, did not require a doctor's certificate stating the child was unfit for vaccination. Applicants' knowledge or ignorance of medical, sanitary, or statistical matters was equally irrelevant. The key point of clarification was that the magistrate did not himself have to agree with the applicant's position as long as the declaration was sincere.

The 1907 Vaccination Act

The problems raised by the implementation of the 1898 act convinced those on both sides of the vaccination question that the first conscience clause seemed to have failed in its objective. Before the bill was passed, the Oldham Chronicle warned that it would not quash resistance but, instead, place the anti-vaccinator in a "position of permanent rebellion."[67] By the turn of the century, it had become clear that the conscience clause had not "mitigated in any way the opposition of anti-vaccinators."[68] Defaulters continued to be prosecuted, and earlier forms of resistance—such as moving or giving false addresses on the registration of birth—persisted. Indeed, in the first year of the 1898 act, only 3.5 percent of births were registered as conscientious objectors. Many anti-vaccinationists argued that paying for a certificate still amounted to a fine for not vaccinating one's children, thus leaving the situation for working people largely unchanged. Indeed, the conscience clause was a form of economic discrimination, according to some agitators, for if a laborer in a country district "wishes to apply for an exemption, he will have to buy a railway ticket, costing, say 2 [shillings]," noted the Liberal M P Arnold Lupton. "He will have to take with him a copy of the birth certificate of his child, costing, say 3 [shillings] 6 [pence]. He must pay the magistrate's clerk's fee, say, 3 [shillings]. He must lose a day's wage, say 2 [shillings] 6 [pence]; making a total cost of 11 [shillings]. How can a poor labourer on 15 [shillings] a week afford such a large sum? And is he likely to make that sacrifice when he knows that there is a strong likelihood of his being refused, when he will come home, without the exemption having lost 8 [shillings] of very hardly earned money?" As it stands, concluded Lupton, the law "gives exemption to the rich and denies it to the poor."[69] In effect, rather than removing the martyrdom produced by fining and imprisonment, the 1898 conscience clause produced a whole new kind of resister: those refused conscientious-objector status. A Home Office circular of 1906 specifically stated that magistrates' misinterpretation of the act had actually "caused the friction which the provisions for exemption were designed to remove."[70]

THE LIBERAL PARTY AND THE STATUTORY DECLARATION   Despite this argument, it was not until the anti-vaccination movement again exercised its political might that any change in vaccination legislation was undertaken. In the 1906 general election, Lupton, who appeared in court in person to defend anti-vaccinators, defeated Henry Chaplin in Lincolnshire.[71] Lupton then persuaded 174 M PS to sign a petition demanding the entire repeal of the vaccination acts. He suggested that many M PS owed their seats to the anti-vaccination vote and warned that, if the government did not act now, it would "go hard with the Liberal Party at the next election."[72] Indeed, the sweeping Liberal victory in 1906 encouraged anti-vaccinationists to pressure the government for total repeal of the compulsory clauses. At the same time, they cautioned agitators against lobbying for a reformed conscience clause. "The Acts will never be repealed so long as we encourage the government to tinker with them," argued a correspondent to *The Individualist*.[73] Once again, the government responded with a compromise rather than with the longed-for abolition of the vaccination acts. It opted for a bill introduced by John Burns, a working-class M P, anti-vaccinator, and newly appointed president of the Local Government Board, that changed only the procedure for obtaining certificates of exemption.

There was relatively little debate in Parliament over the proposition to substitute a statutory declaration for the satisfying of magistrates. Sir Walter Foster, who declared himself to be the "parent in this House of the conscientious objectors—a family which had grown up in the country and had been despitefully used by various Governments and by magistrates," reminded the House of Commons of the turmoil he had predicted in 1898 would occur if the word *satisfy* remained in the act. He and others argued that conscientious objectors had routinely been treated as "quasi-criminals" in the courts and "mulcted of half-a-day's work as well as fees" only to be treated with "contempt"; a statutory declaration would remedy the uneven enforcement of the 1898 act, Foster declared.[74] Although fervent anti-vaccinationists actively lobbied against the bill, seeking instead the repeal of the compulsory clauses, the bill passed. For it served as the perfect political compromise, attempting to satisfy those who maintained the need for compulsory laws and those who decried the treatment of conscientious objectors in the courts.

The new act no longer required the applicant to "satisfy" magistrates. Instead, a parent could obtain the certificate on declaring a conscientious objection to vaccination because it would be prejudicial to the health of the child, without being either questioned or refused. Although one father penned his statement of conscientious objection directly on a vaccination officer's postcard urging him to vaccinate his child (see Figure 11), the government required these statements to be made before a magistrate, a justice of the peace, or a commissioner of oaths. The amount that could be charged for a certificate was also limited to 1–2 shillings; justices of the peace, however, were not supposed to charge anything at all. Although fervent anti-vaccinators continued to protest the new law, the passage of the legislation proved a significant social move, for it acknowledged, in a highly public and legal way, that working-class people could also have a moral life and could make conscientious choices. The new conscience clause effectively

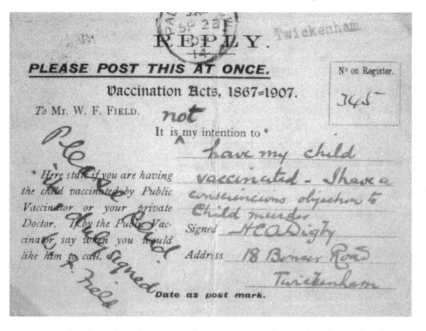

11. Conscientious objection postcard, 1909. *By permission of Denis Vandervelde.*

eradicated class-based biases in the granting of exemptions. However, it provoked new debates about women's role in conscientious objection.

GENDER AND THE CONSCIENCE   While the act resolved one question of equity, it generated another. The willingness of most anti-vaccinators to obtain certificates of exemption curbed accusations that they
were irresponsible parents and bad citizens whose neglect necessitated
state intervention. The new objection raised, however, was that the
wrong parent—namely, the mother—was taking responsibility for such
an important decision. The 1898 act, noted the legal textbook *Fry's Law
of Vaccination*, contained no definition of the word *parent*. By the time
the 1867 act came into force, *Fry's Law* pointed out, the word *parent*
could mean the mother or father of a legitimate child or the mother of
an illegitimate child. According to the 1871 act, the term *parent* referred
to anyone who had custody of the child. It was the father, *Fry's Law*
reasoned, who had custody of the legitimate child, and thus it was he,
not his wife, who must attend to apply for a certificate of exemption.[75]

Conservative politicians who supported compulsory vaccination were outraged at the suggestion that a mother could claim a certificate, for it meant that the child was in her custody. In debates over the 1898 Vaccination Bill, Chaplin had proclaimed that either the father or the mother, whoever had custody of the child, could claim a certificate of conscientious objection. After the passage of the act, the Law Officers of the Crown released a confidential circular specifying that under "ordinary circumstances the father is the only person who can obtain a certificate of conscientious objection. The child is in his custody, not in that of the mother."[76] Anti-vaccinators maintained that this was a ludicrous interpretation of the act. The word *parent* used in relationship to procuring vaccination, they argued, "clearly means 'mother,' " so why should it mean something different in regards to conscientious objection? (See Figure 12.)[77] *Punch*, which was otherwise unsympathetic to the anti-vaccination cause, appeared to agree. In 1901, it quipped: "It seems to ordinary wits / A mother to her son / Is bound to be a parent. It's / Apparent she is none."[78]

Because the act was vague and left the gender identity of the parent undefined, local courts made their own decisions. In some places, women applying for certificates were sent away with the explanation that the father must make the application. In others, mothers were readily accepted as conscientious objectors and appeared in court for exemptions, just as they had when summoned for prosecution. At Keighley in 1898, 95 percent of applicants reportedly were women.[79] This inconsistency sparked some public debate initially at the local level. By the early twentieth century, it proved a divisive issue in the Houses of Parliament. In 1905 and 1906, several M Ps introduced bills proposing that the law be revised to specify that either parent could apply for an exemption. In an anonymous minute, however, it was suggested to the Home Office that it be made clear that in ordinary circumstances only the father could make the statutory declaration. As many parliamentarians maintained, it was a universal proposition of English law that the father be primarily responsible for his child. As the legal guardian, they argued, it was the father's decision to vaccinate or not.[80]

The social questions raised by the conscience clause were contentious. Although the father might be the legal guardian of the child, as

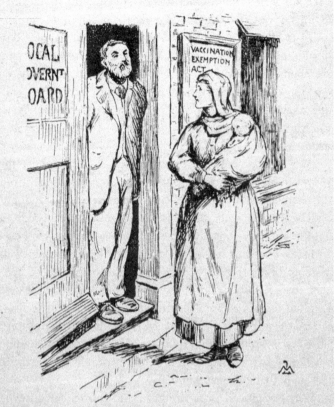

RIGHTS OF WOMEN.

Mother. "Please, Mr. Burns, my baby ain't fit to be vaccinated."

John Burns. "No good for you to come here. Where's your husband?"

Mother. "At sea."

John Burns. "Well, be off with you, mothers don't count as parents."

Printed and Published by the Artists' Suffrage League, 259, King's Road, Chelsea.

12. "Rights of Women," c. 1907. *By permission of the Mary Evans Picture Library and the Women's Library, London.*

one MP suggested, the mother was responsible for the health of the child; thus, it was she who should make the declaration. Mothers were the primary caregivers in most families and generally assumed responsibility for the well-being of the children. It therefore seemed natural to many Liberal and Labour MPs for women to obtain either the vaccination of the child or the exemption certificate. It was also easier for women to apply for exemptions, they argued, for they were not forced to sacrifice a day of work to journey to court.[81] Indeed, it was generally women who appeared in court for violations of the Compulsory Education Acts.[82] The family structure of working people meant that this type of responsibility was usually and appropriately invested in the mother.

Although he was an anti-vaccinator, Burns, as instigator of the 1907 bill, advised that it would be "unwise and bad law and injudicious" to accept the mother as a parent for the purposes of conscientious objection. He reasoned that the most "reverential figure" of the new mother should not be "impose[d]" on so soon after the birth of her child. Women were not physically fit to travel in this condition, he assumed, and should remain at home to care for the infant. Burns also maintained that women should be denied the ability to claim a certificate because it was wrong for the "indifferent or the lazy man to impose on his wife" his own "elementary duty." We must not "sub-let the duty of fathers to mothers," he cautioned.[83]

Burns, an engineer, trade unionist, and former socialist, became president of the Local Government Board in a Liberal cabinet. Significantly, he allied himself to the infant-welfare movement, contending that lowering child mortality was dependent on good mothering; on that basis, he opposed the right of married women to work.[84] As a labor leader, he was in favor of the family wage—hence, his assertion of separate spheres even within a working-class home. Implicit in Burns's position regarding women as applicants for certificates of exemption was both a critique of the working-class husband for allowing his wife to assume his own social role and a suggestion that women belonged at home with children, not in courtrooms staking political rights to conscientious-objector status. Women, he implied, were biological and domestic rather than intellectual and political creatures. It was inappropriate (and perhaps impossible) for them to make conscientious choices.

The debate over women's role in conscientious objection spilled out into the daily and national press, where anti-vaccinationists lobbied fervently for an inclusive interpretation of the word *parent*. An open letter to Burns from Jay Aitchbee, a "professed anti-vaccinator," published in the weekly political, social, and satirical newspaper *Daylight* is typical of the moral outrage Burns's position provoked. Aitchbee attacked Burns for claiming that men who permitted their wives to appear before the magistrates were lazy and indifferent. Men, he argued, worked during the hours when it was convenient for magistrates to hear applications; women generally did not. Burns's sentimentalized worship of childbearing women and his denigration of fathers were patently disingenuous, the letter continued. "[A] man may be as disinterested as you please, so far as the welfare of his family is concerned, and delegate his authority to his wife, except upon this one particular point, and then he is allowed to remain top-dog."[85] Anti-vaccinationists themselves recognized that the issues of class and gender were intimately connected. In evaluating which parent was fit to make a statement of conscientious objection, Aitchbee maintained, Burns also attempted to reorganize gender relations and the division of labor within working-class homes.

The amendment to allow women to claim certificates was passed by a narrow margin of two votes in a Standing Committee, with Burns voting against it. However, to push the new conscience clause through Parliament without further delay, the Liberal-dominated House of Commons eventually agreed to a House of Lords amendment that replaced the words *either parent* with *he*. This meant that only the father could make a statutory declaration.[86] Despite this compromise, the 1907 act inexplicably retained the term *parent* rather than *father*, as did the new Vaccination Order that accompanied it. In effect, this ambiguity left the situation unaltered until the following year, when, in response to a vaccination officer's query, the *Local Government Chronicle* declared the mother to be a parent within the meanings of the act and thus eligible to apply for an exemption.[87] As a result of this interpretation of the new legislation, the first widely acknowledged conscientious objectors were not only predominantly working class but also often female.

The Aftermath of the Act

As it became easier for working-class anti-vaccinators to "opt out" of the compulsory system, many chose to do so regardless of any stigma that might have been attached to what some considered licensed lawbreaking. In the first four years of the new act, only 56.3 percent of births were vaccinated, while the conscientious objections had grown to 25 percent.[88] The Registrar General's reports indicate that the actual number of certificates of conscientious objection almost tripled directly after the passage of the 1907 legislation.[89] In some districts, after 1907, even prosecutions for default had come to an end. By 1907, vaccination was no longer compulsory for all intents and purposes, as anyone could obtain a certificate of exemption on making a statutory declaration. While this still involved some effort and at times a nominal fee, it was no more problematic than taking the child to be vaccinated, which seemed a fair enough manner of establishing legitimate objections.

Securing conscientious-objector status on a secular basis for women and workers was a significant social and political achievement of the anti-vaccination campaign. In allowing all citizens the right to appeal to their consciences, the 1907 act challenged the primacy of the middle-class man as the model of individual subjectivity. World War I, however, reworked the classed and gendered nature of the conscientious objector. While women were heavily involved with the pacifist movement and engaged in acts of civil disobedience, the "conchie" who resisted conscription (which was limited to male soldiers) was by definition male. The No-Conscription Fellowship was heavily identified and allied with the Independent Labour Party, whose constituency was overwhelmingly working-class. But despite the large number of socialists who protested the war, the issue of conscientious objection created deep divisions within working-class culture, and, in the end, Independent Labour Party soldiers outnumbered objectors.[90] Working-class proponents of compulsory vaccination were few and far between, and there is no evidence that any resisted the legalization of conscientious objection to vaccination. In contrast, many working-class soldiers deeply resented the conscientious objector to military service who, despite his often plebeian roots, was frequently depicted as the effete upper-class sissy epitomized by the intellectuals and pacifists of the Bloomsbury Group.[91]

Anti-vaccinationists provided an obvious but contentious legal precedent for conscientious objection to the Military Service Act of 1916. The
government eventually adopted the phrase *conscientious objection* in relation to military service largely because it was already a familiar term,
legally in play since 1898 and more widely associated with the anti-
vaccination movement since at least the 1870s. Thanks in part to the
precedent set by anti-vaccinationists, conscientious objectors to military
service could stake their claim on moral as well as religious grounds.
About 16 percent of conscientious objectors called before the tribunal
responsible for advising on work of national importance claimed to be
either moral or political, rather than religious, conscientious objectors.
It is estimated that moral or political objectors actually outnumbered
the purely religious objectors three to one.[92]

The government, however, returned to methods of evaluating conscientious objectors that the experience of compulsory vaccination had
already proved both offensive and untenable. Anti-conscriptionists in
Parliament pointed to the procedure delineated in the 1907 Vaccination
Act as an example of an effective means of separating shirkers from
legitimate objectors.[93] Nevertheless, the government eventually adopted
a tribunal system similar to that outlined in the largely ineffectual, and
heavily criticized, Vaccination Act of 1898. Walter Long, Conservative
president of the Local Government Board from 1915 to 1916 and the
official in charge of managing the terms of exemptions from military
service, had also headed the Local Government Board from 1900 to 1905
and thus had been responsible for the administration of the first vaccination conscience clause. He defended the actions of magistrates under
the 1898 act that he himself had overseen and promoted the tribunal as
an effective means of weeding out malingerers. The tribunals were
therefore instituted by a man who was intimately familiar with, and yet
undisturbed by, the complete lack of uniformity that had already been
demonstrated by the local and thus inconsistent administration of a
conscience clause. In many respects, then, the administration of conscientious objection to military service self-consciously recapitulated the
terms of the first vaccination conscience clause. This effectively reversed
the Liberal decision to allow statutory declarations in matters of conscience. It returned to a Conservative policy that retained state control
over the meanings of conscientious convictions and, thus, access to
conscientious-objector status.

Conclusion

☞ In a letter to *The Individualist* in 1906, an anti-vaccinator foretold the decline of the movement once conscientious-objector status became readily available. Accepting "half-measures," he argued, "takes the backbone out of the movement and prolongs the life of the evil we are combating, while the use of a Conscience Clause makes any tyranny possible by removing the very man who would fight the oppressor."[1] Conscientious objectors would no longer agitate once they had ceased to be threatened with prosecution, and some of the most fervent and committed anti-vaccinationists, he warned, would be the first to defect from the campaign. Allowing for conscientious objection in effect meant the end of a cohesive movement.

As the 1907 bill was being debated in Parliament, John Brown declared it to be "a very insignificant measure." Indeed, he concluded, "it could not well be smaller."[2] In fact, the reformed conscience clause created severe divisions within the movement, which contributed to its ultimate demise. The "considerable amount of diversity" encountered from different branch leagues regarding the reformulated conscience clause spelled disaster for a unified movement as it opened up fissures in what had once been common ground.[3]

Libertarians and defenders of personal rights remained committed to the anti-vaccination movement because they considered the 1907 act a failure. If the new conscience clause is passed, warned the secretary of the Personal Rights Association, then the anti-vaccination campaign would have "been fought *and lost*."[4] Many working people, however, gladly accepted the concession, obtained their certificates, and ceased to agitate, disenchanted perhaps with the attitude of extremists who refused to concede the benefits of conscientious-objector status to those who suffered financially under the strain of repeated fining. Organized

anti-vaccinationism took the middle ground and accepted the new conscience clause as "an installment toward unconditional liberty." Fearing
dissent within the ranks, the NAVL expressed a desire for anti-vaccinationists to unite on broad principles and to retain a broad platform.
Attempting to please all parties, the league proclaimed itself to be like
"Oliver Twist," having simply "taken what they could get, and impa-
tiently asked for more."[5]

The campaign for total repeal of the vaccination acts declined as the
numbers of conscientious objectors grew each year. By early 1908,
support for the movement was waning precisely because obtaining
exemptions had silenced most of the working-class population that had
provided popular support for the campaign. In March of that year, the
Vaccination Inquirer reported on the parliamentary progress made to
date but admitted that there would now be a "momentary pause," as
anti-vaccinationists were prepared to "stand aside for a little" to allow
other popular grievances to be redressed. In October, the future of the
NAVL was clearly in doubt, as it was patent that many had abandoned
the movement. Those left were uncertain whether they should remain
actively on the offensive or should retreat to a more "watchful and
defensive" stance.[6]

The *Vaccination Inquirer* increasingly began to report on international, Scottish, and Irish news, as the English campaign became less
vibrant and less newsworthy. The *British Medical Journal* noted what it
called the "funeral dirge" tone of the NAVL and reported skirmishes
within the movement. In October, the journal gleefully printed an article on the "The Passing of the Anti-Vaccination League," proclaiming
that "old members are doubtlessly fleeing the sinking ship."[7] In 1909,
the annual meeting of the NAVL witnessed diminished attendance, and
John Bonner, its paid lecturer, announced his retirement.[8] The general
election of 1910 was not as favorable to anti-vaccinators as the previous
one had been. By this time, the movement, along with its prominent
leaders, was largely dead.

Despite its rapid decline in the years after the conscience clause was
passed, the NAVL remained in operation through the 1970s and in this
later period could still claim over 1,000 members.[9] This must be cred-
ited in large part to its secretary, Lily Loat, who retained her post from
1909 until her death in the late 1950s.[10] Throughout the twentieth
century, the league continued to mount campaigns against newly devel-

oped vaccines. In the late 1940s, it even lobbied the United Nations to include the right to refuse vaccination in the charter of human rights.[11] In its last three decades, however, the NAVL focused most of its efforts on helping British travelers circumvent the immunization requirements of other countries. When it received a legacy of 100,000 pounds from a Mrs. Howey in the mid-1970s, the NAVL dissolved to form the Howey Foundation, a wide-ranging environmental agency that remained in operation until 1982, when it folded by mutual decision of its board.[12] After more than 100 years of agitation, the anti-vaccination movement had officially collapsed.

By the end of the twentieth century organized anti-vaccinationism had ceased to pose a threat to the public's health. So, too, had smallpox. After a relationship with humans that lasted over 2,000 years, the last naturally occurring case of *Variola major* was diagnosed on 16 October 1975, on a small island off the coast of Bangladesh. The child survived; the disease did not, falling victim to the World Health Organization's vigorous Smallpox Eradication Program.[13] In 1980, the Thirty-third World Health Assembly accepted the final report of the Global Commission for the Certification of Smallpox Eradication, which proclaimed the disease exterminated from all corners of the globe.[14] Smallpox was dead.

While the complete eradication of smallpox has provided many with an appropriately celebratory end to the triumphant narrative of vaccination, the means by which this eradication was achieved has received little critical attention. Vaccinations were often performed by zealous American epidemiologists from the Centers for Disease Control, at times against the will of the population. A senior World Health Organization physician and epidemiologist maintained that the initial stage of efforts to contain smallpox was marked "by an almost military style attack on infected villages":

> In the hit-and-run excitement of such a campaign, women and children were often pulled out from under beds, from behind doors, from within latrines, etc. People were chased and, when caught, vaccinated. . . . We considered the villagers to have an understandable though irrational fear of vaccination. . . . We just couldn't let people get smallpox and die needlessly. We went from door to door and vaccinated. When they ran, we chased. When they locked their doors, we broke down their doors and vaccinated them.[15]

While Victorian children were only rarely vaccinated against the will of their parents, the assumptions that underlay the nineteenth-century vaccination acts lived on at the end of the twentieth century in "global health" policies. Just as the state enforcement of smallpox vaccination in England targeted mainly the poor and working classes, who were often coerced into the procedure, the Smallpox Eradication Program in action implied that some people's consent to vaccination—in this case, inhabitants of the "Third World"—was less important than that of others.[16]

The tactics of coercion and manipulation are still evident in immunization programs in inner-city America. In Baltimore in 1998, public-health workers conducted a door-to-door campaign to promote immunization among "stubborn cases" of noncompliance: "poor, transient single mothers." "Like detectives, they knock on doors of hundreds of Baltimore families," reported the *Baltimore Sun*, "leave notes when no one answers, and coax their way in when someone does." These mothers responded to these tactics in ways reminiscent of their Victorian counterparts: They associated these public-health workers with the Department of Social Services and were highly suspicious of their intentions. Those who accepted the proffered vaccinations were lauded as model mothers. "It did me good," declared one mother of five intent on finding a "decent home" and a job, reported the *Sun*.[17] In Chicago, the relationship between welfare and immunization has been cemented rather than discouraged. A 1996 initiative required that the parents of unvaccinated children report to local authorities monthly to receive their food vouchers rather than quarterly, as is the norm. During these visits, health workers inform the parents of the dangers of leaving a child unvaccinated and at times provide free shots in the same office. Only once their children are immunized can the parents return to the quarterly distribution system. This is the first time that local immunization efforts have been linked to federal food-distribution programs.[18]

While these initiatives are an attempt to address the problems of what public-health officials see as widespread neglect rather than active resistance, anti-vaccinationism is again on the rise in Britain and North America within both the military and the civilian sectors. In an age preoccupied no longer with nuclear war but with the threat of a "biological event," smallpox has appeared in a new role: as bio-weapon. Whether the Russians have the deadly virus locked away in a freezer, and whether terrorists and "rogue states" have gained access to it, strikes fear into the hearts of Western governments. For the great irony of smallpox today is that its successful eradication has led humans to lose their immunity to the disease and thus to become vulnerable to its ravages once more.[19] Compulsory vaccination has thus re-emerged as an issue, particularly within the military, whose soldiers are most at risk of biological attack, and the health-care community, since medical personnel are most likely to have contact with the first wave of infected persons. But because much of the stored vaccine has now expired, and the potential side effects of smallpox vaccination remain a concern, the issue proves contentious. The tensions between government agencies and local and state health authorities regarding the need for a large-scale vaccination campaign are palpable and underscore the lack of a coherent national program. Indeed, the director of the Centers for Disease Control in Atlanta has declared that the question of mass vaccination is ultimately a state, rather than a federal, decision.[20]

The U.S. government's uneasiness about mandating smallpox vaccination even for key players in the "war on terrorism" stems in part from the negative publicity generated around the anthrax vaccine. That vaccine has caused side effects in a significant minority of those exposed to it, resulting in many members of the military refusing the required shot. The Canadian and American armed forces have responded by initiating disciplinary action against several individuals who have refused to be vaccinated against anthrax for fear of adverse reactions. This type of coercion prompted one Canadian seaman to proclaim, in language that echoed nineteenth-century polemics: "I will never be able to trust my leaders or their politics again, as they have violated my trust and body."[21]

In the late-twentieth and early-twenty-first centuries, a range of fears about the safety and efficacy of vaccination have surfaced, not only in relation to vaccination against diseases that can be used as biological weapons, but also in relation to routine childhood immunization. Anxieties over the safety of the mumps, measles, and rubella (MMR) vaccine has provoked widespread concern in Britain in recent years. Prompted by research published in 1998 by Dr. Andrew Wakefield theorizing a relationship between the MMR vaccine and both autism and chronic bowel conditions, British parents have once again mounted a vigorous campaign against childhood immunization. Groups such as Justice Awareness and Basic Support, or JABS, and The Informed Parent have formed to educate parents about the risks inherent in all vaccines and to provide support to those whose children have allegedly been injured by immunization. While Prime Minister Tony Blair has dismissed the dissemination of this type of material as scaremongering, he also declined to participate personally in the debate, refusing to divulge whether his own newborn was vaccinated with MMR.

This new vaccination controversy has led to a public-health crisis in the United Kingdom as MMR immunization rates have dropped from 93 percent to 87 percent.[22] In large metropolitan areas, the rates may be as low as 80 percent, 15 percent below that required to produce "herd immunity," which protects those too vulnerable to be vaccinated themselves. The government has responded to the alarmingly low rates of immunization by launching its own scientific investigations into Wakefield's research and by mounting a pro-vaccination education campaign, insisting that MMR is safe—indeed, that it is much safer than the single vaccines that many parents are calling for. This campaign has been largely unsuccessful, however, due to profound distrust of the government's motives: Britain's National Health Service is in crisis, and reducing spending on health care is a parliamentary priority. Many parents who left comments at an interactive display at London's Science Museum titled "The MMR Files" criticized the government's reaction to their concerns. "We are told it's safe," one father wrote, "but can you trust central government to tell the truth and not just issue their chosen version of what is true and safe?" While the exhibit aimed to provide a neutral forum for discussing the MMR issue, its bias was clear. A video-game component of the display, presumably aimed at children, required the player to vaccinate as many babies as possible by touching the screen before they died of measles.

The concerns of parents today echo those of their Victorian ancestors. As Elaine Showalter has demonstrated, the fears and fantasies of the nineteenth-century fin de siècle have played out in strikingly familiar ways at the turn of the twenty-first century.[23] A study of English-language anti-vaccination websites published in the *Journal of the American Medical Association* in 2002 reveals that the three major themes of present-day anti-vaccinationists—that vaccines are unsafe and ineffective, that the government is abusing its power, and that alternative health practices are preferable[24]—are little different from the dominant concerns of the nineteenth-century campaign. Contemporary anti-vaccinators consistently maintain that enforced vaccination violates "civil rights" and that it should be "a choice not a mandate."[25] As a former Navy cook who refused the anthrax vaccine insisted, "I didn't raise my hand and give away my civil liberties."[26] Many stress the experimental nature of vaccination. "I didn't sign up to be a guinea pig for these shots," asserted an American aircraft planner.[27] Indeed, smallpox vaccination still harbors associations with government corruption. A recurrent storyline in the immensely popular 1990s television show *The X-Files* depicted smallpox vaccination as part of a government conspiracy to brand and trace its citizens that was linked to Gulf War syndrome and, perhaps less convincingly, to a state-sponsored program for world domination by alien life forms.

While vaccination has provoked widespread shared anxieties over the course of the two centuries in which it has been practiced, contemporary debates in Britain differ from those in the Victorian period, not least because vaccination is no longer compulsory. The success of the nineteenth-century anti-vaccination movement ensured that no other immunizations were ever made compulsory for the civilian population under British law. Indeed, a Ministry of Health publicity campaign to raise diphtheria-immunization rates during and after World War II confirmed that voluntary programs emphasizing democratic engagement and responsibility to the community could be more effective than compulsion.[28] The responsibility of the individual to maintain the health of the social body, however, has waned in recent years. Resistance to vaccination in Britain today exists within the context of state-sponsored medical care. Those who refuse vaccination, or request single shots, lobby from a position that views health care as an entitlement and that assumes that all citizens have a right to demand services that they themselves deem appropriate, regardless of their impact on the public's health or the economy. Although the democratization of access to medical care has not always encouraged the public to consume scarce medical resources responsibly, it is nevertheless one of the great achievements of the modern British state. The public's expectation that the government will provide for the health of the people reveals how profoundly the relationship between the state and its citizens has shifted, particularly in relation to care of the body, since World War II.

While some historians have positioned the National Health Service as the direct descendant of the medical services of the New Poor Law,[29] the Labour initiatives of the post–World War II era dramatically reformulated the meanings of state medicine. The National Health Service for the first time made a comprehensive package of medical services available to all citizens and enabled free choice of practitioner. At the same time, the Labour government attempted to remove the stigma attached to state medical provision by eradicating the Poor Law, returning to a system of outdoor relief. That the "cumbersome and out of date"[30] compulsory vaccination acts were repealed under the same series of legislation reveals the extent to which the postwar Labour government actively sought to distance itself from the coercive and disciplinary medical practices identified with the Poor Law. Compulsory vaccination clearly had no place in this new welfare state, which made free medical care a right without fear of pauperization.[31]

This reconfiguration of the relationship between the citizen and the state, however, was a long-term process. In an account of her 1950s working-class childhood, the historian Carolyn Steedman reveals that the first generation brought up under the National Health Service experienced the intersections of body, class, and state in very different ways from their parents, for whom state medicine retained some of its taint. Steedman distinctly remembers a health visitor, now present under the auspices of the National Health Service, shaming her mother to tears by declaring the house unfit for a baby. Steedman's mother grew up amid the political radicalism of a Lancashire weaving town. But it was this kind of state intervention in health care that helped to transform her into that not so rare breed in the postwar period: a working-class Conservative. However, for Steedman herself—who, it appears, was raised without much parental tenderness—it was precisely the state's involvement in her bodily welfare that affirmed her sense of self-worth. "I think I would be a very different person now," she contends, "if orange juice and milk and dinners at school hadn't told me, in a covert way, that I had a right to exist, was worth something."[32] This new kind of state medicine held out the possibility that, instead of stigmatizing, it could instill a sense of self. In this way, whatever its shortcomings, the National Health Service emerged as a direct reaction against the coercive corporeal policies that compulsory vaccination had epitomized and that nineteenth- and early-twentieth-century anti-vaccinationists had helped to dismantle.

Notes

INTRODUCTION

1 *The Times*, 14 August 1876, 7, 15 August 1876, 4, 18 November 1876, 9.
2 Ibid., 18 November 1876, 9; Beck, "Issues in the Anti-Vaccination Movement in England"; MacLeod, "Law, Medicine and Public Opinion"; Porter and Porter, "The Politics of Prevention"; Lambert, "A Victorian National Health Service"; Williams, "The Implementation of Compulsory Infant Smallpox Vaccination."
3 Poovey, *A History of the Modern Fact*, 307–28.
4 Gibbs, *Fortification by Disease and Its Effect on Infant Life*, 8.
5 Walsh, *The Medical Officer's Vade-Mecum or Poor Law Surgeon's Guide*, 64; *Report of the Medical Officer of the Privy Council, 1858*, app. 1.
6 For a non-Western perspective on this issue, see White, "The Needle and the State," 6.
7 Baldwin, *Contagion and the State in Europe, 1830–1930*, 273–316; Huerkamp, "The History of Smallpox Vaccination in Germany"; Nelson and Rogers, "The Right to Die?"; Hennock, "Vaccination Policy Against Smallpox, 1835–1914"; Arnup, " 'Victims of Vaccination?' "; Leavitt, "Politics and Public Health"; Kaufman, "The American Anti-Vaccinationists and Their Arguments."
8 Arnold, *Colonizing the Body*.
9 White, " 'They Could Make Their Victims Dull.' "
10 McKiernan, "Fevered Measures."
11 Meade, " 'Civilizing Rio de Janeiro.' "
12 Hadwen, *The Case Against Vaccination*, 5.
13 Hall et al., *Defining the Victorian Nation*.
14 Foucault, *The Birth of the Clinic*, *Discipline and Punish*, and *The History of Sexuality: An Introduction*.
15 Hamlin, *Public Health and Social Justice in the Age of Chadwick*, 17.
16 Arnold, *Colonizing the Body*, 7–8. For recent studies of the imperial body-state relationship, see also Vaughan, *Curing Their Ills*; Burke, *Lifebuoy Men, Lux Women*; Comaroff, "The Diseased Heart of Africa"; Pedersen, "National Bodies and Unspeakable Acts."

17 *National Anti-Compulsory Vaccination Reporter*, 1 July 1882, 165.

18 Carroll, "Medical Police and the History of Public Health"; Porter and Porter, "The Enforcement of Health."

19 These vaccination acts applied only to England and Wales; separate and considerably less stringent vaccination acts existed for Scotland and Ireland, which are beyond the scope of this book. On public vaccination in Ireland, see Brunton, "The Problems of Implementation."

20 *The Times*, 21 January 1859, 8.

21 Holmes, *A Letter on Vaccination*, 1.

22 On the revolution in government, see MacDonagh, "The Nineteenth-Century Revolution in Government"; MacLeod, *Government and Expertise.*

23 Mooney, " 'A Tissue of the Most Flagrant Anomalies,' " 263.

24 Burney, *Bodies of Evidence*, 1.

25 General Register Office Smallpox Vaccination Returns, PRO RG 56/3; Swan, *The Vaccination Problem*, 85; see also the Local Government Board Annual Reports and their supplements for the years from 1908 to World War I.

CHAPTER ONE: THE PARLIAMENTARY LANCET

1 Gibbs, *Our Medical Liberties*, 9.

2 Ibid., 35.

3 Porter, *Health for Sale*; Jewson, "Medical Knowledge and the Patronage System in Eighteenth Century England."

4 Loudon, *Medical Care and the General Practitioner, 1750–1850*; Digby, *Making a Medical Living.*

5 Porter, *Health for Sale*, 26–31.

6 Reader, *Professional Men*, 16.

7 Waddington, "General Practitioners and Consultants in Early Nineteenth Century England."

8 Richardson, *Death, Dissection and the Destitute*; Laqueur, "Bodies, Death, and Pauper Funerals."

9 Richardson, *Death, Dissection and the Destitute*, 266.

10 Ibid., xvi.

11 Crowther, *The Workhouse System 1834–1929*, 31–34.

12 Digby, *Pauper Palaces*, 220.

13 Hodgkinson, *The Origins of the National Health Service*, 15, 269.

14 Waddington, *The Medical Profession in the Industrial Revolution.*

15 Peterson, *The Medical Profession in Mid-Victorian London.*

16 Lambert, "A Victorian National Health Service," 1.

17 John Simon, as quoted in Wohl, *Endangered Lives*, 150.

18 Hamlin, *Public Health and Social Justice in the Age of Chadwick*, 288.

19 Mort, *Dangerous Sexualities*.

20 Lambert, *Sir John Simon 1816–1904 and English Social Administration*, 299.

21 *Associated Medical Journal*, 19 August 1853, 718.

22 Brunton, "Pox Britannica."

23 Langdon, *The Life of Roger Langdon*, 14–21.

24 Sanger, *Seventy Years a Showman*, 56–57.

25 *Report of the Section Appointed to Enquire into the Present State of Vaccination*, 29.

26 Ibid., 22.

27 Ibid., 3, 29.

28 Bashford, "Foreign Bodies," 41.

29 *Report of the Section Appointed to Enquire into the Present State of Vaccination*, 29.

30 Smith, *The People's Health, 1830–1910*, 161–62.

31 *Letter from Dr. Edward Seaton to Viscount Palmerston*, 21.

32 *Report on the State of Small-Pox and Vaccination*, 24.

33 Epidemiological Society of London, *The Commemoration Volume*, 7.

34 Hardy, "Smallpox in London."

35 Lambert, *Sir John Simon 1816–1904 and English Social Administration*, 618.

36 As quoted in Mort, *Dangerous Sexualities*, 28.

37 John Snow's famous isolation of contaminated water as the source of a local cholera epidemic was first published in 1849, but his further experiments with the Broad Street water pump were not formulated until 1854. Even then, Snow's ideas were not wholly embraced and took decades to become part of accepted medical theory. See Rosen, *A History of Public Health*, 261–62.

38 *Report on the State of Small-Pox and Vaccination*, 5.

39 As quoted in Lambert, *Sir John Simon 1816–1904 and English Social Administration*, 253.

40 *Hansard*, 12 April 1853, 1002.

41 Ibid., 4 April 1853, 518.

42 Seaton, *On the Protective and Modifying Powers of Vaccination*, 25; *Papers Relating to the History and Practice of Vaccination*, lxx; *Hansard*, 20 July 1853, 473.

43 *Associated Medical Journal*, 15 April 1853, 314, 28 October 1853, 950–51, 9 December 1853, 1093, 27 January 1854, 93; *The Lancet*, 21 May 1853, 476.

44 As noted in John Simon's report published in *Papers Relating to the History and Practice of Vaccination*, lxxvi.

45 *The Lancet*, 28 May 1853, 503. Simon confirmed this in his report: see *Papers Relating to the History and Practice of Vaccination*.

46 Dr. Watts to Poor Law Board, letter, 9 November 1853, PRO MH 12/13963/40656/528; Clerk of Derby Union to Dr. Watts, letter, 27 December 1853, PRO MH 12/13963/47046/528; Joseph Ashbury Smith to Poor Law Board, letter, 12 January 1854, PRO MH 12/2023/1599/73.

47 *Papers Relating to the History and Practice of Vaccination*, app. G, 25.

48 Rees, "Water as a Commodity"; Nicholls, *Homeopathy and the Medical Profession*; Winter, *Mesmerized*; Barrow, "Why Were Most Medical Heretics at Their Most Confident around the 1840s?" 165; Miley and Pickstone, "Medical Botany around 1850," 145; Harrison, "Early Victorian Radicals and the Medical Fringe," 199.

49 Brown, "Social Context and Medical Theory in the Demarcation of Nineteenth-Century Boundaries."

50 Barrow, "Why Were Most Medical Heretics at Their Most Confident around the 1840s?" 166–68.

51 Barrow, *Independent Spirits*; Harrison, "Early Victorian Radicals and the Medical Fringe," 199.

52 Harrison, "Early Victorian Radicals and the Medical Fringe," 200.

53 *Dr. Skelton's Botanic Record and Family Herbal*, 1 May 1852, 1; *Hydropathic Record and Journal of the Water Cure*, January 1869, 57–58.

54 *Dr. Skelton's Botanic Record and Family Herbal*, 7 January 1854, 321, 335; emphasis in the original.

55 Ibid., 3 September 1853, 270.

56 *Botanic Eclectic Review and Medical Tribune*, May 1856, 82.

57 Warner, "Therapeutic Explanation and the Edinburgh Bloodletting Controversy," 241.

58 Coffin, *Medical Botany*, 5.

59 Ibid., 200.

60 Coffin, *Botanic Guide to Health*, xii.

61 Morison, *Morisonia*, iii–iv.

62 As quoted in Brown, "Social Context and Medical Theory in the Demarcation of Nineteenth-Century Boundaries," 220–21.

63 Barrow, *Independent Spirits*, 146–212.

64 *Dr. Skelton's Botanic Record and Family Herbal*, 3 July 1852, 35.

65 Brown, "Nineteenth-Century American Health Reformers and the Early Nature Cure Movement in Britain," 174–75.

66 Coffin, *Medical Botany*, 153.

67 Stevens, *Medical Reform*, xiii.

68 Harrison, *The Common People of Great Britain*, 271; Briggs, "Samuel Smiles."

69 Nichols, *A Woman's Work in Water Cure and Sanitary Education*, 138.

70 *Dr. Skelton's Botanic Record and Family Herbal*, 2 December 1854, 501; emphasis in the original.

71 Stevens, *Medical Reform*, xii.

72 *Family Physician or People's Medical Adviser*, February 1866, 20.

73 White, *The Story of a Great Delusion*, 580–89.

74 Gibbs, *Our Medical Liberties*, 6; emphasis in the original.

75 *Letter dated 30 June 1855*, 27.

76 *A Bill to Consolidate and to Amend the Laws Relating to Vaccination*, 513; Lambert, *Sir John Simon 1816–1904 and English Social Administration*, 256.

77 *Hansard*, 1 July 1857, 722.

78 Gibbs, *Compulsory Vaccination Briefly Considered in Its Scientific, Religious, and Political Aspects*, 23.

79 See *Hydropathic Record and Journal of the Water Cure*, May 1869, back cover.

80 *Dr. Skelton's Botanic Record and Family Herbal*, 2 September 1854, 454.

81 *Botanic Eclectic Review and Medical Tribune*, May 1856, 82.

82 See his *Eclectic Medical Journal*, published in 1858.

83 *Hygiest or Medical Reformer*, 1 January 1855, 3.

84 *Coffin's Botanical Journal and Medical Reformer*, 9 August 1856, 101.

85 *Hygiest or Medical Reformer*, 2 June 1856, 137.

86 *Vaccination as the Cause of Fever and Consumption*; Rose, *How to Cure and Prevent Small-Pox*, 4.

87 Pickering, *The Smallpox Epidemic in Gloucester and the Water Cure*; *Gloucester Journal*, 23 May 1896, 3. See also *Human Nature*, November 1867, 448, for hydropathic cures for smallpox.

CHAPTER TWO: FIGHTING THE "BABIES' BATTLE"

1 French, *Antivivisection and Medical Science in Victorian Society*; Harrison, *Drink and the Victorians*; Walkowitz, *Prostitution and Victorian Society*; MacLeod, "Law, Medicine and Public Opinion."

2 Figures for league membership are difficult to come by. In 1889, the Oldham league claimed 693 members; in 1890, the Nelson league claimed 336. At its peak in 1878, the Keighley league claimed 244 members. See *Oldham Standard*, 9 November 1889, in LSHTM, Milnes Collection, vol. 17, 26; *Nelson Chronicle*, 28 February 1890, in Milnes Collection, vol. 18, 39; Keighley and District Anti-Compulsory Vaccination League Register of Members, BK 33/6.

3 White, *The Story of a Great Delusion*, 543.

4 *Co-operator and Anti-Vaccinator*, 3 December 1870, 781, 15 April 1871, 237; *Report from the Select Committee on the Vaccination Act (1867)*, 161, Q. 2894.

5 *National Anti-Compulsory Vaccination League Occasional Circular*, February 1876, 12; *East London Observer*, 21 October 1876, 6.

6 Hume-Rothery, *What Smallpox and Vaccination and the Vaccination Acts*

Really Are, 12–13; *National Anti-Compulsory Vaccination Reporter*, 1 September 1882, 195.

7 *Anti-Vaccinator and Public Health Journal*, 1 February 1873, 314. See also *National Anti-Compulsory Vaccination Reporter*, 1 January 1878, 63, 1 March 1878, 120.

8 MacLeod, "Law, Medicine and Public Opinion," 189.

9 *British Medical Journal*, 18 December 1948, 1073.

10 *National Anti-Compulsory Vaccination Reporter*, 1 July 1878, 198, 1 February 1884, 90; *Fourth Report of the Royal Commission Appointed to Inquire into the Subject of Vaccination*, 240, Q. 15, 153; *Vaccination Inquirer*, 1 May 1888, 25, June 1886, 41; *Co-operator and Anti-Vaccinator*, 8 July 1871, 429, 19 November 1870, 744; *Anti-Vaccinator and Public Health Journal*, 15 November 1872; *The Anti-Vaccinator*, 11 September 1869, 59, 62; Hume-Rothery, *150 Reasons for Disobeying the Vaccination Law*; Vaccination Officers' Birth Books (Enfield District, Edmonton Union), LMA BG/E/166–BG/E/175; Registers of Successful Vaccination, Tewkesbury District of Tewkesbury Union, GRO TBR B62/1, B62/6–B62/8.

11 Crossick, *The Lower Middle Class in Britain*; Crossick, *An Artisan Elite in Victorian Society*; Gray, *The Labour Aristocracy in Victorian Edinburgh*; Bailey, "White Collars, Gray Lives?"

12 Edwards, *No Gold on My Shovel*, 8; Goss, "My Boyhood at the Turn of the Century," 8–9.

13 *The Month*, 454.

14 *Nineteenth Century*, June 1883, 1080.

15 Brown, *The Case for Vaccination*, 2.

16 *National Anti-Compulsory Vaccination Reporter*, 1 February 1884, 79–80.

17 Orwell, *The Road to Wigan Pier*, 147.

18 *Co-operator and Anti-Vaccinator*, 8 April 1871, 216.

19 Watson, "Autobiography," Tameside Local Studies Library.

20 Turner, *About Myself 1863–1930*.

21 Vaccination Officers' Birth Books (Enfield District, Edmonton Union), LMA BG/E/166–BG/E/175.

22 *Vaccination Inquirer*, October 1885, 119; *Leicester Daily Mercury*, 23 March 1885, 3.

23 *Vaccination Inquirer*, 1 January 1904, 199.

24 Pickstone, "Establishment and Dissent in Nineteenth-Century Medicine, 165–89.

25 *National Anti-Compulsory Vaccination Reporter*, 7 October 1880, 3; *National Anti-Compulsory Vaccination League Occasional Circular*, 1 February 1876, 12; *East London Observer*, 21 October 1876, 6; *National Anti-Compulsory Vaccination Reporter*, 1 August 1877, 2.

26 Larsen, *Friends of Religious Equality*.

27 Register of Successful Vaccination, Tewkesbury District, Tewkesbury Union, TBR B62/6; Vaccination Officers' Birth Books (Enfield District, Edmonton Union), LMA BG/E/166, BG/E/173; Paul, *The Vaccination Problem in 1903*, 28; *Vaccination Inquirer*, March 1885, 234; *Co-operator and Anti-Vaccinator*, 27 May 1871, 323.

28 *The Anti-Vaccinator*, 25 September 1869, 85; *National Anti-Compulsory Vaccination Reporter*, 1 April 1882, 122; *Vaccination Inquirer*, May 1884, 22, 1 July 1907, 71; *Co-operator and Anti-Vaccinator*, 1 July 1871, 409; *Vaccination Inquirer*, 1 May 1887, 31, 1 November 1887, 139, 1 January 1902, 190.

29 *Personal Rights Journal*, July 1887, 70, October 1887, 84. See also the preface in Young, *Vaccination Tracts*, 30.

30 Bristow, *Vice and Vigilance*, 76.

31 Hughes, *The Rev. Hugh Price Hughes on Vaccination*.

32 Langdon, *The Life of Roger Langdon*, 18–19.

33 *Vaccination Inquirer*, February 1885, 212; Brown, *Compulsory Vaccination in Scotland*, 22.

34 For example, *Human Nature*, November 1867, 448, May 1868, 213–15; *Medium and Daybreak* 14, 1879, 43; Hunt, *Vaccination Brought Home to the People*. On spiritualism and anti-vaccination, see Barrow, *Independent Spirits*, 186–88; Owen, *The Darkened Room*, 131–32.

35 Dixon, *Divine Feminine*, 121–51.

36 For examples, see *Shafts*, 14 January 1893, 162, October 1893, 155, March 1897, 72; *Women's Penny Paper*, 7 September 1889, 6, 19 October 1889, 5; Scott, "Physical Purity Feminism and State Medicine in Late Nineteenth-Century England," 625–51.

37 *Co-operator and Anti-Vaccinator*, 13 May 1871, 297.

38 *Daylight*, 24 August 1907, 9.

39 *Vaccination Inquirer*, 1 March 1887, 188; *The Anti-Vaccinator*, 23 September 1871, 608.

40 At least 6,000 copies of the first edition of the *Anti-Vaccinator and Public Health Journal* were printed. See *Anti-Vaccinator and Public Health Journal*, 1 May 1872, 32.

41 Birmingham Anti-Variole League for the Repeal of Compulsory Vaccination, *Annual Report*, 4.

42 J. H. Lynn to A. E. Schoon, letter, 18 December 1889, Keighley Library, BK 33/17; *Fourth Report of the Royal Commission*, 209, Q. 14,347; *National Anti-Compulsory Vaccination Reporter*, 1 March 1879, 114; *Vaccination Inquirer*, November 1889, 129, 1 October 1892, 114.

43 Linkman, *The Victorians*.

44 *The Times*, 31 December 1875, 10.

45 Hart, *The Truth about Vaccination*, 1.

46 Thompson, *The Rise of Respectable Society*, 303.

47 Biggs, *Leicester*, III.

48 Ibid., 108. On Thomas Cook and temperance meetings, see Harrison, *Drink and the Victorians*, 319.

49 For a complete account of the Leicester demonstration, see Biggs, *Leicester*, chap. 25.

50 *National Anti-Compulsory Vaccination Reporter*, 1 November 1880, 32, 1 December 1876, 24.

51 Storch, " 'Please to Remember the Fifth of November.' "

52 See, for example, *National Anti-Compulsory Vaccination Occasional Circular*, 1 August 1876, 9; *Banbury Guardian*, 1 March 1877, 8; *Manchester Guardian*, 2 October 1876, 7.

53 *National Anti-Compulsory Vaccination Reporter*, 1 March 1881, 99–102.

54 Steedman, *Policing the Victorian Community*, 8, 15.

55 Over twenty policemen are listed as refusing to vaccinate their children in the Vaccination Officers' Birth Books for the Enfield District of the Edmonton Union, Middlesex, in the 1890s (LMA BG/E/169–BG/E/175). On sympathetic policemen, see Turner, *About Myself*, 72–73. In fact, once conscientious objection became possible, enough policemen applied for exemptions to create a controversy within the Metropolitan Police Force: see *Vaccination Inquirer*, 1 March 1901, 199. Eleven policemen were granted exemption certificates between 1899 and 1909 in Enfield (LMA BG/E/176–BG/E/188). In the Fulham district of London in 1907–09, seven policeman took out certificates of conscientious objection (Register of Vaccinations, Hammersmith and Fulham Archives and Local History Centre, FBG/1/56–FBG/1/64).

56 Harvey Whiston, clerk to the Justices of Derby, to the Secretary of State, letter, 10 February 1887, PRO HO 45/9670/A46403/1.

57 Enforcement of Distress Warrant in Vaccination Cases, PRO HO 45/10044/A61858/20.

58 *Sheffield Telegraph*, 11 May 1889, in Milnes Collection, vol. 15, 55.

59 Gomm, "Water under the Bridge," 16.

60 *The Times*, 10 May 1887, 12.

61 *Gravesend Standard*, 18 February 1893, in Milnes Collection, vol. 35, 71.

62 *Stroud Journal*, 24 November 1893, ibid., vol. 39, 27.

63 Harvey Whiston, Clerk to the Justices of Derby, to the Secretary of State, letter, 10 February 1887, PRO, HO 45/9670/A46403/1; Enforcement of Distress Warrant in Vaccination Cases, PRO, HO 45/10044/A61858.

64 *Public Health* 9 (1896–97): 148–49.

65 West, *The Kent Occasional Eye Opener on the Ill Effects and Inutility of Compulsory Vaccination*, 24–25.

66 Ibid.

67 *National Anti-Compulsory Vaccination Reporter*, 1 January 1884, 62.

68 *Vaccination Inquirer*, July 1886, 61, 1 November 1899, 104; *The Co-operator*, 30 April 1870, 282.

69 *Anti-Vaccinator and Public Health Journal*, 15 August 1872, 139.

70 Duxbury, *Vaccination Rhymes*, 11.

71 *National Anti-Compulsory Vaccination Reporter*, 1 November 1880, 35.

72 Ibid., 1 December 1880, 45–47.

73 *Killed by Vaccination*, 2; *The Pioneer*, 16 June 1883, in Milnes Collection, vol. 1, 57.

74 *Insurance Against Vaccination*, 4.

75 *Vaccination Inquirer*, 1 December 1903, 168.

76 *Blackburn Standard*, 24 September 1898, in Milnes Collection, vol. 51, 26.

77 See James Furness Marson's testimony in *Report from the Select Committee on the Vaccination Act (1867)*, Q: 4,174–6.

78 Scott, *The Kensington Protest against Vaccination*, 1; *Anti-Vaccinator and Public Health Journal*, 15 August 1872, 133; Loane, *The Next Street but One*, 214.

79 *Some Leading Arguments against Compulsory Vaccination*, 6.

80 *The Anti-Vaccinator*, 21 August 1869, 2.

81 *Anti-Vaccinator and Public Health Journal*, 1 February 1873, 309.

82 *Herald of Health*, May 1879, 200.

83 Younger, *The Magnetic and Botanic Family Physician*, 456.

84 *Sixth Report of the Royal Commission Appointed to Inquire into the Subject of Vaccination*, 188, Q. 22,792.

85 *Co-operator and Anti-Vaccinator*, 8 April 1871, 216.

86 *Vaccination Inquirer*, June 1881, 49.

87 *To Members of Parliament*, 8; Newman, *To Parents and Citizens of Gloucester*, 1.

88 *Hackney Express*, 29 September 1896, in Milnes Collection, vol. 48, 18; Hume-Rothery, *Women and Doctors*, 2; *Vaccination Inquirer*, June 1880, 41.

89 *The Times*, 11 September 1869, 9; *Anti-Vaccinator and Public Health Journal*, 15 August 1872, 135; *National Anti-Compulsory Vaccination Reporter*, May 1881, 130; emphasis in the original.

90 *Anti-Vaccinator and Public Health Journal*, 2 December 1872, 271.

91 *Leicester Daily Mercury*, 23 March 1885, 3.

92 *The Hampstead Hospital*.

93 *National Anti-Compulsory Vaccination Reporter*, 1 June 1878, 172.

94 Thomas, *The Safety-Valve of Life*, 4.

95 *National Anti-Compulsory Vaccination Reporter*, 1 April 1880, 114.

96 *Vaccination: A Folly and a Crime*.

97 *Vaccination Inquirer*, September 1885, 104.

98 *National Anti-Compulsory Vaccination Reporter*, 5 October 1878, 17; *Vaccination Inquirer*, April 1885, 4.

99 Jeremiah 31:15; Matthew 2:18. While this particular envelope circulated in Canada, its origin was undoubtedly English: See Vandervelde, "British Anti-Vaccination Propaganda," 378.

100 *National Anti-Compulsory Vaccination Reporter*, 1 September 1881, 208; Wilkinson, *Herodian Decree of the Local Government Board.*

101 *Vaccination Inquirer*, January 1885, 193

102 *National Anti-Compulsory Vaccination Reporter*, September 1884, 198.

103 Davin, "Imperialism and Motherhood," 204.

104 *Daylight*, 24 August 1907, 9.

105 On the politics of maternalism, see Koven and Michel, *Mothers of a New World.*

106 Walkowitz, *Prostitution and Victorian Society*; Summers, "*The Constitution Violated*"; Tickner, *The Spectacle of Women*, 104–8.

107 *Vaccination: A Folly and a Crime*; *Vaccination Inquirer*, April 1885, 4; *Leicester Daily Mercury*, 23 March 1885, 3. This may have been the same banner remembered in different ways.

108 *National Anti-Compulsory Vaccination Reporter*, 5 October 1878, 17.

109 *To Members of Parliament*, 8; *The Anti-Vaccinator*, 2 October 1869, 111; *Vaccination Inquirer*, April 1879, 9; *Co-operator and Anti-Vaccinator*, 10 June 1871, 362; Clark, "Manhood, Womanhood, and the Politics of Class in Britain, 1790–1845," 273.

110 Homans, *Royal Representations*, 17–32; *Herald of Health*, May 1879, 200.

111 *The Anti-Vaccinator*, 27 November 1869, 233.

112 *National Anti-Compulsory Vaccination Reporter*, 1 September 1884, 195; Hume-Rothery, *Women and Doctors*, 14.

113 *Return of the Number of Prosecutions in Respect of England and Wales*, PP 1880 (146).

114 *Insurance Against Vaccination*, 12.

115 *Vaccination Inquirer*, 1 October 1896, 119; *Berkshire Chronicle*, 10 October 1896, in Milnes Collection, vol. 48, 22.

116 Ross, *Love and Toil*; Pennybacker, *A Vision for London, 1889–1914*; Lewis, *Labour and Love*; Behlmer, *Friends of the Family.*

117 Registers of Children Not Vaccinated, Fulham Union, Fulham Sub-District, Hammersmith and Fulham Archives and Local History Centre, FBG/1/4.

118 *Anti-Vaccinator and Public Health Journal*, 1 August 1872, 115.

119 Vaccination Officers' Report Books, Fulham Union, Fulham Sub-District, Hammersmith and Fulham Archives and Local History Centre, FBG/2/16/1.

120 *National Anti-Compulsory Vaccination Reporter*, 5 October 1878, 17.

121 *Vaccination Inquirer*, 1 February 1889, 188; Burne, "Kentish Anti-Vaccinators."

122 *Report from the Select Committee on the Vaccination Act (1867)*, 133, Q. 2370.

123 *The Star*, 10 June 1891, in Milnes Collection, vol. 26, 38; *East London Observer*, 27 June 1903, 3.

124 Goss, "My Boyhood at the Turn of the Century," 43–46. The expression is generally "cocking a snook."

125 Fox, *The Question of Compulsory Vaccination*, 7; *Vaccination Inquirer*, August 1879, 71–72.

126 [Allinson], *How Parents May Protect Their Offspring from the Dangers and Injuries of Vaccination*, 2.

127 *Vaccination Inquirer*, January 1887, 155.

128 Ibid., 1 April 1891, 2, June 1881, 49.

129 Pickering, *Which?* 165.

130 *National Anti-Compulsory Vaccination Reporter*, January 1881, 71.

131 *Vaccination Inquirer*, 1 January 1887, 164.

132 *Anti-Vaccinator and Public Health Journal*, 15 April 1873, 398.

CHAPTER THREE: POLITICS OF VICTORIAN LIBERALISM

1 Fawcett, *The Vaccination Act of 1898*. Fawcett was playing on the Whig Bishop William Magee's 1870 quote, "[I]t would be better that England should be free than that England should be compulsorily sober": see Harrison, *Drink and the Victorians*.

2 *Report from the Select Committee on the Vaccination Act (1867)*, 120, Q. 2015.

3 Hume-Rothery, "Men, not Slaves."

4 *Co-operator and Anti-Vaccinator*, 8 April 1871, 299.

5 Milnes, *What about Vaccination?* 191.

6 *Report of the Sixth Annual Meeting of the London Society for the Abolition of Compulsory Vaccination*, 3.

7 Biagini, *Liberty, Retrenchment and Reform*, 51.

8 Hume-Rothery, *Vaccination and the Vaccination Laws*, 16.

9 Walkowitz, *Prostitution and Victorian Society*, 108. See also Peterson, *The Medical Profession in Mid-Victorian London*.

10 *Vaccination Inquirer*, 1 September 1891, 93.

11 *East London Observer*, 27 May 1876, 7. The term *policing of parents* is drawn from Behlmer, *Friends of the Family*.

12 Hadwen, *The Vaccination Delusion*, 4. On Hadwen, see Kidd and Richards, *Hadwen of Gloucester*.

13 *South Western Star*, 6 October 1883, in Milnes Collection, vol. 2, 66.

14 *National Anti-Compulsory Vaccination Reporter*, 1 October 1883, 4; *Vaccination Inquirer*, 1 April 1904, 19.

15 "Historical and Critical Summary in Three Parts, Part Three," in Young, *Vaccination Tracts*, 23.

16 Wilkinson, *Compulsory Vaccination*, 15; *Reynold's Newspaper*, 20 March 1898, in Milnes Collection, vol. 50, 72.

17 As quoted in Harrison, *Drink and the Victorians*, 210.

18 Scott, *The Kensington Protest against Vaccination*, 1.

19 *South Western Star*, 8 December 1883, in Milnes Collection, vol. 3, 38.

20 Fox, *Compulsory Vaccination*, 10.

21 *Vaccination Inquirer*, December 1885, 146.

22 *National Anti-Compulsory Vaccination Reporter*, 1 April 1883, 116.

23 *The Knell of Compulsory Vaccination*.

24 *National Anti-Compulsory Vaccination Reporter*, 7 October 1882, 14; *Authoritative Opinions Adverse to Vaccination or Its Compulsory Enforcement*, 9.

25 *Co-operator and Anti-Vaccinator*, 13 May 1871, 290.

26 *The Pioneer*, 16 June 1883, in Milnes Collection, vol. 1, 57.

27 *Vaccination Inquirer*, 1 March 1898, 168.

28 Gibbs, *Compulsory Vaccination Briefly Considered in Its Scientific, Religious, and Political Aspects*, 3; *National Anti-Compulsory Vaccination Reporter*, 1 August 1882, 187.

29 Johnson, *Essay upon Compulsory Vaccination*, 23.

30 Hume, *A Word for the Baby*. See also *National Anti-Compulsory Vaccination Reporter*, 1 April 1880, 122; Sexton, *Vaccination Useless and Injurious*, 6–7; Watson, *An Essay on Vaccination*, 44.

31 Wilkinson, *Smallpox and Vaccination*, 40.

32 *Vaccination Inquirer*, 1 July 1887, 71; *Hansard*, 17 June 1887, 398.

33 *Vaccination Inquirer*, 1 July 1903, 74.

34 Loane, *An Englishman's Castle*, 8. See also Behlmer, *Friends of the Family*.

35 *National Anti-Compulsory Vaccination Reporter*, 1 November 1881, 34.

36 *Vaccination Inquirer*, 1 November 1899, 99.

37 Ibid., 1 March 1899, 151, June 1886, 52; Malings, *Narrative of Three Prosecutions Under the Vaccination Act*, 3.

38 Vernon, *Why Little Children Die*, 144; Ladies' Sanitary Association, *When Were You Vaccinated*, 15.

39 *Wanted!* 2.

40 *Anti-Vaccinator and Public Health Journal*, 15 April 1872, 3.

41 *East London Observer*, 15 April 1876, 2.

42 Stobbs, *To the Fathers and Mothers of Great Britain*.

43 *National Anti-Compulsory Vaccination Reporter*, 1 April 1878, 125.

44 Tebb, *A Personal Statement of the Results of Vaccination*, 4.

45 *The Anti-Vaccinator*, 21 August 1869, 16; *The Cornishman*, 3 April 1890, in Milnes Collection, vol. 19, 16.

46 *Vaccination Inquirer*, 1 June 1887, 47–48. The *Vaccination Inquirer* published an Irish issue in May 1905. On vaccination in Ireland, see Brunton, "The Problems of Implementation."

47 Vernon, *Politics and the People*, 295–330.

48 Guttery, *Anti-Compulsory Vaccination*, 3–4.

49 "The Vaccination Laws a Scandal to Public Honesty and Religion," in Young, *Vaccination Tracts*, 7. See also Newman, *The Coming Revolution*, 10; Gibbs, *Compulsory Vaccination Briefly Considered in Its Scientific, Religious, and Political Aspects*, 52.

50 Vernon, *Politics and the People*; Fox, *The Question of Compulsory Vaccination*, 6.

51 *An Appeal to Passive Resisters*.

52 Gibbs, *Compulsory Vaccination Briefly Considered in Its Scientific, Religious, and Political Aspects*, 53; emphasis in the original.

53 *Northampton Daily Reporter*, 26 September 1891, in Milnes Collection, vol. 28, 8.

54 *The Knell of Compulsory Vaccination*; Gibbs, *Our Medical Liberties*, 36; Hume-Rothery, *Women and Doctors*, 15.

55 *Wiltshire Times*, 19 September 1896, in Milnes Collection, vol. 48, 11.

56 Sexton, *Vaccination Useless and Injurious*, 5; Allen, *Vaccination and the Vaccination Act*, 14. See Thompson, *The Making of the English Working Class*.

57 *National Anti-Compulsory Vaccination Reporter*, 1 June 1881, 163, 1 August 1881, 193.

58 Fraser, *An Attempt to Prove that Vaccination with Its Compulsory Law, Instead of Being a General Blessing, Is a Universal Curse*, 56.

59 Gibbs, *Our Medical Liberties*, 39.

60 Wilkinson, *Compulsory Vaccination*, 34.

61 *National Anti-Compulsory Vaccination Reporter*, 1 September 1882, 195.

62 *Vaccination Inquirer*, 1 March 1897, 206.

63 Arnold, *Colonizing the Body*. According to Arnold (personal communication), Indians also paid little attention to the anti-vaccination movement in England.

64 Ibid.; Burke, *Lifebuoy Men, Lux Women*; Vaughan, *Curing Their Ills*; Pedersen, "National Bodies and Unspeakable Acts"; *Vaccination Inquirer*, November 1882, 123.

65 *Vaccination Inquirer*, October 1885, 115. The countess generously donated 100 pounds to the *Vaccination Inquirer* fund in 1887.

66 Ibid., 1 August 1887, 96.

67 Ibid., November 1879, 118.

68 Ibid., 1 January 1894, 160.

69 Ibid., 1 August 1892, 91; Hume-Rothery, *What Smallpox and Vaccination and the Vaccination Acts Really Are*, 12; Heath, *Vaccination*, 35.

70 Burton, "States of Injury," 339.

71 *Vaccination Inquirer*, 1 August 1893, 77.

72 Ibid., 1 October 1895, 89–90.

73 Thorne, " 'The Conversion of Englishmen and the Conversion of the World Inseparable' "; Nord, "The Social Explorer as Anthropologist," 123–24.

74 Hollis, "Anti-Slavery and British Working-Class Radicalism in the Years of Reform," 296.

75 Gray, *The Factory Question and Industrial England, 1830–1860*.

76 *Dr. Skelton's Botanic Record and Family Herbal*, 4 March 1854, 357, 1 January 1853, 138; *Hygiest or Medical Reformer*, 1 July 1857, 204.

77 Behlmer, "Grave Doubts," 230.

78 Tebb, *Sanitation, not Vaccination*, 12. See also his *The Results of Vaccination and the Inequity and Injustice of Its Enforcement*, 19; *Vaccination Inquirer*, 1 June 1887, 35, June 1882, 40.

79 Tebb, *Compulsory Vaccination in England*, 12; *Vaccination Inquirer*, 1 July 1897, 56.

80 *National Anti-Compulsory Vaccination Reporter*, 1 January 1884, 62.

81 *Third Report of the Royal Commission Appointed to Inquire into the Subject of Vaccination*, 174, Q. 10, 323.

82 *The Echo*, 25 January 1884, in Poor Law Unions and Local Authorities, PRO MH 12/6493/1884/1311/239.

83 *National Anti-Compulsory Vaccination Reporter*, 1 April 1884, 114.

84 Ibid., 1 September 1879, 209, 7 October 1882, 10.

85 *Vaccination Inquirer*, June 1884, 46.

86 Brebner, "Laissez Faire and State Intervention in Nineteenth-Century Britain"; Taylor, *Laissez-Faire and State Intervention in Nineteenth-Century Britain*.

87 [Tebb], *Government Prosecutions for Medical Heresy*, 35; *Report of the Sixth Annual Meeting of the London Society for the Abolition of Compulsory Vaccination*, 40.

88 *The Individualist*, February 1905, 16.

89 Hutton, *The Vaccination Question*, 92.

90 Levy, *State Interference in the Vaccination Controversy*, 2.

91 *National Anti-Compulsory Vaccination Reporter*, 7 October 1880, 9.

92 As quoted in Lupton, *Vaccination and the State*, 58.

93 Bradley, *The Optimists*, 225.

94 *Personal Rights Journal*, 1 December 1886, 94.

95 Taylor, *Personal Rights*, 55.

96 Eastes, *Concerning Vaccination*, 61.

97 "History and Practice of Vaccination" (1857), in Simon, *Public Health Reports*, vol. 1, 281.

98 Weiler, *The New Liberalism*; Freeden, "The New Liberalism and Its Aftermath."

99 *Report from the Select Committee on the Vaccination Act (1867)*, 142, Q. 2548; Hume-Rothery, *Vaccination and the Vaccination Laws*, 16.

100 Pennybacker, *A Vision for London 1889–1914*.

101 Behlmer, *Child Abuse and Moral Reform in England, 1870–1908*, 64, 74–75; *Vaccination Inquirer*, 1 November 1900, 119; Sykes, *The Rise and Fall of British Liberalism, 1776–1988*, 131; Swan, *The Vaccination Problem*, 37n.

102 *Pall Mall Gazette*, 17 June 1893, in Milnes Collection, vol. 37, 52; emphasis in the original.

103 *Anti-Vaccinator and Public Health Journal*, 15 August 1872, 142.

104 Newman, *The Political Side of the Anti-Vaccination System*, 8.

CHAPTER FOUR: BODY POLITICS OF CLASS FORMATION

1 *National Anti-Compulsory Vaccination Reporter*, 1 February 1882, 92.

2 *Fourth Report of the Royal Commission Appointed to Inquire into the Subject of Vaccination*, 169, Q. 13,456.

3 Tebb, *Compulsory Vaccination in England*, 7.

4 *Daily Mail*, 21 November 1905, in Enforcement of Distress Warrant in Vaccination Cases, Registered Papers, PRO HO 45/10044/A61858/61.

5 *Co-operator and Anti-Vaccinator*, 16 September 1871, 580.

6 Hainsworth, *Results of an Investigation into the Sheffield Small-Pox Epidemic of 1887*.

7 Hadwen, *The Gloucester Epidemic of Smallpox, 1895–96*, 22–23; *Vaccination Inquirer*, 1 January 1904, 191–201.

8 Swan, "Why I Am an Anti-Vaccinist," 4.

9 *Vaccination Inquirer*, 2 November 1908, 123.

10 "Opinions of Statesmen, Politicians, Publicists, Statisticians, and Sanitarians No. 1" in Young, *Vaccination Tracts*, 6; "Fellow Electors of the Keighley Parliamentary Division," Smallpox Collection, MS 55, Box 1, University of California, Los Angeles, Biomedical Library.

11 *Vaccination Inquirer*, 1 October 1903, 143.

12 As quoted in Kean, *Animal Rights*, 133.

13 Denham, *The Extinction of Small-Pox and Diseases of Vaccination by a Practical Process*, 18.

14 Richardson, *Death, Dissection, and the Destitute*.

15 Hardy, *The Epidemic Streets*, 118.

16 Scott, "Smallpox and Vaccination," 72.

17 Blackbook of Complaints Against Medical Practitioners, PRO MH 155; Bromley Local Government Board Correspondence, Bromley Central Library G/By ACa 54/74.

18 Poor Law Board to Clerk of Cambridge Board of Guardians, letter, 30 June 1869, PRO MH 12/575/1869/31919/26; Poor Law Board to J. L. Lee, relieving officer for Lutterworth Union, letter, 6 December 1864, PRO MH 12/6552/1864/44240/241.

19 Barrow, "In the Beginning Was the Lymph," 206–7.

20 Rumsey, *On the Amendment of the Vaccination Laws in England*, 3.

21 *Hansard*, 12 April 1853, 1008.

22 Poor Law Board to Plomesgate Union Clerk, letter, 18 February 1854, PRO MH 12/11940/6035/441; Medical Officer of Health, Priors Marston, to Poor Law Board, letter, 10 November 1860, PRO MH 12/13497/1860/39188/502; Poor Law Board to Clerk to Plymouth Guardians, letter, 16 January 1866, PRO MH 12/2432/1866/1191/87.

23 *Manchester Guardian*, 24 May 1902, 5.

24 *Western Daily Mercury*, 23 January 1891, in Milnes Collection, vol. 28, 58.

25 *The Anti-Vaccinator*, 21 August 1869, 15.

26 *Vaccination Inquirer*, 1 May 1890, 27.

27 *The Anti-Vaccinator*, 4 December 1869, 245; emphasis in the original.

28 *Vaccination Inquirer*, 2 December 1901, 155.

29 Toye, *Vaccination Condemned by Medical Men*, iv.

30 *Vaccination Inquirer*, 1 December 1886, 146.

31 *National Anti-Compulsory Vaccination Reporter*, 1 April 1882, 113.

32 *Second Report of the Royal Commission Appointed to Inquire into the Subject of Vaccination*, 218, Q. 6662.

33 *National Anti-Compulsory Vaccination Reporter*, 1 April 1882, 113; emphasis in the original.

34 *The Lancet*, 23 May 1863, 596.

35 Handbill, in Milnes Collection, vol. 9, 58–59; White, *Sir Lyon Playfair Taken to Pieces and Disposed of*, 44; *Medical Herbalist: A Monthly Circular of Organic Medicine, Hygiene, Household Hints*, June 1885, 1.

36 *Oldham Evening Express*, 20 October 1885, in Milnes Collection, vol. 10, 9.

37 Longman, *Fifteen Years Fight against Compulsory Vaccination*, 2.

38 *East London Observer*, 29 October 1881, 5.

39 Vaccination Officers' Birth Books (Enfield District, Edmonton Union), LMA BG/E/166–75.

40 *The Co-operator*, 30 July 1871, 491.

41 *Insurance against Vaccination*, 21.

42 *Defence Fund, Reminder Notice*.

43 On this type of saving, see Reeves, *Round about a Pound a Week*. On defense funds, see McWilliam, "Radicalism and Popular Culture," 51.

44 Abdiel, *Vaccination and Smallpox*, 7–8.

45 Young, *The Tyranny of the Vaccination Acts*; on the Hayward case, see Registered Papers, Supplementary, PRO HO 144/469/X9911.

46 *Berkshire Chronicle*, 10 October 1896, in Milnes Collection, vol. 48, 21.

47 *Vaccination Inquirer*, 1 November 1900, 116.

48 Hume-Rothery, *Vaccination and the Vaccination Laws*, I; *Anti-Vaccinator and Public Health Journal*, 15 August 1872, 139; *Oldham Chronicle*, 29 July 1871, 3; *Anti-Vaccinator and Public Health Journal*, 15 March 1873, 354.

49 *Vaccination Inquirer*, December 1884, 168.

50 *Kettering Observer*, 5 October 1883, in Milnes Collection, vol. 2, 65.

51 Hume-Rothery, "Men, not Slaves"; *Fourth Report of the Royal Commission Appointed to Inquire into the Subject of Vaccination*, 154, Q. 13,033, 240, Q. 15,153.

52 Clark, *The Struggle for the Breeches*; Bailey, " 'Will the Real Bill Banks Please Stand Up?,' " 338.

53 *Echo*, 21 March 1883, in Milnes Collection, vol. 1, 14.

54 Ross, " 'Not the Sort That Would Sit on the Doorstep' "; Roberts, *The Classic Slum*; Davidoff and Hall, *Family Fortunes*.

55 *Vaccination Inquirer*, 1 January 1896, 140.

56 *Anti-Vaccinator*, 23 October 1869, 146; *Vaccination Inquirer*, May 1888, 25.

57 Ibid., May 1888, 25; *The Anti-Vaccinator*, 23 October 1869, 146; Hunter, *No More Vaccination!* 8.

58 *Compulsory Vaccination*, 3.

59 *The Anti-Vaccinator*, 23 October 1869, 146.

60 Hunter, *No More Vaccination!* 8.

61 *Sixth Report of the Royal Commission Appointed to Inquire into the Subject of Vaccination*, 188, Q. 22,792.

62 Wiener, *Reconstructing the Criminal*, 332–33.

63 Ibid., 330–31.

64 *Vaccination Inquirer*, December 1884, 168.

65 *Second Report of the Royal Commission Appointed to Inquire into the Subject of Vaccination*, 219, Q. 6702–6708.

66 *Fifth Report of the Royal Commission Appointed to Inquire into the Subject of Vaccination*, 2–3.

67 *West Cumberland Times*, 15 August 1887, in Milnes Collection, vol. 12, 63.

68 *Fourth Report of the Royal Commission Appointed to Inquire into the Subject of Vaccination*, 182, Q. 13,652; *Vaccination Inquirer*, 1 November 1886, 130; *Recent Utterances on the Vaccination Question*; *Co-operator and Anti-Vaccinator*, 8 July 1871, 422.

69 Milnes, *What about Vaccination?* 16; *Vaccination Inquirer*, 1 October 1888, 128.

70 *The Times*, 15 December 1875, 11.

71 *Hansard*, 19 April 1898, 454.

72 *Vaccination Inquirer*, 1 December 1903, 168.

73 *The Anti-Vaccinator*, 4 December 1869, 249.

74 Stephen, *How Leicester Won "Home Rule,"* 4.

75 *Stroud Journal*, 24 November 1893, in Milnes Collection, vol. 39, 27.

76 *Vaccination Inquirer*, 1 February 1904, 218.

77 Gibbs, *More Words on Vaccination*, 30.

78 *The News*, 22 March 1884, in Milnes Collection, vol. 5, 5. On Craigen, see Holton, "Silk Dresses and Lavender Kid Gloves."

79 Pitman, *Prison Thoughts on Vaccination Part 2*, 3–4.
80 Reid, "Interpreting the Festival Calendar."
81 Pickering, "White Skin, Black Masks," 84–85.

CHAPTER FIVE: THE VICTORIAN BODY

1 Duxbury, *Vaccination Rhymes*, 4–5.
2 *Vaccination Inquirer*, June 1881, 50.
3 *National Anti-Compulsory Vaccination Reporter*, 1 June 1877, 4.
4 Hurley, *The Gothic Body*, 3–4.
5 *The Anti-Vaccinator*, 23 October 1869, 147.
6 Bland, *Dr. Francis T. Bond Very Much "Over the Border,"* 5; *Anti-Vaccinator and Public Health Journal*, 15 June 1872, 76; Halket, *Compulsory Vaccination!* 9; *Vaccination Inquirer*, 1 April 1903, 3, May 1882, 25, 2 July 1906, 64, 1 April 1908, 18, 1 June 1892, 54, 1 April 1904, 16, October 1879, 98, 1 May 1894, 17; *National Anti-Compulsory Vaccination Reporter*, 1 September 1878, 231; *Reading Observer*, 23 July 1898, 8; *Vaccination as the Cause of Fever and Consumption and as a Transmitter of All Kinds of Disease*, 11; Mc-Cormick, *Is Vaccination a Disastrous Delusion?* 31; *Co-operator and Anti-Vaccinator*, 21 January 1871, 38, 16 September 1871, 581; West, *The Kent Occasional Eye Opener on the Ill Effects and Inutility of Compulsory Vaccination*, 24; Vernon, *Politics and the People*, 318.
7 *National Disease*, 3–10.
8 *The Hampstead Hospital*; *British Medical Journal*, 19 December 1863, 661.
9 *East London Observer*, 28 October 1876, 5; *Vaccination Inquirer*, 1 March 1887, 183.
10 Blakewell, "Is It Expedient to Make Vaccination Compulsory?" 640; Shortt, *A Popular Lecture on Vaccination*, 1–2.
11 *Killed by Vaccination*, 13.
12 *East London Observer*, 26 October 1895, 5.
13 *National Anti-Compulsory Vaccination Reporter*, 1 April 1877, 20.
14 Connell, *My Experience of Vaccination*, 11.
15 *Preston Chronicle*, 23 February 1884, in Milnes Collection, vol. 4, 65; Hurley, *The Gothic Body*.
16 Younger, *The Magnetic and Botanic Family Physician*, 457.
17 *The Anti-Vaccinator and Public Health Journal*, 1 July 1872, 89.
18 Halket, *Compulsory Vaccination!* 13.
19 *Hydropathic Record and Journal of the Water Cure*, November 1868, 12.
20 *National Anti-Compulsory Vaccination Reporter*, 1 September 1881, 202–3, 1 September 1882, 196, 1 October 1876, 8.
21 Brown, *The Captured World*, 5–7, 43.

22 "The Vaccination Laws a Scandal to Public Honesty and Religion," in Young, *Vaccination Tracts*, 6; Hume-Rothery, *150 Reasons for Disobeying the Vaccination Law*, 12.

23 As quoted in *Vaccination Inquirer*, 1 March 1904, 236. On the idea of nature in anti-vaccinationist thought, see Scarpelli, " 'Nothing in Nature That is Not Useful.' "

24 *National Anti-Compulsory Vaccination Reporter*, 1 December 1883, 52, 5 October 1878, 5.

25 Ibid., 1 June 1878, 165.

26 While I have been unable to locate either of these pamphlets, the first is cited in Sexton, *Vaccination Useless and Injurious*, 5; the second is listed in London Society for the Abolition of Compulsory Vaccination, *Catalogue of Anti-Vaccination Literature Issued by the Society*, 12. See also [Foster], *Murder and Mutilation!* 10; *Vaccination Inquirer*, April 1884, 4.

27 Leviticus 19:28. See Longman, *Fifteen Years Fight against Compulsory Vaccination*; Pickering, *Which?* 5.

28 Winterburn, *The Value of Vaccination*, 145. Although this was an American pamphlet, it also circulated in Britain.

29 *Anti-Vaccinator and Public Health Journal*, 1 February 1873, 309.

30 Schieferdecker, *Dr. C. G. G. Nittinger's Evils of Vaccination*, 43–49; *Vaccination Inquirer*, 1 May 1888, 33, 35; Fraser, *An Attempt to Prove That Vaccination with Its Compulsory Law, Instead of Being a General Blessing, Is a Universal Curse*, 28. On the Swedish campaign, see Nelson and Rogers, "The Right to Die?"

31 *Vaccination Inquirer*, June 1879, 40.

32 Hume-Rothery, *What Smallpox and Vaccination and the Vaccination Acts Really Are*, 7.

33 *National Disease*, 48.

34 Deuteronomy 12:23. See *Vaccination as the Cause of Fever and Consumption and as a Transmitter of All Kinds of Disease*, 11.

35 Morison, *The Truth Hygiean Manifesto*; Fraser, *An Attempt to Prove That Vaccination with Its Compulsory Law, Instead of Being a General Blessing, Is a Universal Curse*, 2.

36 Port, *Precaution Against Small-Pox*, 13.

37 *Family Doctor and People's Medical Adviser*, 31 May 1890, 221; *East London Observer*, 16 August 1873, 3, 11 June 1887, 2; *Reading Mercury*, 9 July 1898, 3.

38 Colley, *Vaccination a Moral Evil*, 5, 8; "Vaccination a Sign of Decay of the Political and Medical Conscience," in Young, *Vaccination Tracts*, 15.

39 *Vaccination Inquirer*, April 1885, 4.

40 Ibid., April 1879, 2; Hume-Rothery, *Vaccination and the Vaccination Laws*, 3; White, *The Story of a Great Delusion*, 594; Newman, *The Coming Revolution*, 8; *National Anti-Compulsory Vaccination Reporter*, 1 September 1880, 200.

41 Barrow, *Independent Spirits*, 89; Scott, "Physical Purity Feminism and State Medicine in Late Nineteenth-Century England."

42 *The Anti-Vaccinator*, 18 September 1869, 79.

43 Ibid., 28 August 1869, 22.

44 Belchem, " 'Temperance in all Things' "; Leneman, "The Awakened Instinct"; Behlmer, "Grave Doubts," 229–30; *Vaccination Inquirer*, 1 August 1901, 94.

45 *The Anti-Vaccinator*, 21 August 1869, 8.

46 Furnival, *The Conscientious Objector*, 16.

47 *Vaccination Inquirer*, 1 April 1890, 2.

48 *Dietetic Reformer and Vegetarian Messenger*, April 1872, 61; Collinson, *What It Costs to Be Vaccinated*, 32–34; Abdiel, *Vaccination and Smallpox*, 22; W. D. Stokes, "A Startling Revelation" in Contemporary Medical Archives Collection, Wellcome Institute for the History of Medicine, SA/BMA, box 206, item F.59; *Vaccination Inquirer*, 1 July 1905, 74–75, April 1907, 6.

49 *Herald of Health*, May 1879, 200.

50 Bashford, "Foreign Bodies."

51 *Sixth Report of the Royal Commission Appointed to Inquire into the Subject of Vaccination*, 158, Q. 21,839.

52 *Vaccination Inquirer*, 1 September 1890, 97–98.

53 *Gloucester Epidemic of Smallpox, 1895–96*, 14; *Evening Standard*, 4 February 1891, in Milnes Collection, vol. 23, 52.

54 Gomm, "Water Under the Bridge," 15.

55 Gibbs, *Our Medical Liberties*, 8; *The Danger and Injustice of Compulsory Vaccination*, 4; *Fourth Report of the Royal Commission Appointed to Inquire into the Subject of Vaccination*, app. 3, table 4, case 206.

56 "The Vaccination Laws a Scandal to Public Honesty and Religion," in Young, *Vaccination Tracts*, 5.

57 Eadon, *Vaccination*, 1; Wilder, *Vaccination a Medical Fallacy*, 25.

58 Hadwen, *The Vaccination Delusion*, 26.

59 *Vaccination Inquirer*, 1 January 1898, 129.

60 Wilkinson, *Smallpox and Vaccination*, 42.

61 Halket, *Compulsory Vaccination!* 8.

62 *The Anti-Vaccinator*, 21 August 1869, 13; Fraser, *An Attempt to Prove That Vaccination with Its Compulsory Law, Instead of Being a General Blessing, Is a Universal Curse*, 22; Colley, *Vaccination a Moral Evil*, 5.

63 Wilkinson, *Smallpox and Vaccination*, 21.

64 *Family Doctor and People's Medical Adviser*, 2 December 1893, 216; Barrow, "In the Beginning Was the Lymph," 207; Makuna, ed., *Transactions of the Vaccination Inquiry*, 66.

65 *The Echo*, 23 June 1891, in Milnes Collection, vol. 26, 49; *Vaccination Inquirer*, 1 June 1891, 52, 1 July 1891, 63.

66 *National Anti-Compulsory Vaccination League Occasional Circular*, 2 August 1875, 2, 1 July 1875, 3; *International Herald*, 16 November 1872, 4; Tebb, *The Spread of Leprosy*; McCormick, *Is Vaccination a Disastrous Delusion?* 11; *National Anti-Compulsory Vaccination Reporter*, 1 April 1881, 111; Gairdner, *A Remarkable Experience Concerning Leprosy*; *The Anti-Vaccinator*, 21 August 1869, 16; *The Times*, 31 December 1875, 10.

67 *National Anti-Compulsory Vaccination Reporter*, 1 June 1881, 164.

68 Bright, *An Evil Law Unfairly Enforced*, 2.

69 Seaton, *A Handbook of Vaccination*, 106; Purvis, *Statistics of Vaccination at the Greenwich Public Vaccination Station*, 13; Russell and Wheeler, *A Night's Debate on Vaccination*, 37; Davidson, *Special Report on the Recent Outbreak of Small-Pox in Congleton by the Medical Officer of Health to the Urban Sanitary Authority*, 13.

70 *The Anti-Vaccinator*, 21 August 1869, 15; Tebb, *The Results of Vaccination and the Inequity and Injustice of Its Enforcement*, 22.

71 *Vaccination Inquirer*, June 1886, 52.

72 Ibid., 2 January 1893, 166.

73 *The Anti-Vaccinator*, 21 August 1869, 15.

74 Burnett, *Destiny Obscure*, 90.

75 Gomm, "Water under the Bridge," 16.

76 Bayard, *Extract from an Essay on Vaccination*, 22.

77 Nichols, *A Woman's Work in Water Cure and Sanitary Education*, 72; *Fourth Report of the Royal Commission Appointed to Inquire into the Subject of Vaccination*, app. 3, table 4, cases 154, 198.

78 Wilkinson, *Compulsory Vaccination*, 5; *The Co-operator*, 26 June 1869, 471; Wilkinson, *Extract from a Book Just Published on Human Science and on Divine Revelation*, 3.

79 *Vaccination Inquirer*, April 1880, 2.

80 Hume-Rothery, *150 Reasons for Disobeying the Vaccination Law*, 12; *National Anti-Compulsory Vaccination Reporter*, 1 February 1880, 70.

81 As quoted in *The Anti-Vaccinator*, 4 December 1869, 245.

82 *Vaccination Inquirer*, 1 July 1907, 71; Colley, *Vaccination a Moral Evil*, 5; *National Anti-Compulsory Vaccination League Occasional Circular*, 1 June 1876, 9–10; *National Anti-Compulsory Vaccination Reporter*, 1 July 1884, 167; Baldwin, *Contagion and the State in Europe, 1830–1930*, 289.

83 Young, *A Warning to Parents*, 3.

84 Creighton, *The Natural History of Cow-Pox and Vaccinal Syphilis*, 143, 155; G. R., *Cow-Pox and Vaccinal Syphilis*; *Eclectic Journal and Medical Free Press*, 1 May 1866, 76.

85 *The Doctor's Baby*; *Vaccinal Syphilis*; Wallace, *Vaccination Proved Useless and Dangerous from Forty-five Years of Registration Statistics*, 23; Taylor, *Compulsory Vaccination*, 5; Health and Liberty League, *Does Compulsory*

Education Justify Compulsory Vaccination? 5; "The Propagation of Syphilis to Infants and Adults by Vaccination and Revaccination," in Young, *Vaccination Tracts*, 16; Cassel, *The Secret Plague*, 33.

86 *Weekly Star and Vegetarian Restaurant Gazette*, 7 September 1889, 139.

87 Spongberg, *Feminizing Venereal Disease*, 143.

88 *Vaccination Inquirer*, 1 December 1886, 142.

89 *Some Leading Arguments Against Compulsory Vaccination*, 17.

90 Colley, *Vaccination a Moral Evil*, 4–5.

91 Hume-Rothery, "Men, not Slaves."

92 *Vaccination Inquirer*, 1 December 1886, 142. For a similar case, see *Report from the Select Committee on the Vaccination Act (1867)*, 136, Q. 2413.

93 Collinson, *What It Costs to Be Vaccinated*, 39–40.

94 *Disease by Law*, 6.

95 Pick, *Faces of Degeneration*; Chamberlain and Gilman, *Degeneration*.

96 *Hygiest or Medical Reformer*, 2 June 1856, 137.

97 *The Anti-Vaccinator*, 21 August 1869, 5. See also *International Herald*, 22 March 1873, 5; Halket, *Compulsory Vaccination!* 7.

98 *Vaccination Inquirer*, April 1907, 13, 2 July 1906, 54.

99 *Hackney Examiner*, 3 November 1883, in Milnes Collection, vol. 3, 12.

100 Hume-Rothery, *What Smallpox and Vaccination and the Vaccination Acts Really Are.*

101 *Anti-Vaccinator and Public Health Journal*, 1 July 1872, 91.

102 *Vaccination and Physical Deterioration*; Gilbert, "Health and Politics."

103 *The Co-operator*, 30 April 1870, 281.

104 Bayard, *Extracts from an Essay on Vaccination*, i.

105 *British Medical Journal*, 13 June 1903, 1394.

106 *National Anti-Compulsory Vaccination League Occasional Circular*, 15 March 1876, 11.

107 Kingscote, *The English Baby in India*, 41–42; Stoler, *Race and the Education of Desire*, 50. Bashford's *Imperial Hygiene* unfortunately appeared too late for me to adequately address her compelling argument about the colonial implications of anti-vaccinationists' concern with corporeal boundaries.

108 *British Medical Journal*, 14 March 1896, 699.

109 Allinson, *Medical Essays Reprinted from the "Weekly Times and Echo,"* 7, 94.

110 Scott, "Physical Purity Feminism and State Medicine in Late Nineteenth-Century England," 638–39.

111 Wilkinson, *The Vaccination Vampire.*

112 Leatherdale, *Dracula*, 46; Gelder, *Reading the Vampire.*

113 Rymer, *Varney the Vampire.* There is some debate over whether *Varney* was written by Rymer or by Thomas Peckett Prest, author of *Sweeney Todd, the Demon Barber of Fleet Street.*

114 *Coffin's Botanical Journal and Medical Reformer*, 28 September 1850, 220.

115 *Vaccination Inquirer*, August 1885, 78.

116 Pelis, "Transfusion, with Teeth," and "Blood Clots."

117 Braddon, "The Good Lady Ducayne."

118 Halket, *Compulsory Vaccination!* 13.

119 Baldick, *In Frankenstein's Shadow*, 17.

120 Punter, *The Literature of Terror*, 119, 257–58.

121 *Dr. Skelton's Botanic Record and Family Herbal*, 5 November 1853, 298.

122 Walkowitz, *Prostitution and Victorian Society*, 108. See also Peterson, *The Medical Profession in Mid-Victorian London*.

123 Quoted in Gelder, *Reading the Vampire*, 21.

124 Tucker, *The Marx–Engels Reader*, 362–63.

125 Auerbach, *Our Vampires, Ourselves*, 31. On Marx's vampires, see Baldick, *In Frankenstein's Shadow*, 121–40.

126 *Vaccination Inquirer*, 1 November 1897, 107; *Manchester Guardian*, 14 November 1897, in Milnes Collection, vol. 49, 35.

127 Purdy, *Smallpox*, 34; *Rye Press*, 29 November 1890, in Milnes Collection, vol. 23, 6; Hume-Rothery, *What Smallpox and Vaccination and the Vaccination Acts Really Are*, 12.

128 *National Anti-Compulsory Vaccination Reporter*, 5 October 1878, 17, 1 August 1877, 10; Oswald, *Vaccination a Crime*, 96.

129 This concern with the undead also manifested itself in debates over premature burial. By the 1890s, premature burial was a frequent topic in the popular press and had even been raised as an issue in Parliament. The anti-vaccinators William Tebb, Walter Hadwen, A. Phelps, J. M. Peebles, Alexander Wilder, J. R. Williamson, and Carlo Ruata were all members of the London Association for the Prevention of Premature Burial (founded in 1896) and supported a variety of burial reforms to deal with what they considered a real and pressing problem: see Behlmer, "Grave Doubts."

130 His brother George was physician to the Lyceum, where Bram Stoker was Henry Irving's stage manager. George Stoker was involved in a minor vaccination scandal, accused by the LSACV of poisoning the blood of the famous actress Ellen Terry through a botched vaccination: *Vaccination Inquirer*, August 1884, 91, November 1884, 139; Belford, *Bram Stoker*, 128.

131 A range of *Dracula* criticism analyzes these themes. See Carter, *Dracula*; Pick, " 'Terrors of the Night' "; Spencer, "Purity and Danger."

132 Punter, *The Literature of Terror*, 240.

133 Roth, "Suddenly Sexual Women in Bram Stoker's *Dracula*"; Bentley, "The Monster in the Bedroom"; Craft, " 'Kiss Me with Those Red Lips' "; Halberstam, "Technologies of Monstrosity"; Zanger, "A Sympathetic Vibration"; Arata, "The Occidental Tourist."

134 Richards, "Anaesthetics, Ethics, and Aesthetics," 165.

135 Kean, *Animal Rights*, 100, 103.

136 On anti-vivisection, see French, *Antivivisection and Medical Science in Victorian Society*; Kean, "The 'Smooth Cool Men of Science' "; Lansbury, *The Old Brown Dog*; Elston, "Women and Anti-Vivisection in Victorian England 1870–1900," 259–86; Weinbren, "Against *All* Cruelty." Frances Power Cobbe in fact poached Hadwen to be an anti-vivisection spokesman after she saw him speak at an anti-vaccination rally.

137 *Vaccination Inquirer*, 1 July 1895, 46.

138 Ibid., 1 August 1904, 88; Hume, *The Mind-Changers*, 194; Kidd and Richards, *Hadwen of Gloucester*, 142.

139 As quoted in Kean, *Animal Rights*, 103.

140 Halket, *Compulsory Vaccination!* 12.

141 *Family Physician or People's Medical Adviser*, February 1866, 12; *Killed by Vaccination*, 2.

142 As quoted in Kean, *Animal Rights*, 102.

143 Oswald, *Vaccination a Crime*, 4; *Co-operator and Anti-Vaccinator*, 23 September 1871, 599, 13 May 1871, 290; "Historical and Critical Summary in Three Parts, Part Three," in Young, *Vaccination Tracts*, 26; Purdy, *Smallpox*, 12; Hume-Rothery, *What Smallpox and Vaccination and the Vaccination Acts Really Are*, 12; *National Anti-Compulsory Vaccination Reporter*, 1 September 1882, 198.

144 Ross, *Love and Toil*, 174.

145 As quoted in Lansbury, *The Old Brown Dog*, 92.

146 As quoted in White, *The Story of a Great Delusion*, xxxi; "Preface and Supplement," in Young, *Vaccination Tracts*, 3; Hume-Rothery, *Women and Doctors*, 1; "Vaccination Laws a Scandal to Public Honesty and Religion," in Young, *Vaccination Tracts*, 6–7.

147 *The Times*, 9 March 1865, 11.

148 London Society for the Abolition of Compulsory Vaccination, *Vaccination Unveiled* (c. 1884), in PRO MH 12/6493/1884/40617/239.

149 *Vaccination Inquirer*, July 1886, 56, October 1886, 109–10. See also *East Grinstead Observer*, 14 December 1901, 5.

150 See Walkowitz, *City of Dreadful Delight*; McLaren, *A Prescription for Murder*; *Phonetic Journal*, 12 January 1883, in Milnes Collection, vol. 3, 23; *Anti-Vaccinator and Public Health Journal*, 1 October 1872, 178; *Bath Argus*, 16 February 1888, in Milnes Collection, vol. 14, 27–28; Cobbe quoted in Elston, "Women and Anti-Vivisection in Victorian England, 1870–1900," 281.

151 Walkowitz, *City of Dreadful Delight*, 81–134; *Vaccination Inquirer*, 1 April 1908, 18.

152 See Scott, "Physical Purity Feminism and State Medicine in Late Nineteenth-Century England." Lansbury has drawn connections between the devices used to restrain women during examinations or surgery and

those deployed to hold women for sexual purposes in late-nineteenth- and early-twentieth-century pornography. While I am not convinced of the extent to which the tropes of pornography entered the cultural imagination at this historical moment, the connections are worth noting: see Lansbury, *The Old Brown Dog*; Purdy, *Smallpox*, 12; [Foster], *Murder and Mutilation!*; Walkowitz, *City of Dreadful Delight*, 192.

153   On the image of the scientist, see Haynes, *From Faust to Strangelove*; MacAndrew, *The Gothic Tradition in Fiction*, 173–79.

154   Wells, *The Island of Doctor Moreau*, 46.

155   Collinson, *What It Costs to Be Vaccinated*, 9–10.

156   Tebb, *Sanitation, not Vaccination*, 17.

157   *Eclectic Journal and Medical Free Press*, 1 July 1869, 289.

158   *Hansard*, 19 July 1898, 381; *Vaccination Inquirer*, 1 September 1900, 85.

159   *Vaccination Inquirer*, 1 February 1902, 196.

160   Ibid., 1 August 1904, 86. A history of human experimentation in Britain is yet to be written. For the American case, see Lederer, *Subjected to Science*.

161   *Preston Chronicle*, 23 February 1884, in Milnes Collection, vol. 4, 65.

162   Linebaugh, "The Tyburn Riot against the Surgeons"; Richardson, *Death, Dissection and the Destitute*.

163   Morison, *Morisonia*, iii–iv.

164   Wilkinson, *War, Cholera and the Ministry of Health*, 51.

165   Halsted, *Doctor in the Nineties*, 25.

166   *The Individualist*, May 1903, 38.

167   Woodward, *Jipping Street*, 27.

168   Kean, *Animal Rights*, 154.

169   *National Anti-Compulsory Vaccination Reporter*, 1 May 1881, 126, 7 October 1882, 22, 1 April 1883, 123. The Liverpool Society for the Prevention of Cruelty to Children, the first organization of its kind in the United Kingdom, was founded in 1883: see Behlmer, *Child Abuse and Moral Reform in England, 1870–1908*.

170   *Vaccination Inquirer*, 1 January 1894, 146, 1 April 1905, 10. On the relationship between Victorians and their animals, see Turner, *Reckoning with the Beast*.

171   Glover, *Vampires, Mummies, and Liberals*, 71.

CHAPTER SIX: GERMS, DIRT, AND THE CONSTITUTION

1   *National Anti-Compulsory Vaccination Reporter*, 1 March 1882, 111.

2   Hamlin, "Predisposing Causes and Public Health in Early Nineteenth-Century Medical Thought."

3 *Co-operator and Anti-Vaccinator*, 20 May 1871, 312.

4 Tebb, *Sanitation, not Vaccination*, 13.

5 Dickens, *Bleak House*, chap. 46.

6 Porter, "Public Health."

7 Hamlin, "Providence and Putrefaction," 386.

8 Worboys, *Spreading Germs*, 35.

9 Hume-Rothery, *What Smallpox and Vaccination and the Vaccination Acts Really Are*, 4.

10 Pickering, *Anti-Vaccination*, 33.

11 Wilkinson, *Smallpox and Vaccination*, 22; *Vaccination Inquirer*, July 1884, 71.

12 Medicus, *Compulsory Vaccination*, 6.

13 *Testimonies of Medical Men on the Protection Supposed to Be Afforded by Vaccination, 1805–81*, 20; emphasis in the original.

14 *Vaccination Inquirer*, 1 January 1894, 160.

15 *Family Doctor and People's Medical Adviser*, 18 September 1886, 39.

16 *Echo*, 30 April 1883, in Milnes Collection, vol. 1, 30; Collins, *Sir Lyon Playfair's Logic*, 20; *Vaccination Inquirer*, September 1885, 93, April 1885, 4, July 1890, 53, May 1890, 23; Gibbs, *More Words on Vaccination*, 22.

17 Porter and Porter, "The Politics of Prevention," 252; MacLeod, "Law, Medicine and Public Opinion," 211.

18 *East London Observer*, 15 June 1907, 6.

19 Collinson, *What It Costs to be Vaccinated*, 10.

20 Hamlin, *Public Health and Social Justice in the Age of Chadwick*, 8–15; Sigsworth and Worboys, "The Public's View of Public Health in Mid-Victorian Britain."

21 MacLeod, "Law, Medicine and Public Opinion," 108–9; Porter and Porter, "The Politics of Prevention," 251–52.

22 Tomes and Warner, "Introduction to Special Issue on Rethinking the Reception of the Germ Theory of Disease," 10.

23 Weindling, "The Immunological Tradition"; Martin, *Flexible Bodies*.

24 Worboys, *Spreading Germs*, 109.

25 As quoted in *Vaccination Inquirer*, 1 December 1909, 181; *Hydropathic Record and Journal of the Water Cure*, February 1869, 77.

26 *Vaccination Inquirer*, 1 November 1899, 97.

27 *National Anti-Compulsory Vaccination Reporter*, 1 July 1882, 172, 1 October 1880, 12, 1 June 1877, 16.

28 MacLeod, "Law, Medicine and Public Opinion," 108; Porter and Porter, "The Politics of Prevention," 245; Stevenson, "Science Down the Drain."

29 See Crookshank, *The Prevention of Small-Pox with Special Reference to the Origin and Development of the Stamping-Out System*; E. M. Crookshank, *History and Pathology of Vaccination*; Cook, "Charles Creighton (1847–

1927)"; and the following works by Creighton: *Exit Dr. Jenner; Jenner and Vaccination; The Natural History of Cow-Pox and Vaccinal Syphilis;* and "Vaccination."

30 Alfred Russel Wallace, however, was an exception. Involved in spiritualism, socialism, pacifism, and women's rights, he was marginalized by the scientific community despite his achievements in evolutionary theory: see Scarpelli, " 'Nothing in Nature That Is Not Useful.' "

31 Worboys, *Spreading Germs,* 143; Makuna, *Transactions of the Vaccination Inquiry,* 23; *Vaccination Inquirer,* 1 July 1901, 73.

32 Porter and Porter, "What Was Social Medicine?" 97.

33 McVail, *Vaccination Vindicated; Papers Relating to the History and Practice of Vaccination.* For a mortality table detailing this decline (except in epidemic years), see *Vaccination Inquirer,* 1 March 1889, 201.

34 Leighton, *The People of Dewsbury and Vaccination,* 5.

35 Ackerknecht, *A Short History of Medicine,* 180.

36 Worboys, *Spreading Germs,* 211.

37 As quoted in *National Anti-Compulsory Vaccination Reporter,* 1 June 1884, 151; *Daily News,* 1 April 1904, 5; *Light of Day,* August 1891, 24.

38 Young, *The Toadstool Millionaires,* 144–62; *The Times,* 19 November 1891, 3; William Radam, *To Intelligent Searchers after Truth,* c. 1893, in University of Oxford, Bodleian Library, John Johnson Collection, Patent Medicines Box 3.

39 Worboys, *Spreading Germs,* 244, 3.

40 *National Anti-Compulsory Vaccination Reporter,* 1 June 1881, 148.

41 *The Echo,* 16 September 1896, in Milnes Collection, vol. 44, 20.

42 Baker, *A Battling Life,* 83; Hadwen, *The Follies and Cruelties of Vivisection,* 9.

43 Sykes, *Smallpox, Vaccination and the Glycerination of Vaccine Lymph,* 50; Farrar, *On the Present Condition of Our Knowledge of the Aetiological Agent in Vaccinia and Variola,* 3.

44 Copeman, *Vaccination,* 153; *Vaccination Inquirer,* 1 February 1898, 144; MacNalty, "The Prevention of Smallpox."

45 *Vaccination Inquirer,* 1 February 1905, 210, 1 February 1895, 169; *East London Observer,* 25 December 1897, 7; *Personal Rights Journal,* 15 January 1898, 8; *Vaccination Inquirer,* 1 November 1898, 108.

46 *Vaccination Inquirer,* 1 September 1891, 96, 1 September 1888, 106.

47 Hadwen, *The Follies and Cruelties of Vivisection,* 10.

48 Tomes, *The Gospel of Germs,* 245.

49 Bashford, *Purity and Pollution,* 136; Barnes, *The Making of a Social Disease,* 41.

50 Abdiel, *Vaccination and Smallpox,* 12.

51 Wallace, *The Wonderful Century,* 213.

52 *Vaccination Inquirer*, 1 April 1898, 3; *National Anti-Compulsory Vaccination Reporter*, 1 April 1883, 129.

53 Moon, *The Secret of Perfect Health.*

54 *National Anti-Compulsory Vaccination Reporter*, 1 June 1881, 148.

55 MacLeod, "Law, Medicine and Public Opinion," 118, n. 44; Jervoise, *Infection*, 63.

56 *Vaccination Inquirer*, 1 March 1893, 203.

57 *A Report on Vaccination and Its Results Based on the Evidence Taken by the Royal Commission 1889–97*, 338–478.

58 Fraser, "Leicester and Smallpox"; Ross, "Leicester and the Anti-Vaccination Movement 1853–1889."

59 *Vaccination Inquirer*, 1 May 1903, 32.

60 Allinson, *Medical Essays Reprinted from the "Weekly Times and Echo,"* 93.

61 *Health*, 23 April 1886, in Milnes Collection, vol. 10, 57.

62 Perry, *Small-Pox and Vaccination*, 6.

63 Dougall, *The Artificial Cultivation of Vaccine Lymph*, 4.

64 *The People*, 25 May 1884, in Milnes Collection, vol. 5, 30.

65 *Sixth Report of the Royal Commission Appointed to Inquire into the Subject of Vaccination*, 11, Q. 18,269.

66 *Family Medical Adviser*, 285.

67 Younger, *The Magnetic and Botanic Family Physician*, 450; *Vaccination Inquirer*, 1 November 1899, 97; *National Anti-Compulsory Vaccination Reporter*, 7 October 1882, 17; *Vaccination*, 4.

68 *Vaccination Inquirer*, 1 November 1897, 132.

69 Hadwen, *The Follies and Cruelties of Vivisection*, 10.

70 Marginal notation on W. J. Collins's copy of Klein, *Micro-organisms and Disease*, 249, on file, Woodward Library, University of British Columbia, Vancouver.

71 *Saturday Review*, 5 October 1901, 422.

72 *Newcastle Daily Chronicle*, 11 July 1891, in Milnes Collection, vol. 27, 21.

73 *Vaccination Inquirer*, 1 November 1907, 132.

74 Wallace, *The Wonderful Century*, 145.

75 Tomes, *The Gospel of Germs*, 33–34; Worboys, *Spreading Germs*, 32.

76 Goss, "My Boyhood at the Turn of the Century," 43.

77 Baldwin, *Contagion and the State in Europe, 1830–1930*, 534–35.

CHAPTER SEVEN: THE CONSCIENTIOUS OBJECTOR

1 *Vaccination Inquirer*, 1 March 1900, 151.

2 *Return of Statement Showing the Number of Certificates of Conscientious Objection . . . Received by the Vaccination Officers in the Year 1899*, 2; *Vac-*

cination Inquirer, 1 February 1899, 148; General Register Office Smallpox Vaccination Returns, PRO RG 56/1.

3 Vaccination Officers' Birth Books (Enfield District, Edmonton Union), LMA BG/E/176–BG/E/188; Register of Vaccinations, Hammersmith and Fulham Archives and Local History Centre, FBG/1/35–FBG/1/61.

4 *Vaccination Inquirer*, 2 January 1899, 8.

5 *Dr. Skelton's Botanic Record and Family Herbal*, 2 September 1854, 453; Gibbs, *Our Medical Liberties*, 7; *Eclectic Medical Journal*, 1 September 1858, 180; *British Medical Journal*, 19 November 1870, 570; *The Times*, 5 December 1870, 11; *Co-operator and Anti-Vaccinator*, 1 July 1871, 413; Case of Charles Hayward, PRO HO 144/469/X9911; *Vaccination Inquirer*, 1 October 1892, 122; *Keighley News*, 27 February 1875, 3; [Allinson], *How Parents May Protect Their Offspring from the Dangers and Injuries of Vaccination*, 1; Hume-Rothery, *Vaccination and the Vaccination Laws*, 1; *Co-operator and Anti-Vaccinator*, 17 June 1871, 371; *Vaccination Inquirer*, August 1880, 74.

6 Handbill, in Milnes Collection, vol. 9, 58–59.

7 Fraser, *An Attempt to Prove that Vaccination with Its Compulsory Law, Instead of Being a General Blessing, Is a Universal Curse*, 56; *National Anti-Compulsory Vaccination Reporter*, 1 September 1881, 203; *Vaccination Inquirer*, 1 February 1904, 218, June 1884, 39.

8 In 1893, the Oxford English Dictionary defined *conscience* as "[t]he internal acknowledgment or recognition of the moral quality of one's motives and actions; the sense of right and wrong as regards things for which one is responsible."

9 *Vaccination Inquirer*, November 1884, 137.

10 *Shafts*, March 1897, 72.

11 Guttery, *Anti-Compulsory Vaccination*, 6–7.

12 Braithwaite, "Conscience in Conflict with the Law."

13 Braithwaite, "Legal Problems of Conscientious Objection to Various Compulsions under British Law."

14 *Vaccination Inquirer*, 1 April 1904, 15; *An Appeal to Passive Resisters*.

15 Notes on Prison Rules, May 1889, PRO HO 45/9704/A50333B/1.

16 Rutter, *Is It Right to Try to Force Parents to Have Their Children Vaccinated against Their Judgment and Conscience?*; Health and Liberty League, *Does Compulsory Education Justify Compulsory Vaccination?* 6–7; *Hydropathic Record and Journal of the Water Cure*, November 1868, 15.

17 MacLeod, "Medico-Legal Issues in Victorian Medical Care."

18 Furnival, *The Conscientious Objector*, 3.

19 *Daylight*, 10 August 1907, 9.

20 *Vaccination Inquirer*, 1 February 1908, 194.

21 Hardy, "Smallpox in London."

22 *A Report on Vaccination and Its Results Based on the Evidence Taken by the*

Royal Commission 1889–97, 292, para. 512; *Report of the Medical Officer of Health for Mile End*, 1896, 16; *Report of the Medical Officer of Health for Coventry*, 1895, 21.

23 *Vaccination Inquirer*, 1 May 1906, 28.

24 Ibid., 1 April 1898, 2. On the trials and tribulations of this bill, see Mac-Leod, "In the Interests of Health"; *Reynold's Newspaper*, 20 March 1898, in Milnes Collection, vol. 50, 72.

25 *Hansard*, 19 July 1898, 345–47.

26 Ibid., 20 July 1898, 449–52, 466.

27 MacLeod, "In the Interests of Health," 156.

28 *Reading Observer*, 16 July 1898, 8.

29 On the events in Reading, see Swan, *The Vaccination Problem*, 70; Hume, *The Mind-Changers*, 193; *Reading Mercury*, 30 July 1898, 3; *Reading Observer*, 23 July 1898, 8, 30 July 1898, 2.

30 Braithwaite, "Legal Problems of Conscientious Objection to Various Compulsions Under British Law."

31 *Shaw's Manual of the Vaccination Law*, 36–37.

32 *Vaccination Inquirer*, 1 July 1898, 49.

33 Ibid., 1 April 1896, 9, 1 January 1897, 165–66, 1 August 1898, 63.

34 *Oldham Chronicle*, 3 December 1898, 3.

35 *Kettering Guardian*, 2 December 1898, in Milnes Collection, vol. 52, 31; *Vaccination Inquirer*, 1 September 1898, 75.

36 *The Times*, 13 September 1898, 13.

37 *Vaccination Inquirer*, 1 October 1898, 86–87.

38 Ibid., 1 December 1898, 117, 1 October 1898, 88.

39 *Report of the Medical Officer of Health for Paddington*, 1898, 12.

40 *St. James' Gazette*, 22 August 1898, 38, in Milnes Collection, vol. 51, 38.

41 *Vaccination Inquirer*, 1 September 1898, 84.

42 *The Times*, 1 September 1898, 10.

43 Christ and Jordan, *Victorian Literature and the Victorian Visual Imagination*; Crary, *Techniques of the Observer*; Tucker, "Science Illustrated." On similar nineteenth-century problems of the visible, see Owen, *The Darkened Room*; Barrow, "An Imponderable Liberator," 89–117.

44 *Morning Leader*, 4 October 1898, in Milnes Collection, vol. 51, 72. The Roentgen ray was an early term for the X-ray.

45 *East London Observer*, 17 November 1900, 7.

46 Behlmer, *Friends of the Family*, 181–82.

47 *The Times*, 25 January 1900, 14.

48 Ibid., 28 December 1898, 2. On diphtheria, see Hardy, *The Epidemic Streets*, 80–109; *Manchester Guardian*, 27 September 1898, 9; Sherton Watson to Local Government Board, letter, 27 August 1898, PRO HO 45/9937/B27667/12.

49 *Vaccination Inquirer*, 1 October 1898, 88.

50 *Manchester Guardian*, 26 December 1898, 7; *The Times*, 12 January 1900, 14, 17 October 1901, 13; *East London Observer*, 1 December 1900, 2; *Manchester Guardian*, 12 March 1902, 11.

51 *Saturday Review*, 5 October 1901, 423.

52 Davis, "A Poor Man's System of Justice"; *East London Observer*, 1 December 1900, 2; Minute from Home Secretary, n.d., PRO HO 45/10322/129038/59; *The Lancet*, 8 October 1898, 953.

53 Edwards, *The Small-Pox Epidemic and Its Treatment*, 5; Swan, *Why I Am an Anti-Vaccinist*, 4.

54 *East London Observer*, 28 August 1902, 6; *Vaccination Inquirer*, 2 December 1901, 165; *The Star*, 5 November 1898, in Milnes Collection, vol. 52, 18.

55 *British Medical Journal*, 13 June 1903, 1394.

56 Fawcett, *The Vaccination Act of 1898*, 24; *Holloway Press*, 3 September 1898, in Milnes Collection, vol. 51, 54.

57 *Blackburn Standard*, 24 September 1898, in Milnes Collection, vol. 51, 26.

58 Gibbs, *Small-Pox and Vaccination*, 7; emphasis in the original.

59 *The Lancet*, 8 October 1898, 960; *British Medical Journal*, 23 February 1907, 457.

60 *Oldham Chronicle*, 3 December 1898, 3, 10 December 1898, 5; *Yorkshire Daily Post*, 13 December 1898; *Manchester Courier*, 14 December 1898, in Milnes Collection, vol. 52, 43–44.

61 Turner, *About Myself 1863–1930*, 73–74; *British Medical Journal*, 5 November 1898, 1443.

62 *The Lancet*, 5 January 1907, 57; *The Times*, 20 October 1902, 2.

63 *East London Observer*, 26 November 1898, 3.

64 *British Medical Journal*, 29 August 1903, 482–83; *East London Observer*, 8 September 1906, 6.

65 National Anti-Vaccination League, *How to Avoid Vaccination*, c. 1898, in John Johnson Collection, Societies Box 5, University of Oxford, Bodleian Library; *Vaccination Inquirer*, 1 October 1898, 88; *The Star*, 7 October 1898, in Milnes Collection, vol. 51, 56.

66 Memorandum on Vaccination Act, 1898, Conscientious Objectors, 23 March 1904, PRO HO 45/10297/115475/7; Memorandum from M. D. Chalmers, 1 September 1904, LMA PS/LAM/HI/4/137.

67 *Oldham Chronicle*, 30 April 1898, 5.

68 Greenwood, *The Law Relating to the Poor Law Medical Service and Vaccination*, 53.

69 *Bedford Times*, 17 December 1898, in Milnes Collection, vol. 52, 48; *Grantham Times*, 17 December 1898, ibid., 53; *Vaccination Inquirer*, 1 October 1898, 87; *South Wales Daily News*, 11 October 1898, in Milnes Collec-

tion, vol. 52, 7; *Oldham Chronicle*, 3 December 1898, 3; *British Medical Journal*, 24 December 1898, 1905; *Vaccination Inquirer*, 1 October 1898, 87; *Westminster Gazette*, 27 September 1898, in Milnes Collection, vol. 51, 68; Lupton, *Vaccination and the State*, 52.

70 Memorandum from M. D. Chalmers, 1 September 1904, LMA PS/LAM/H1/4/137.

71 *Manchester Guardian*, 13 December 1907, 10; *Vaccination Inquirer*, 1 February 1906, 218.

72 *Hansard*, 14 February 1907, 401–3.

73 *The Individualist*, June 1906, 60.

74 *Hansard*, 15 February 1907, 439–43, 453, 24 May 1907, 1279.

75 Vulliamy, *Fry's Law of Vaccination*, 79, nn. g, h.

76 *Hansard*, 25 July 1898, 1137; Confidential Circular on the Vaccination Acts of 1867 to 1898, PRO HO 45/10368/157384/49.

77 Holmes, *A Letter on Vaccination*.

78 As quoted in *Vaccination Inquirer*, 1 August 1901, 85.

79 *Buxton Chronicle*, 3 March 1899, in Milnes Collection, vol. 50, 4; *Vaccination Inquirer*, 1 July 1901, 72, 2 April 1906, 16; *British Medical Journal*, 23 February 1907, 457, 5 November 1898, 1443.

80 Vaccination Bill, 1905, PRO HO 45/10297/115475/91; Anonymous Minute, 28 May 1907, PRO HO 45/10358/152844/1; *Hansard*, 8 August 1907, 286.

81 *Hansard*, 22 August 1907, 1202–4.

82 Auerbach, " 'In the Courts and Alleys.' "

83 *Vaccination Inquirer*, 1 July 1907, 65.

84 Brown, *John Burns*, 155; Kent, *John Burns*, 200, 250; Lewis, "The Working-Class Wife and Mother and State Intervention, 1870–1918," 106; Dwork, *War Is Good for Babies and Other Young Children*, 114.

85 *Daylight*, 31 August 1907, 16.

86 *Hansard*, 22 August 1907, 1200–1207; *British Medical Journal*, 31 August 1907, 546.

87 *Local Government Chronicle*, 25 January 1908, 86, 7 March 1908, 233; *Vaccination Inquirer*, 2 March 1908, 204; Vaccination Act 1907, H. Booth to the President of the Board of Trade, letter, 8 January 1908, PRO HO 45/10368/157384/19.

88 Swan, *The Vaccination Problem*, 85; *Vaccination Inquirer*, 1 November 1909, 170.

89 General Register Office Smallpox Vaccination Returns, PRO RG 56/3.

90 Millman, *Managing Domestic Dissent in First World War Britain*, 11.

91 Rae, *Conscience and Politics*, 81. See also Martin, *Pacifism*; Kennedy, "Public Opinion and the Conscientious Objector, 1915–1919."

92 Rae, *Conscience and Politics*, 29, app. C ; Graham, *Conscription and Conscience*, 173.

93 Kennedy, *The Hound of Conscience*, 84; Graham, *Conscription and Conscience*, 58.

CONCLUSION

1   *The Individualist*, August 1906, 76.
2   *East London Observer*, 13 July 1907, 3.
3   *Vaccination Inquirer*, 1 June 1907, 45.
4   *The Individualist*, May 1907, 34.
5   *Vaccination Inquirer*, 1 June 1907, 45, 1 October 1907, 110–11, 1 November 1907, 132.
6   Ibid., 2 March 1908, 197, 1 October 1908, 105–6.
7   *British Medical Journal*, 18 April 1908, 950, 17 October 1908, 1205; *Vaccination Inquirer*, 2 November 1908, 134.
8   *Vaccination Inquirer*, 1 March 1909, 193, 204. Despite his proclaimed retirement, Bonner continued to lecture into the 1910s.
9   In some respects, the late-twentieth-century members of the NAVL resembled their Victorian counterparts. Some still practiced naturopathic medicine, while others shared similar religious beliefs. Allinson's family, makers of whole-meal bread, remained involved with the league until its demise. In the 1960s, the *Vaccination Inquirer* catered to a readership concerned also with vegetarianism, yoga, and anti-fluoridation. A retired employee of the NAVL recalled with some discomfort that at one point in its recent history, the NAVL also had fascist and anti-Semitic connections. Not an anti-vaccinationist himself, he remembered the league as a bunch of "maniacs."
10 Little is known about Loat except that she became converted to anti-vaccinationism in 1898 through reading the *Vaccination Inquirer* while working for the British Union for the Abolition of Vivisection: see Hume, *The Mind-Changers*.
11 *Vaccination Inquirer*, January–February 1947, 1.
12 The papers of the NAVL no longer exist; they were destroyed in 1982 when the league closed its doors. Much of the information on the league from the 1950s onward was gleaned from an interview with a former employee who has asked to remain unidentified. This interview was conducted on 21 October 1997 in the presence of Chris Kohler.
13 Greenough, "Intimidation, Coercion and Resistance in the Final Stages of the South Asian Smallpox Eradication Campaign, 1973–1975."
14 Hopkins, *Princes and Peasants*, 317.
15 As quoted in Greenough, "Intimidation, Coercion and Resistance in the Final Stages of the South Asian Smallpox Eradication Campaign, 1973–1975," 635–36.

16 White, "The Needle and the State," 15.

17 Sugg, "Baltimore Children Getting Their Shots," A1.

18 Noble, "Incentive Program Raises Immunization Rates," A14.

19 Preston, "The Demon in the Freezer," 59.

20 Connolly, "Focus on Smallpox Threat Revived," A3.

21 Blanchfield, "I Will Never Be Able to Trust My Leaders Again," A3.

22 Carroll, "Researchers Deal New Blow to Vaccination," 7.

23 Showalter, *Sexual Anarchy*.

24 Wolfe et al., "Content and Design Attributes of Antivaccination Web Sites," 3247.

25 Pollak, "Doctors Fighting Backlash over Vaccines," D7.

26 Crawley, "Take Vaccine or Risk Loss of Jobs, Some Employees to Military Told," B1.

27 Ibid.

28 Boon, "Campaigning for Consent"; *Hansard*, 14 March 1946, 250. This, however, is not to say that immunizations were generally accepted in the twentieth century, for as Lucinda Beier has documented, many working-class mothers still objected to "putting something in your body that shouldn't be there anyway": see Beier, "Contagion, Policy, Class, Gender, and Mid-Twentieth-Century Lancashire Working-Class Health Culture," 16.

29 Hodgkinson, *The Origins of the National Health Service*.

30 *Vaccination Inquirer*, January–February 1947, 3. For objections raised, see *Hansard*, 2 May 1946, 357; *British Medical Journal*, 1 June 1946, 851–52.

31 The National Health Service Act nevertheless retained a two-tier system, allowing for private practice and thus for the wealthy few to purchase what many considered a higher standard of health care. Ironically, then, while introducing socialized medicine, the National Health Service Act in some respects perpetuated class-based divisions in the provision of state medicine. For a somewhat polemical analysis of class and the National Health Service, see Navarro, *Class Struggle, the State and Medicine*.

32 Steedman, *Landscape for a Good Woman*, 122.

Bibliography

ARCHIVAL SOURCES

Bromley Central Library, Bromley, England

Vaccination Registers 1907–1910
Local Government Board Correspondence

Brunel University Library, London

Gomm, Amy Frances. "Water under the Bridge." Unpublished typescript, June 1975, on file.
Goss, Frank. "My Boyhood at the Turn of the Century. An Autobiography." Unpublished typescript, on file.

Contemporary Medical Archives Centre, Wellcome Institute for the History of Medicine, London

British Medical Association Files. SA/BMA Box 206

Gloucestershire Record Office (GRO), Gloucester, England

Registers of Successful Vaccinations
Vaccination Officers' Report Book

Hammersmith and Fulham Archives and Local History Centre, London

Registers of Children Not Vaccinated
Registers of Successful Vaccinations
Register of Vaccinations
Vaccination Officers' Report Books

Keighley Library, Keighley, England

Keighley and District Anti-Compulsory Vaccination League
Register of Members
Keighley and District Anti-Compulsory Vaccination League Correspondence

London Metropolitan Archives (LMA), London

Vaccination Officers' Birth Books, Enfield District, Edmonton Union
Summary of Vaccination Officer's Proceedings, Edmonton Union
Bow Street Magistrates Court, Summary Jurisdictions
Clerks Registered Papers, Lambeth Police Court
Edmonton Petty Sessions
Thames Street Police Court Registers
West London Police Court Registers

London School of Hygiene and Tropical Medicine (LSHTM), London

Alfred Milnes collection of newspaper cuttings and other material on
vaccination and smallpox, 1881–1902.

Public Record Office (PRO), London

HO 45 Registered Papers
HO 144 Registered Papers, Supplementary
MH 12 Poor Law Unions and Local Authorities
MH 155 Ministry of Health and Predecessors: Register of Official Inquiries into
Charges Against Officers
RG 56 General Register Office Smallpox Vaccination Returns

Southwark Local Studies Library, London

Vaccination Registers, Southwark Union
Vaccination Officer's Report Book

Tameside Local Studies Library, Stalybridge, England

Watson, Lewis. "Autobiography." Unpublished typescript, on file.

University of California, Los Angeles, Biomedical Library, Los Angeles

Smallpox Collection MS 55 Box 1

University of Oxford, Bodleian Library, John Johnson Collection, Oxford

Societies Box 5
Patent Medicines Boxes 3 and 6

NEWSPAPERS AND PERIODICALS

The Anti-Vaccinator, 1869
Anti-Vaccinator and Public Health Journal, 1872–73
Associated Medical Journal, 1853–56
Botanic Eclectic Review and Medical Tribune, 1855–56
British Medical Journal, 1857–1908, 1946–48
The Co-operator, 1860–70
Co-operator and Anti-Vaccinator, 1870–71
Coffin's Botanical Journal and Medical Reformer, 1847–59
Dietetic Reformer and Vegetarian Messenger, 1861–81
Dr. Skelton's Botanic Record and Family Herbal, 1852–55
East London Observer, 1857–1908
Eclectic Journal and Medical Free Press, 1866–67
Family Doctor and People's Medical Adviser, 1885–95
Family Physician or People's Medical Adviser, 1866
Hansard, 1853–1907, 1946–48
Herald of Health, 1879–84
Human Nature, 1867–69
Hydropathic Record and Journal of the Water Cure, 1868–69
Hygiest or Medical Reformer, 1855–63, 1866–67
The Individualist, 1903–8
Journal of the Vigilance Association, 1881–86
The Lancet, 1853–1908, 1946–48
Manchester Guardian, 1871–1907
National Anti-Compulsory Vaccination League Occasional Circular, 1874–76
National Anti-Compulsory Vaccination Reporter, 1876–84
Oldham Chronicle, 1854, 1867, 1871, 1898, 1907
Personal Rights Journal, 1886–1902
Public Health, 1888–1908
The Times, 1853–1907
Vaccination Inquirer, 1879–1910

OFFICIAL PAPERS AND PUBLICATIONS

Published Government Reports

A Report on Vaccination and Its Results Based on the Evidence Taken by the Royal Commission 1889–97, vol. 1. London: New Sydenham Society, 1898.
Fifth Report of the Royal Commission Appointed to Inquire into the Subject of Vaccination; with Minutes of Evidence and Appendices. London: HMSO, 1892.

Final Report of the Royal Commission Appointed to Inquire into the Subject of Vaccination; with Minutes of Evidence and Appendices. London: HMSO, 1896.

First Report of the Royal Commission Appointed to Inquire into the Subject of Vaccination; with Minutes of Evidence and Appendices. London: HMSO, 1889.

Fourth Report of the Royal Commission Appointed to Inquire into the Subject of Vaccination; with Minutes of Evidence and Appendices. London: HMSO, 1893.

Local Government Board Annual Reports.

Medical Officer of Health Annual Reports (various districts).

"Memorial Presented in 1855 to Sir Benjamin Hall, Then President of the Board of Health, by the President and Council of the Epidemiological Society, on a Proper State Provision for the Prevention of Smallpox and the Extension of Vaccination." In *Papers Relating to the History and Practice of Vaccination.* London: HMSO, 1857.

Papers Relating to the History and Practice of Vaccination. London: HMSO, 1857.

Registrar General Annual Reports.

Report from the Select Committee on the Vaccination Act (1867); Together with the Proceedings of the Committee, Minutes of Evidence, Appendix and Index. London: HMSO, 1871.

Report of the Medical Officer to the Privy Council, 1858. London: HMSO, 1859.

Return of Statement Showing the Number of Certificates of Conscientious Objection . . . Received by the Vaccination Officers in the Year 1899. London: HMSO, 1900.

Return of Statement Showing the Number of Certificates of Conscientious Objection . . . Received by the Vaccination Officers in Each of the Years 1900 and 1901. London: HMSO, 1902.

Second Report of the Royal Commission Appointed to Inquire into the Subject of Vaccination; with Minutes of Evidence and Appendices. London: HMSO, 1890.

Sixth Report of the Royal Commission Appointed to Inquire into the Subject of Vaccination; with Minutes of Evidence and Appendices. London: HMSO, 1897.

Third Report of the Royal Commission Appointed to Inquire into the Subject of Vaccination; With Minutes of Evidence and Appendices. London: HMSO, 1890.

Parliamentary Papers

A Bill to Consolidate and to Amend the Laws Relating to Vaccination. PP 1856 VI (67).

An Amended Return for Returns Showing the Number of Persons Who Have Been Imprisoned or Fined for Non-compliance with the Provision of the Act Relating to the Vaccination of Children. PP 1881 LXXVI (289).

Letter Dated 30 June 1855, Addressed to the President of the Board of Health, by John Gibbs, Esquire, Entitled "Compulsory Vaccination Briefly Considered in Its Scientific, Religious, and Political Aspects." PP 1856 LII (109).

Letter from Dr. Edward Seaton to Viscount Palmerston, with Enclosed Copy of a Report on the State of Small Pox and Vaccination in England and Wales and Other Countries, and on Compulsory Vaccination, with Tables and Appendices, Presented to the President and Council of the Epidemiological Society by the Small Pox and Vaccination Committee, the 26th Day of March 1851. PP 1852–3 CI (434).

Report on the State of Small-Pox and Vaccination in England and Wales and Other Countries, and on Compulsory Vaccination, with Tables and Appendices, Presented to the President and Council of the Epidemiological Society by the Small-Pox and Vaccination Committee, the 26th Day of March 1853. PP 1852–53 XVIII (HL 256).

Return of the Number of Prosecutions in Respect of England and Wales since 1st Day of January 1875 to the 1st Day of January 1879, under the Vaccination Act, 1867. PP 1880 (146).

Returns Showing the Number of Persons Who Have Been Imprisoned or Fined for Non-compliance with the Provision of the Acts Relating to the Vaccination of Children. PP 1890 LIX (104).

OTHER PUBLISHED PRIMARY SOURCES

Major collections of anti-vaccination pamphlets can be found at the British Library; the University of California, Los Angeles, Biomedical Library; the Institute for the History of Medicine, Johns Hopkins University; and the National Library of Medicine in Bethesda. For reasons of space, only cited materials appear here.

Abdiel [William Thomas Wiseman]. *Vaccination and Smallpox.* London: G. Hill, 1882.

Allen, (Rev.) Munderford. *Vaccination and the Vaccination Act: A Paper Read at Exeter Hall.* Cheltenham: G. F. Poole, 1874.

[Allinson, Thomas R.] *How Parents May Protect Their Offspring from the Dangers and Injuries of Vaccination.* n.p., c. 1878.

Allinson, Thomas R. *Medical Essays Reprinted from the "Weekly Times and Echo,"* vol. 1. London: Renshaw, 1887.

———. *How to Avoid Vaccination.* London, 1888.

An Appeal to Passive Resisters. London: National Anti-Vaccination League, 1905.

Authoritative Opinions Adverse to Vaccination or Its Compulsory Enforcement. London: Miller, Son and Company, 1902.

Baker, Thomas. *A Battling Life, Chiefly in the Civil Service.* London: Kegan Paul, Trench and Company, 1885.

Bayard (Dr.). *Extracts from an Essay on Vaccination, after Thirty-five Years*

Observation and Experience. Trans. by George S. Gibbs. London: Ladies'
Sanitary Association, 1870.

Biggs, J. T. *Leicester: Sanitation versus Vaccination.* London: National Anti-
Vaccination League, 1912.

Birmingham Anti-Variole League for the Repeal of Compulsory Vaccination.
Annual Report. 1890.

Blakewell, R. H. "Is It Expedient to Make Vaccination Compulsory?"
Transactions of the New Zealand Institute 24 (1891): 636–41.

Bland, Samuel. *Dr. Francis T. Bond Very Much "Over the Border."* Gloucester:
privately published, 1898.

Bright, Ursula M. *An Evil Law Unfairly Enforced.* London: Health and Liberty
League, 1884.

Brown, E. *The Case for Vaccination.* London: Balliere, Tindall, and Cox, 1902.

Brown, John. *Compulsory Vaccination in Scotland.* Kilmarnock: Kilmarnock
Anti-Compulsory Vaccination League, 1897.

Coffin, Albert Isaiah. *Medical Botany: A Course of Lectures Delivered at Sussex
Hall During 1850.* London: W. B. Ford, 1851.

——. *Botanic Guide to Health,* 13th ed. London: British Medico-Botanic
Establishment, 1855.

Colley (Ven. Archdeacon). *Vaccination a Moral Evil, a Physical Curse and a
Psychological Wrong.* Leicester: National Anti-Compulsory Vaccination
League, 1882.

Collins, W. J. *Sir Lyon Playfair's Logic.* London: E. W. Allen, 1883.

Collinson, Joseph. *What It Costs to Be Vaccinated: The Pains and Penalties of an
Unjust Law.* London: Humanitarian League, 1896.

Compulsory Vaccination. n.p., c. 1866.

Connell, Ira. *My Experience of Vaccination: Its Influence and Results, by Ira
Connell, a Sufferer and a Victim to Vaccination for the Space of Twenty-two
Years.* London: F. Pitman, 1869.

Copeman, Sydney Monckton. *Vaccination: Its Natural History and Pathology.*
London: Macmillan, 1899.

Creighton, Charles. *The Natural History of Cow-Pox and Vaccinal Syphilis.*
London: Cassell and Company, 1887.

——. "Vaccination." *Encyclopedia Britannica,* 9th ed. London: Adam and
Charles Black, 1888.

——. *Jenner and Vaccination.* London: Sonnenschein, 1889.

——. *Exit Dr. Jenner.* London: National Anti-Vaccination League, 1906.

Crookshank, Edgar. *The Prevention of Small-Pox with Special Reference to the Origin
and Development of the Stamping-Out System.* London: H. K. Lewis, 1894.

The Danger and Injustice of Compulsory Vaccination. London: Mothers' Anti-
Compulsory Vaccination League, 1873.

Davidson, P. M. *Special Report on the Recent Outbreak of Small-Pox in Congleton by the Medical Officer of Health to the Urban Sanitary Authority.* London: Hansard, 1889.

Defence Fund, Reminder Notice. London: National Anti-Vaccination League, 1898.

Denham, W. H. *The Extinction of Small-Pox and Diseases of Vaccination by a Practical Process.* London: Gould and Son, 1881.

Dickens, Charles. *Bleak House.* Oxford: Oxford University Press, 1966.

Disease by Law: An Indictment of Compulsory Vaccination. London: E. W. Allen, 1884.

The Doctor's Baby. London: William Young, 1883.

Dougall, J. *The Artificial Cultivation of Vaccine Lymph.* Glasgow: Alex Macdougall, 1886.

Duxbury, Thomas. *Vaccination Rhymes.* Blackburn: self-published, 1884.

E. M. Crookshank, History and Pathology of Vaccination, a Review. London: E. W. Allen, 1890.

Eadon, Samuel. *Vaccination; or Infant Poisoning and Murdering by Act of Parliament, Chapter II.* n.p., 1880.

Eastes, G. *Concerning Vaccination: A Critical Exposition of the Subject for Non-Professional Readers.* London: Robert Hardwicke, 1871.

Edwards, Ifan. *No Gold on My Shovel.* London: Porcupine Press, 1947.

Edwards, William Henry. *The Small-Pox Epidemic and Its Treatment: A Plea for Common Sense. Some Reasons Why the Death-Rate from Small-Pox Has Increased.* Boscombe: A. Sutton, c. 1903.

Epidemiological Society of London. *The Commemoration Volume.* London: Bedford Press, 1900.

Family Medical Adviser: A Practical Treatise on Hygiene, Diet and Medical Treatment at Home. London: Ward, Lock, and Company, 1888.

Farrar, Reginald. *On the Present Condition of Our Knowledge of the Aetiological Agent in Vaccinia and Variola.* Reprint. from *Public Health*, July 1901.

Fawcett, Mrs. Henry [Millicent Garrett]. *The Vaccination Act of 1898: Reasons Why Parliament Was Right to Relax the Compulsory Clauses of Previous Vaccination Acts.* Women's Printing Society, n.d. Reprint. from *Contemporary Review*, March 1899, with some additions.

[Foster, E.] *Murder and Mutilation! A Trial in a British Court of Justice.* Stockport: John Moss, c. 1873.

Fox, Charles. *The Question of Compulsory Vaccination, Illustrated by Fifty-six Unpublished Cases of Illness and Death.* London: E. W. Allen, 1890.

Fox, John Makinson. *Compulsory Vaccination: An Explanatory Catechism.* London: National Health Society, 1877.

Fraser, John. *An Attempt to Prove That Vaccination with Its Compulsory Law, Instead of Being a General Blessing, Is a Universal Curse.* London: British College of Health, 1871.

Furnival, W. J. *The Conscientious Objector: Who He Is! What He Has! What He Wants! And Why!* Stone: W. J.Furnival, 1902.

Gairdner, W. T. *A Remarkable Experience Concerning Leprosy: Involving Certain Facts and Statement Bearing on the Question—Is Leprosy Communicative Through Vaccination?* London: British Medical Association, 1887.

Gibbs, George S. *Small-Pox and Vaccination. A Letter Addressed to Major Graham, Registrar General of Births, Marriages and Deaths in England and Wales.* Darlington: Mothers' Anti-Compulsory Vaccination League, 1874.

——. *Fortification by Disease and Its Effect on Infant Life.* London: Mothers' Anti-Compulsory Vaccination League, 1877.

Gibbs, John. *Our Medical Liberties.* London: Sotheran, Son and Draper, 1854.

——. *Compulsory Vaccination Briefly Considered in Its Scientific, Religious, and Political Aspects.* London: Sotheran and Willis, 1856.

——. *More Words on Vaccination.* London: Willis and Sotheran, 1856.

Gloucester Epidemic of Smallpox, 1895–96. Report of the Committee Appointed by the Board of Guardians to Organize and Carry out the General Vaccination of the City and District. Gloucester, 1896.

Greenwood, M. *The Law Relating to the Poor Law Medical Service and Vaccination.* London: Balliere, Tindall and Cox, 1901.

Guttery, (Rev.) A. T. *Anti-Compulsory Vaccination, An Address.* Oldham: John Owen and Sons, 1889.

Hadwen, W. R. *The Case against Vaccination.* Gloucester: Gloucester Anti-Vaccination League, 1896.

——. *The Gloucester Epidemic of Smallpox, 1895–96. The Case for the Anti-Vaccinationists.* Weston-super-Mare: Weston-super-Mare and District Anti-Compulsory Vaccination Society, 1896.

——. *The Vaccination Delusion.* Liverpool: Liverpool Anti-Vaccination League, 1902.

——. *The Follies and Cruelties of Vivisection.* London, 1905.

Hainsworth, Robert. *Results of an Investigation into the Sheffield Smallpox Epidemic of 1887.* Leeds: Oldfield, Brooke and Company, c. 1889.

Halket, W. *Compulsory Vaccination! A Crime Against Nature.* London: J. Burns, n.d.

The Hampstead Hospital: Great Meeting on the Heath. London: Frederick C. Mathieson, c. 1875.

Hart, Ernest. *The Truth about Vaccination: An Examination and Refutation of the Assertions of the Anti-Vaccinators.* London: Smith, Elder and Company, 1880.

Health and Liberty League. *Does Compulsory Education Justify Compulsory Vaccination?* London: E. W. Allen, 1887.

Heath, Edward. *Vaccination; or, Blood Poisoning with Animal Diseases.* London: Heath and Company, 1898.

Holmes, J. R. *A Letter on Vaccination.* London: National Anti-Vaccination League, 1898.

Hughes, Hugh Price. *The Rev. Hugh Price Hughes on Vaccination.* Reprint. from *Vaccination Inquirer,* 1 November 1899.

Hume, A. *A Word for the Baby.* Walthamstow, 1879.

Hume, E. Douglas. *The Mind-Changers.* Letchworth: Hume Books Trust, 1939.

Hume-Rothery, Mary. *Women and Doctors: Or Medical Despotism in England.* Manchester: Abel Heywood, 1871.

———. *150 Reasons for Disobeying the Vaccination Law, by Persons Prosecuted Under It.* Cheltenham: George F. Poole, 1878.

———. *What Smallpox and Vaccination and the Vaccination Acts Really Are.* Leicester: E. Lamb, 1880.

Hume-Rothery, William. *Vaccination and the Vaccination Laws: A Physical Curse, and a Class-Tyranny,* 2nd ed. Manchester: W. Tolley, 1873.

———. "Men, not Slaves" (letter to the editor). *The Indicator,* 5 January 1875.

Hunt, Chandos Leigh. *Vaccination Brought Home to the People.* London: James Burns, c. 1876.

Hunter, A. S. *No More Vaccination!* Manchester: S. Clarke, 1905.

Hutton, Arthur Wollaston. *The Vaccination Question.* London: Methuen, 1894.

Insurance Against Vaccination: A Project, Correspondence, and Referendum. London: London Society for the Abolition of Compulsory Vaccination, 1884.

Jervoise, (Sir) J. Clarke. *Infection.* London: Vacher and Sons, 1882.

Johnson, Horace. *Essay upon Compulsory Vaccination.* Brighton: Fleet and Son, 1856.

Kidd, Beatrice E., and M. Edith Richards. *Hadwen of Gloucester: Man, Medico, Martyr.* London: John Murray, 1933.

Killed by Vaccination, 2nd ed. London: William Young, 1887.

Kingscote, Mrs. Howard. *The English Baby in India.* London: Churchill, 1893.

Klein, E. *Micro-organisms and Disease.* Reprint. from *The Practitioner,* October 1884.

The Knell of Compulsory Vaccination. London: Anti-Compulsory Vaccination and Mutual Protection Society, 1874.

Ladies' Sanitary Association. *When Were You Vaccinated.* London: Ladies' Sanitary Association, c. 1860.

Langdon, Roger. *The Life of Roger Langdon.* London: Elliot Stock, 1909.

Leighton, A. *The People of Dewsbury and Vaccination: A Letter to William Chambers.* London: W. Kent and Company, 1876.

Levy, J. H. *State Interference in the Vaccination Controversy.* London: Personal Rights Association, 1887.

Loane, M. E. *The Next Street But One.* London: Edward Arnold, 1907

———. *An Englishman's Castle.* London: Edward Arnold, 1909.

London Society for the Abolition of Compulsory Vaccination. *Catalogue of Anti-Vaccination Literature Issued by the Society,* 2nd ed. London: E. W. Allen, 1895.

Longman, F. *Fifteen Years Fight against Compulsory Vaccination*. London, 1900.

Lupton, Arnold. *Vaccination and the State*. London: P. S. King and Son, 1906.

Makuna, Montague D., ed. *Transactions of the Vaccination Inquiry*. Leicester: W. H. Lead, 1883.

Malings, Joseph Edward. *Narrative of Three Prosecutions under the Vaccination Act*. London: J. Burns, 1873.

McCormick, Ernest. *Is Vaccination a Disastrous Delusion?* London: National Anti-Vaccination League, 1905.

McVail, John. *Vaccination Vindicated: Being an Answer to the Leading Anti-Vaccinators*. London: Cassell and Company, 1887.

Medicus. *Compulsory Vaccination*. London: Billing, 1871.

Milnes, Alfred. *What about Vaccination? And Other Contributions*, 3rd ed. London: National Anti-Vaccination League, c. 1902.

The Month. London: Cassell and Company, 1896. Reprint. from *The Practitioner*, May 1896.

Moon, Walter. *The Secret of Perfect Health: Disease Rendered Preventable and Removable by Washing Its Germs Out of the Body*. London: Sanitary Engineering, c. 1890.

Morison, John. *Morisonia; or Family Adviser of the British College of Health*. 4th ed., vol. 1. London: British College of Health, 1833.

———. *The Truth-Hygiean Manifesto*. London: British College of Health, 1867.

National Disease: Remarks upon the Prevailing Epidemic of Smallpox. London: Longmans, Green, Reader and Dyer, 1871.

Newman, F. W. *The Political Side of the Vaccination System*, 4th ed. Leicester: National Anti-Compulsory Vaccination League, c. 1874.

———. *The Coming Revolution: An Anti-Vaccination Pamphlet*. Nottingham: Stevenson, Bailey and Smith, 1882.

Newman, George. *To Parents and Citizens of Gloucester*. Gloucester: Gloucester and District Branch of the National Anti-Vaccination League, 1896.

Nichols, Mary Gove. *A Woman's Work in Water Cure and Sanitary Education*. London: Hygienic Institute, 1874.

Oswald, Felix. *Vaccination a Crime*. New York: Physical Culture Publishing, 1901.

Paul, Alexander. *The Vaccination Problem in 1903*. London: P. S. King and Son, 1903.

Perry, (Rev.) Jevon J. Muschamp. *Smallpox and Vaccination*. Reprint. from *St. Paul's Parish Magazine*, December 1898.

Pickering, John. *Anti-Vaccination: The Statistics of the Medical Officers to the Leeds Smallpox Hospital Exposed and Refuted in a Letter to the Leeds Board of Guardians*. Leeds: McCorquodale and Company, 1876.

———. *Which? Sanitation and Sanatory Remedies or Vaccination and the Drug Treatment?* London: E. W. Allen, 1892.

———. *The Smallpox Epidemic in Gloucester and the Water Cure*. London: E. W. Allen, 1896.

Pitman, Henry. *Prison Thoughts on Vaccination, Part 2*. Manchester: John Heywood, 1876.

Port, Henry. *Precaution Against Smallpox*. Birmingham: Midland Anti-Compulsory Vaccination Protection Society, 1881.

Purdy, W. *Smallpox: A Practical Treatise on the Smallpox Epidemic. Vaccination: Its Merits and Demerits*. London: John Heywood, 1888.

Purvis, John Prior. *Statistics of Vaccination at the Greenwich Public Vaccination Station, from February 23, 1870 to September 29, 1875*. London: Churchill, 1876.

R., G. *Cow-Pox and Vaccinal Syphilis*. London: Mile End Branch of the National Anti-Vaccination League, c. 1896.

Recent Utterances on the Vaccination Question. London: William Young, 1885.

Reeves, Maud Pember. *Round about a Pound a Week*. London: Virago, 1979.

Report of the Section Appointed to Enquire into the Present State of Vaccination as Read at the Anniversary Meeting of the Provincial Medical and Surgical Association. London: William Clowes and Sons, 1840.

Report of the Sixth Annual Meeting of the London Society for the Abolition of Compulsory Vaccination. London: E. W. Allen, 1886.

Rose, Charles. *How to Cure and Prevent Small-Pox*. London: F. Pitman, 1882.

Rumsey, Henry. *On the Amendment of the Vaccination Laws in England*. London: Faithfull and Head, 1867.

Russell, A. G., and Alexander Wheeler. *A Night's Debate on Vaccination*. London: E. W. Allen, 1889.

Rutter, Clarence E. *Is It Right to Force Parents to Have Their Children Vaccinated against Their Judgment and Conscience?* Wincanton: Fred Shepherd, 1894.

Rymer, James Malcolm. *Varney the Vampire, or The Feast of Blood*. New York: Arno Press, 1970.

Sanger, Lord George. *Seventy Years a Showman*. London: J. M. Dent and Sons, 1927.

Schieferdecker, C. C. *Dr. C. G. G. Nittinger's Evils of Vaccination*. Philadelphia: [H. B. Ashmead], 1856.

Scott, Benjamin. *The Kensington Protest Against Vaccination, Backed by the Un-English Compulsory Law*. Liverpool, 1876.

Scott, John. "Smallpox and Vaccination." in *Health Lectures for the People*, vol. 5, 35–72. London: John Heywood, 1882.

Seaton, Edward. *On the Protective and Modifying Powers of Vaccination*. London: T. Richards, 1857.

———. *A Handbook of Vaccination*. London: Macmillan, 1868.

Sexton, George. *Vaccination Useless and Injurious*. London: G. Howe, 1870.

Shaw's Manual of the Vaccination Law, 6th ed. London: Shaw and Son, 1898.

Shortt, John. *A Popular Lecture on Vaccination.* Madras: Gantz Brothers, 1865.

Simon, John. *Public Health Reports.* London: Sanitary Institute, 1887.

Some Leading Arguments against Compulsory Vaccination. London: E. W. Allen, 1887.

Stephen, J. Thomson. *How Leicester Won "Home Rule": An Example and a Warning.* Leicester: W. Willson, c. 1880.

Stevens, John. *Medical Reform; or, Physiology and Botanic Practice for the People,* 6th ed. London: Collins, 1854.

Stobbs, Robert. *To the Fathers and Mothers of Great Britain, and All Who Groan Beneath the Yoke of a Medical Despotism.* n.p., 1886.

Swan, Joseph. P. "Why I Am an Anti-Vaccinist." Prize Essay reprint. from *Reynold's Newspaper,* 29 November 1903.

——. *The Vaccination Problem.* London: C. W. Daniel Company, 1936.

Sykes, Mark L. *Smallpox, Vaccination and the Glycerination of Vaccine Lymph.* Reprint. from *Transactions and Annual Report of the Manchester Microscopical Society,* 1900.

Taylor, P. A. *Compulsory Vaccination: A Speech in the House of Commons on the Second Reading of the Vaccination Act (Ireland) Amendment Bill, April 7th, 1879.* London: William Young, 1879.

——. *Personal Rights, Speeches of P. A. Taylor.* London: Vigilance Association for the Defense of Personal Rights, 1884.

[Tebb, William]. *Government Prosecutions for Medical Heresy: A Verbatim Report of the Case Regina v. Tebb.* London: E. W. Allen, c. 1879.

Tebb, William. *Sanitation, not Vaccination, The True Protection against Small-Pox.* London: London Society for the Abolition of Compulsory Vaccination, 1881.

——. *The Results of Vaccination and the Inequity and Injustice of Its Enforcement.* London: E. W. Allen, 1887.

——. *Compulsory Vaccination in England: With Incidental References to Foreign States.* London: E. W. Allen, 1889.

——. *The Spread of Leprosy: A West Indian Complaint.* Reprint. from *Homoeopathic World,* 1889.

——. *A Personal Statement of the Results of Vaccination.* London: London Society for the Abolition of Compulsory Vaccination, 1891.

Testimonies of Medical Men on the Protection Supposed to Be Afforded by Vaccination, 1805–81. London: London Society for the Abolition of Compulsory Vaccination, c. 1881.

Thomas, William. *The Safety-Valve of Life.* London: E. W. Allen, 1885.

To Members of Parliament. n.p. , c. 1879.

Toye, E. W. *Vaccination Condemned by Medical Men; and Medical Men Condemned by Vaccination.* London: Charity Record Office, 1884.

Turner, Ben. *About Myself 1863–1930.* London: Humphrey Toulmin, 1930.

Vaccinal Syphilis. London: Mother's Anti-Compulsory Vaccination League, 1873.

Vaccination. Reprint. from *Herald of Health,* March 1878.

Vaccination: A Folly and a Crime. An Appeal to Parents. London: William Young, 1871.

Vaccination and Physical Deterioration. London: National Anti-Vaccination League, c. 1905.

Vaccination as the Cause of Fever and Consumption and as a Transmitter of All Kinds of Disease: Dialogue between a Mother and a Daughter. London: British College of Health, 1868.

Vernon, H. H. *Why Little Children Die.* London: John Heywood, c. 1878.

Vulliamy, A. F. *Fry's Law of Vaccination,* 7th ed. London: Knight and Company, 1899.

Wallace, Alfred Russel. *Vaccination Proved Useless and Dangerous from Forty-five Years of Registration Statistics,* 2nd ed. London: E. W. Allen, 1889.

———. *The Wonderful Century.* Toronto: George Morang, 1898.

Walsh, Nugent Charles. *The Medical Officer's Vade-Mecum or Poor Law Surgeon's Guide.* London: Renshaw, 1866.

Wanted! Wanted! Wanted! Members of Parliament, Noblemen, Government Officers, Judges, Lawyers, Parsons, Councilors, etc. Whose Moral Characters ARE GOOD! n.p., c. 1889.

Watson, J. H. *An Essay on Vaccination.* London: East Post Printing Works, 1869.

Wells, H. G. *The Island of Doctor Moreau.* Athens: University of Georgia Press, 1993.

West, (Mrs.) S. J. *The Kent Occasional Eye Opener on the Ill Effects and Inutility of Compulsory Vaccination.* Rochester, 1877.

White, William. *Sir Lyon Playfair Taken to Pieces and Disposed of; Likewise Sir Charles Dilke.* London: E. W. Allen, 1884.

———. *The Story of a Great Delusion.* London: E. W. Allen, 1885.

Wilder, Alexander. *Vaccination a Medical Fallacy.* n.p., n.d [c. 1870].

Wilkinson, J. J. Garth. *War, Cholera and the Ministry of Health.* London: Robert Theobold, 1854.

———. *Smallpox and Vaccination.* London: F. Pitman, 1871.

———. *Compulsory Vaccination: Its Wickedness to the Poor.* London: F. Pitman, 1873.

———. *Extract from a Book Just Published on Human Science and on Divine Revelation by Dr. Garth Wilkinson.* London: Mother's Anti-Compulsory Vaccination League, 1876.

———. *Herodian Decree of the Local Government Board.* London, 1881.

———. *The Vaccination Vampire.* London: n.p., 1881. Reprint from *National Anti-Compulsory Vaccination Reporter,* February 1881.

Winterburn, G. W. *The Value of Vaccination*. Philadelphia: Hahnemann Publishing, 1886.

Woodward, Kathleen. *Jipping Street*. London: Harper and Brothers, 1928.

Young, William. *A Warning to Parents—Wholesale Propagation of Syphilis by Vaccination*. London: National Anti-Compulsory Vaccination League, 1877.

——. *Vaccination Tracts*. London: William Young, 1879.

——. *The Tyranny of the Vaccination Acts*. London: London Society for the Abolition of Compulsory Vaccination, 1888.

Younger, D. *The Magnetic and Botanic Family Physician*. London: E. W. Allen, 1887.

SECONDARY SOURCES

Ackerknecht, Erwin. *A Short History of Medicine*. Baltimore: Johns Hopkins University Press, 1982.

Arata, Stephen D. "The Occidental Tourist: *Dracula* and the Anxiety of Reverse Colonization." *Victorian Studies* (summer 1990): 621–45.

Arnold, David. *Colonizing the Body: State Medicine and Epidemic Disease in Nineteenth Century India*. Berkeley: University of California Press, 1993.

Arnup, Katherine. " 'Victims of Vaccination?': Opposition to Compulsory Immunization in Ontario, 1900–90." *Canadian Bulletin of Medical History* 9 (1992): 159–76.

Auerbach, Alexander. " 'In the Courts and Alleys': The Enforcement of the Laws on Children's Education and Labor in London, 1870–1904." Ph.D. diss., Emory University, Atlanta, 2001.

Auerbach, Nina. *Our Vampires, Ourselves*. Chicago: University of Chicago Press, 1995.

Bailey, Peter. " 'Will the Real Bill Banks Please Stand Up?': Towards a Role Analysis of Mid-Victorian Respectability." *Journal of Social History* 12(3) (1979): 336–53.

——. "White Collars, Gray Lives? The Lower Middle Class Revisited." *Journal of British Studies* 38(3) (1999): 273–90.

Baldick, Chris. *In Frankenstein's Shadow: Myth, Monstrosity, and Nineteenth-Century Writing*. Oxford: Clarendon Press, 1987.

Baldwin, Peter. *Contagion and the State in Europe, 1830–1930*. Cambridge: Cambridge University Press, 1999.

Barnes, David S. *The Making of a Social Disease: Tuberculosis in Nineteenth Century France*. Berkeley: University of California Press, 1995.

Barrow, Logie. *Independent Spirits: Spiritualism and English Plebeians, 1850–1910*. London: Routledge, 1986.

——. "An Imponderable Liberator: J. J. Garth Wilkinson." 89–117 in *Studies in the History of Alternative Medicine*, ed. by Roger Cooter. New York: St. Martin's Press, 1988.

——. "Why Were Most Medical Heretics at Their Most Confident around the 1840s? (The Other Side of Mid-Victorian Medicine)." 165–85 in *British Medicine in an Age of Reform*, ed. by Roger French and Andrew Wear. London: Routledge, 1991.

——. "In the Beginning Was the Lymph: The Hollowing of Stational Vaccination in England and Wales, 1840–1898." 205–23 in *Medicine, Health and the Public Sphere in Britain, 1600–2000*, ed. by Steve Sturdy. London: Routledge, 2002.

Bashford, Alison. *Purity and Pollution: Gender, Embodiment and Victorian Medicine*. Houndsmills: Macmillan, 1998.

——. "Foreign Bodies: Vaccination, Contagion, and Colonialism in the Nineteenth Century." 39–60 in *Contagion: Historical and Cultural Studies*, ed. by Alison Bashford and Claire Hooker. London: Routledge, 2001.

——. *Imperial Hygiene: A Critical History of Colonialism, Nationalism and Public Health*. Handsmills: Palgrave, 2004.

Beck, Ann. "Issues in the Anti-Vaccination Movement in England." *Medical History* 4 (1960): 310–21.

Behlmer, George K. *Child Abuse and Moral Reform in England, 1870–1908*. Stanford, Calif.: Stanford University Press, 1982.

——. *Friends of the Family: The English Home and Its Guardians, 1850–1940*. Stanford, Calif.: Stanford University Press, 1998.

——. "Grave Doubts: Victorian Medicine, Moral Panic, and the Signs of Death." *Journal of British Studies* 42(2) (2003): 206–35.

Beier, Lucinda M. "Contagion, Policy, Class, Gender, and Mid-Twentieth Century Lancashire Working-Class Health Culture." *Hygiea Internationalis* 2(1) (2001): 7–23.

Belchem, John. " 'Temperance in All Things': Vegetarianism, the Manx Press and the Alternative Agenda of Reform in the 1840s." 149–62 in *Living and Learning: Essays in Honour of J. F. C. Harrison*, ed. by Malcolm Chase and Ian Dyck. Aldershot: Scolar Press, 1996.

Belford, Barbara. *Bram Stoker*. New York: Knopf, 1996.

Bentley, Christopher. "The Monster in the Bedroom: Sexual Symbolism in Bram Stoker's *Dracula*." 24–34 in *Dracula: The Vampires and the Critics*, ed. by Margaret L. Carter. Ann Arbor, Mich.: UMI Research Press, 1988.

Biagini, Eugenio. *Liberty, Retrenchment and Reform*. Cambridge: Cambridge University Press, 1992.

Blanchfield, Mike. "I Will Never Be Able to Trust My Leaders Again." *Ottawa Citizen*, 27 February 2000.

Boon, Timothy. "Campaigning for Consent: The Ministry of Health, Medical Officers of Health, Parents, and Diphtheria Immunisation, 1920–1945."

Unpublished paper, presented at Caring for the Body, Reshaping the Self
conference, 2 May 1998.

Braddon, Mary Elizabeth. "The Good Lady Ducayne." 125–50 in *The Dracula
Book of Great Vampire Stories*, ed. by Leslie Shepard. Secaucus, N.J.: Citadel
Press, 1977.

Bradley, Ian. *The Optimists*. London: Faber and Faber, 1980.

Braithwaite, Constance. "Conscience in Conflict with the Law: The History of
Two Struggles." *Durham University Journal*, New Series 18(2) (1957): 62–
69.

———. "Legal Problems of Conscientious Objection to Various Compulsions
Under British Law." *Journal of the Friends' Historical Society* 52 (1) (1968): 3–
18.

Brebner, J. Bartlet. "Laissez Faire and State Intervention in Nineteenth-
Century Britain." *Journal of Economic History* 8, supp. (1948): 59–73.

Briggs, Asa. "Samuel Smiles: The Gospel of Self-Help." 85–96 in *Victorian
Values: Personalities and Perspectives in Nineteenth Century Society*, ed. by
Gordon Marsden. London: Longman, 1990.

Bristow, Edward J. *Vice and Vigilance: Purity Movements in Britain Since 1700*.
Dublin: Gill and Macmillan, 1977.

Brown, Kenneth D. *John Burns*. London: Royal Historical Society, 1977.

Brown, P. S. "Social Context and Medical Theory in the Demarcation of
Nineteenth-Century Boundaries." 216–33 in *Medical Fringe and Medical
Orthodoxy 1750–1850*, ed. by W. F. Bynum and Roy Porter. London: Croom
Helm, 1987.

———. "Nineteenth Century American Health Reformers and the Early Nature
Cure Movement in Britain." *Medical History* 32(2) (1988): 174–94.

Brown, Penny. *The Captured World: The Child and Childhood in Nineteenth-
Century Women's Writing in England*. New York: Harvester Wheatsheaf,
1993.

Brunton, Deborah. "Pox Britannica: Smallpox Inoculation in Britain, 1721–
1830." Unpublished Ph.D. diss., University of Pennsylvania, Philadelphia,
1990.

———. "The Problems of Implementation: The Failure and Success of Public
Vaccination Against Smallpox in Ireland, 1840–1873." 138–57 in *Medicine,
Disease and the State in Ireland, 1650–1940*, ed. by Elizabeth Malcolm and
Greta Jones. Cork: Cork University Press, 1999.

Burke, Timothy. *Lifebuoy Men, Lux Women: Commodification, Consumption, and
Cleanliness in Modern Zimbabwe*. Durham: Duke University Press, 1996.

Burne, John. "Kentish Anti-Vaccinators." *Bygone Kent* 18(1) (1997): 29–34.

Burnett, John, ed. *Destiny Obscure: Autobiographies of Childhood, Education and
Family from the 1820s to the 1920s*. London: Penguin, 1982.

Burney, Ian. *Bodies of Evidence: Medicine and the Politics of the English Inquest,
1830–1926*. Baltimore: Johns Hopkins University Press, 2000.

Burton, Antoinette. "States of Injury: Josephine Butler on Slavery, Citizenship, and the Boer War." *Social Politics* 5(3) (1998): 338–61.

Carroll, Patrick. "Medical Police and the History of Public Health." *Medical History* 46(4) (2002): 461–94.

Carroll, Rory. "Researchers Deal New Blow to Vaccination" *The Guardian*, 2 June 1999.

Carter, Margaret L., ed. *Dracula: The Vampires and the Critics*. Ann Arbor, Mich.: UMI Research Press, 1988.

Cassel, Jay. *The Secret Plague: Venereal Disease in Canada, 1838–1939*. Toronto: University of Toronto Press, 1987.

Chamberlain, J. Edward, and Sander L. Gilman, eds. *Degeneration: The Dark Side of Progress*. New York: Columbia University Press, 1985.

Christ, Carol T., and John O. Jordan, eds. *Victorian Literature and the Victorian Visual Imagination*. Berkeley: University of California Press, 1995.

Clark, Anna. *The Struggle for the Breeches: Gender and the Making of the British Working Class*. Berkeley: University of California Press, 1995.

——. "Manhood, Womanhood, and the Politics of Class in Britain, 1790–1845." 263–79 in *Gender and Class in Modern Europe*, ed. by Laura L. Frader and Sonya O. Rose. Ithaca, N.Y.: Cornell University Press, 1996.

Comaroff, Jean. "The Diseased Heart of Africa." 305–29 in *Knowledge, Power and Practice*, ed. by Shirley Lindenbaum and Margaret Lock. Berkeley: University of California Press, 1993.

Connolly, Ceci. "Focus on Smallpox Threat Revived." *Washington Post*, 17 July 2003.

Cook, G. C. "Charles Creighton (1847–1927): Eminent Medical Historian but Vehement Anti-Jennerian." *Journal of Medical Biography* 8 (2000): 83–88.

Craft, Christopher. " 'Kiss Me with Those Red Lips': Gender and Inversion in Bram Stoker's *Dracula*." 167–94 in *Dracula: The Vampires and the Critics*, ed. by Margaret L. Carter. Ann Arbor, Mich.: UMI Research Press, 1988.

Crary, Jonathan. *Techniques of the Observer: On Vision and Modernity in the Nineteenth Century*. Cambridge, Mass.: MIT Press, 1990.

Crawley, James. "Take Vaccine or Risk Loss of Jobs, Some Employees to Military Told" *San Diego Union-Tribune*, 12 March, 2000.

Crossick, Geoffrey. *An Artisan Elite in Victorian Society*. London: Croom Helm, 1978.

Crossick, Geoffrey, ed. *The Lower Middle Class in Britain*. London: Croom Helm, 1978.

Crowther, M. A. *The Workhouse System 1834–1929*. Athens: University of Georgia Press, 1982.

Davidoff, Leonore, and Catherine Hall. *Family Fortunes: Men and Women of the English Middle Class, 1780–1850*. London: Hutchinson, 1987.

Davin, Anna. "Imperialism and Motherhood." 203–35 in *Patriotism: The*

Making and Unmaking of British National Identity. Volume 1, History and Politics, ed. by Raphael Samuel. London: Routledge, 1989.

Davis, Jennifer. "A Poor Man's System of Justice: The London Police Courts in the Second Half of the Nineteenth Century." *Historical Journal* 27(2) (1984): 309–35.

Digby, Anne. *Pauper Palaces*. London: Routledge and Kegan Paul, 1978.

——. *Making a Medical Living: Doctors and Patients in the English Market for Medicine, 1720–1911*. Cambridge: Cambridge University Press, 1994.

Dixon, Joy. *Divine Feminine: Theosophy and Feminism in England*. Baltimore: Johns Hopkins University Press, 2001.

Dwork, Deborah. *War Is Good for Babies and Other Young Children*. London: Tavistock, 1987.

Elston, Mary Ann. "Women and Anti-Vivisection in Victorian England, 1870–1900." 259–94 in *Vivisection in Historical Perspective*, ed. by Nicolaas A. Rupke. London: Routledge, 1987.

Foucault, Michel. *The Birth of the Clinic*. New York: Pantheon, 1973.

——. *Discipline and Punish*. New York: Pantheon, 1977.

——. *History of Sexuality, Volume 1: An Introduction*. New York: Vintage Books, 1990.

Fraser, Stuart M. F. "Leicester and Smallpox: The Leicester Method." *Medical History* 24 (1980): 315–32.

Freeden, Michael. "The New Liberalism and Its Aftermath." 175–92 in *Victorian Liberalism*, ed. by Richard Bellamy. London: Routledge, 1990.

French, Richard D. *Antivivisection and Medical Science in Victorian Society*. Princeton, N.J.: Princeton University Press, 1975.

Gelder, Ken. *Reading the Vampire*. London: Routledge, 1994.

Gilbert, Bentley B. "Health and Politics: The British Physical Deterioration Report of 1904." *Bulletin of the History of Medicine* 39(2) (1965): 143–53.

Glover, David. *Vampires, Mummies, and Liberals: Bram Stoker and the Politics of Popular Fiction*. Durham: Duke University Press, 1996.

Graham, John W. *Conscription and Conscience*. New York: Garland, 1971.

Gray, Robert Q. *The Factory Question and Industrial England, 1830–1860*. Cambridge: Cambridge University Press, 1996.

Green, David G. *Working-Class Patients and the Medical Establishment: Self-Help in Britain from the Mid-Nineteenth Century to 1948*. London: Temple Smith, Gower, 1985.

Greenough, Paul. "Intimidation, Coercion and Resistance in the Final Stages of the South Asian Smallpox Eradication Campaign, 1973–1975." *Social Sciences and Medicine* 41(5) (1995): 633–45.

Halberstam, Judith. "Technologies of Monstrosity: Bram Stoker's *Dracula*." *Victorian Studies* 36(3) (1993): 332–52.

Hall, Catherine, Keith McClelland, and Jane Rendall. *Defining the Victorian*

Nation: Class, Race, Gender and the Reform Act of 1867. Cambridge: Cambridge University Press, 2000.

Halsted, D. G. *Doctor in the Nineties.* London: Christopher Johnson, 1959.

Hamlin, Christopher. "Providence and Putrefaction: Victorian Sanitarians and the Natural Theology of Health and Disease." *Victorian Studies* (spring 1985): 381–411.

——. "Predisposing Causes and Public Health in Early Nineteenth-Century Medical Thought." *Social History of Medicine* 5(1) (1992): 43–70.

——. *Public Health and Social Justice in the Age of Chadwick: Britain, 1800–1854.* Cambridge: Cambridge University Press, 1998.

Hardy, Anne. "Smallpox in London: Factors in the Decline of the Disease in the Nineteenth Century." *Medical History* 27 (1983): 111–38.

——. *The Epidemic Streets: Infectious Disease and the Rise of Preventive Medicine, 1856–1900.* Oxford: Clarendon Press, 1993.

Harrison, Brian. *Drink and the Victorians: The Temperance Question in England, 1815–1872.* 2nd ed. Keele: Keele University Press, 1994.

Harrison, J. F. C. *The Common People of Great Britain.* Bloomington: Indiana University Press, 1985.

——. "Early Victorian Radicals and the Medical Fringe." 198–215 in *Medical Fringe and Medical Orthodoxy, 1750–1850,* ed. by W. F. Bynum and Roy Porter. London: Croom Helm, 1987.

Haynes, Roslynn D. *From Faust to Strangelove: Representations of the Scientist in Western Literature.* Baltimore: Johns Hopkins University Press, 1994.

Hennock, E. P. "Vaccination Policy Against Smallpox, 1835–1914: A Comparison of England with Prussia and Imperial Germany." *Social History of Medicine* 11(1) (1998): 49–71.

Hodgkinson, Ruth G. *The Origins of the National Health Service: The Medical Services of the New Poor Law, 1834–71.* Berkeley: University of California Press, 1967.

Hollis, Patricia. "Anti-Slavery and British Working-Class Radicalism in the Years of Reform." 297–311 in *Anti-Slavery, Religion, and Reform,* ed. by Christine Bolt and Seymour Drescher. Folkestone: Dawson, 1980.

Holton, Sandra Stanley. "Silk Dresses and Lavender Kid Gloves: The Wayward Career of Jessie Craigen, Working Suffragist." *Women's History Review* 5(1) (1996): 129–49.

Homans, Margaret. *Royal Representations: Queen Victoria and British Culture, 1837–1876.* Chicago: University of Chicago Press, 1998.

Hopkins, Donald R. *Princes and Peasants: Smallpox in History.* Chicago: University of Chicago Press, 1983.

Huerkamp, Claudia. "The History of Smallpox Vaccination in Germany: A First Step in the Medicalization of the General Public." *Journal of Contemporary History* 20 (1985): 617–35.

Hurley, Kelly. *The Gothic Body: Sexuality, Materialism, and Degeneration at the Fin de Siècle*. Cambridge: Cambridge University Press, 1996.

Jewson, N. D. "Medical Knowledge and the Patronage System in Eighteenth Century England." *Sociology* 8 (1974): 369–85.

Kaufman, Martin. "The American Anti-Vaccinationists and Their Arguments." *Bulletin of the History of Medicine* 41 (1967): 463–78.

Kean, Hilda, "The 'Smooth Cool Men of Science': The Feminist and Socialist Response to Vivisection." *History Workshop Journal* 40 (1995): 16–38.

——. *Animal Rights*. London: Reaktion Books, 1998.

Kennedy, Thomas C. "Public Opinion and the Conscientious Objector, 1915– 1919." *Journal of British Studies* 12(2) (1973): 105–19.

——. *The Hound of Conscience: A History of the No-Conscription Fellowship, 1914– 1919*. Fayetteville: University of Arkansas Press, 1981.

Kent, William. *John Burns: Labour's Lost Leader*. London: Williams and Norgate, 1950.

Koven, Seth, and Sonya Michel. *Mothers of a New World: Maternalist Politics and the Origins of Welfare States*. London: Routledge, 1993.

Lambert, Royston J. "A Victorian National Health Service: State Vaccination 1855–71." *Historical Journal* 5(1) (1962): 1–18.

——. *Sir John Simon 1816–1904 and English Social Administration*. London: Macgibbon and Kee, 1963.

Lansbury, Coral. *The Old Brown Dog: Women, Workers, and Vivisection in Edwardian England*. Madison: University of Wisconsin Press, 1985.

Laqueur, Thomas. "Bodies, Death, and Pauper Funerals." *Representations* 1(1) (1983): 109–31.

Larsen, Timothy. *Friends of Religious Equality: Nonconformist Politics in Mid-Victorian England*. Woodbridge, Suffolk: Boydell Press, 1999.

Leatherdale, Clive. *Dracula: The Novel and the Legend*. Wellingborough: Aquarius Press, 1985.

Leavitt, Judith. "Politics and Public Health: Smallpox in Milwaukee, 1894–5." *Bulletin of the History of Medicine* 50 (1976): 553–68.

Lederer, Susan. *Subjected to Science*. Baltimore: Johns Hopkins University Press, 1995.

Leneman, Leah. "The Awakened Instinct: Vegetarianism and the Women's Suffrage Movement in Britain." *Women's History Review* 6(2) (1997): 271–87.

Lewis, Jane. "The Working-Class Wife and Mother and State Intervention, 1870–1918." 99–120 in *Labour and Love: Women's Experience of Home and Family, 1850–1940*, ed. by Jane Lewis. Oxford: Basil Blackwell, 1986.

Lewis, Jane, ed. *Labour and Love: Women's Experience of Home and Family, 1850– 1940*. Oxford: Basil Blackwell, 1986.

Linebaugh, Peter. "The Tyburn Riot Against the Surgeons." 65–117 in *Albion's*

Fatal Tree, ed. by Douglas Hay, Peter Linebaugh, and E. P. Thompson. London: Allan Lane, 1975.

Linkman, Audrey. *The Victorians: Photographic Portraits*. London: Tauris Parke Books, 1993.

Loudon, Irvine. *Medical Care and the General Practitioner, 1750–1850*. Oxford: Clarendon Press, 1986.

MacAndrew, Elizabeth. *The Gothic Tradition in Fiction*. New York: Columbia University Press, 1979.

MacDonagh, Oliver. "The Nineteenth-Century Revolution in Government: A Reappraisal." *Historical Journal* 1(1) (1958): 52–67.

MacLeod, Roy M. "In the Interests of Health: State Medicine, Social Policy and the Power of Public Opinion in the Late-Victorian Vaccination Services 1871–1907." Unpublished B.A. thesis, Harvard University, Cambridge, Mass., 1963.

——. "Medico-Legal Issues in Victorian Medical Care." *Medical History* 10 (1966): 44–49.

——. "Law, Medicine and Public Opinion: The Resistance to Compulsory Health Legislation 1870–1907." *Public Law* (summer 1967): 107–28, 189–211.

MacLeod, Roy M., ed. *Government and Expertise: Specialists, Administrators and Professionals, 1860–1919*. Cambridge: Cambridge University Press, 1988.

MacNalty, Arthur Salusbury. "The Prevention of Smallpox: From Edward Jenner to Monckton Copeman." *Medical History* 12(1) (1968): 1–18.

Martin, David A. *Pacifism: An Historical and Sociological Study*. New York: Schocken Books, 1966.

Martin, Emily. *Flexible Bodies: The Role of Immunity in American Culture from the Days of Polio to the Age of AIDS*. Boston: Beacon Press, 1994.

McKiernan, John Raymond. " 'Fevered Measures: Race, Communicable Disease, and Community Formation on the Texas Mexico Border, 1880–1923." Unpublished Ph.D. diss., University of Michigan, Ann Arbor, 2002.

McLaren, Angus. *A Prescription for Murder: The Victorian Serial Killings of Dr. Thomas Neill Cream*. Chicago: University of Chicago Press, 1993.

McWilliam, Rohan. "Radicalism and Popular Culture: The Tichborne Case and the Politics of 'Fair Play,' 1867–1886." 44–64 in *Currents of Radicalism*, ed. by Eugenio F. Biagini and Alastair J. Reid. Cambridge: Cambridge University Press, 1991.

Meade, Teresa. " 'Civilizing Rio de Janeiro': The Public Health Campaign and the Riot of 1904." *Journal of Social History* 20(2) (1986): 301–22.

Miley, Ursula, and John V. Pickstone. "Medical Botany around 1850: American Medicine in Industrial Britain." 140–54 in *Studies in the History of Alternative Medicine*, ed. by Roger Cooter. New York: St. Martin's Press, 1988.

Millman, Brock. *Managing Domestic Dissent in First World War Britain*. London: Frank Cass, 2000.

Mooney, Graham. " 'A Tissue of the Most Flagrant Anomalies': Smallpox Vaccination and the Centralization of Sanitary Administration in Nineteenth-Century London." *Medical History* 41 (1997): 261–90.

Mort, Frank. *Dangerous Sexualities: Medico-Moral Politics in England Since 1830*. London: Routledge, 1987.

Navarro, Vicente. *Class Struggle, the State and Medicine*. New York: Prodist, 1978.

Nelson, Marie Clark, and John Rogers. "The Right to Die? Anti-Vaccination Activity and the 1874 Smallpox Epidemic in Stockholm." *Social History of Medicine* 5(3) (1992): 369–88.

Nicholls, Phillip. *Homeopathy and the Medical Profession*. London: Croom Helm, 1988.

Noble, Holcomb B. "Incentive Program Raises Immunization Rates." *New York Times*, 7 October 1998.

Nord, Deborah. "The Social Explorer as Anthropologist: Victorian Travellers among the Urban Poor." 122–34 in *Visions of the Modern City*, ed. by William Sharpe and Leonard Wallock. Baltimore: Johns Hopkins University Press, 1987.

Orwell, George. *The Road to Wigan Pier*. New York: Berkley Publishing, 1961.

Owen, Alex. *The Darkened Room: Women, Power, and Spiritualism in Late Victorian England*. Philadelphia: University of Pennsylvania Press, 1990.

Pedersen, Susan. "National Bodies and Unspeakable Acts: The Sexual Politics of Colonial Policy-Making." *Journal of Modern History* 63(4) (1991): 648–79.

Pelis, Kim. "Blood Clots: The Nineteenth-Century Debate over the Substance and Means of Transfusion in Britain." *Annals of Science* 54 (1997): 331–60.

——. "Transfusion, with Teeth." 1–29 in *Manifesting Medicine: Bodies and Machines*, ed. by Robert Bud, Bernhard Finn, and Helmuth Trischler. Amsterdam: Harwood, 1999.

Pennybacker, Susan D. *A Vision for London 1889–1914: Labour, Everyday Life and the LCC Experiment*. London: Routledge, 1995.

Peterson, M. Jeanne. *The Medical Profession in Mid-Victorian London*. Berkeley: University of California Press, 1978.

Pick, Daniel. " 'Terrors of the Night': *Dracula* and 'Degeneration' in the Late Nineteenth Century." *Critical Quarterly* 30(4) (1988): 71–87.

——. *Faces of Degeneration: A European Disorder, c. 1848–c. 1918*. Cambridge: Cambridge University Press, 1989.

Pickering, Michael. "White Skin, Black Masks: 'Nigger' Minstrelsy in Victorian England." 70–91 in *Music Hall: Performance and Style*, ed. by J. S. Bratton. Milton Keynes: Open University Press, 1986.

Pickstone, John. "Establishment and Dissent in Nineteenth-Century Medicine: An Exploration of Some Correspondence and Connections Between Religious and Medical Belief-Systems in Early Industrial England." 165–89 in *The Church and Healing*, vol. 19, ed. by W. J. Sheils. Oxford: Basil Blackwell, 1982.

Pollak, Michael. "Doctors Fighting Backlash over Vaccines." *New York Times*, 27 April 1999.

Poovey, Mary. *A History of the Modern Fact*. Chicago: University of Chicago Press, 1998.

Porter, Dorothy. "Public Health." 1231–61 in *Companion Encyclopedia of the History of Medicine*, ed. by W. F. Bynum and Roy Porter. London: Routledge, 1993.

Porter, Dorothy, and Roy Porter. "The Enforcement of Health: The British Debate." 97–120 in *AIDS: The Burdens of History*, ed. by Elizabeth Fee and Daniel M. Fox. Berkeley: University of California Press, 1988.

——. "The Politics of Prevention: Anti-Vaccinationism and Public Health in Nineteenth-Century England." *Medical History* 32 (1988): 231–52.

——. "What Was Social Medicine? An Historiographical Essay." *Journal of Historical Sociology* 1(1) (1988): 90–106.

Porter, Roy. *Health for Sale*. Manchester: Manchester University Press, 1989.

Preston, Richard. "The Demon in the Freezer." *New Yorker*, 12 July 1999.

Punter, David. *The Literature of Terror*. London: Longman, 1980.

Rae, John. *Conscience and Politics*. Oxford: Oxford University Press, 1970.

Reader, W. J. *Professional Men: The Rise of the Professional Classes in Nineteenth Century England*. London: Weidenfeld and Nicholson, 1966.

Rees, Kelvin. "Water as a Commodity: Hydropathy in Matlock." 28–45 in *Studies in the History of Alternative Medicine*, ed. by Roger Cooter. New York: St. Martin's Press, 1988.

Reid, Douglas A. "Interpreting the Festival Calendar: Wakes and Fairs as Carnivals." 125–53 in *Popular Culture and Custom in Nineteenth-Century England*, ed. by Robert D. Storch. London: Croom Helm, 1982.

Richards, Stewart. "Anaesthetics, Ethics, and Aesthetics: Vivisection in the Late Nineteenth-Century British Laboratory." 142–69 in *The Laboratory Revolution in Medicine*, ed. by Andrew Cunningham and Perry Williams. Cambridge: Cambridge University Press, 1992.

Richardson, Ruth. *Death, Dissection and the Destitute*. London: Routledge, 1987.

Roberts, Robert. *The Classic Slum*. Manchester: Manchester University Press, 1971.

Rosen, George. *A History of Public Health*. Baltimore: Johns Hopkins University Press, 1993.

Ross, Dale L. "Leicester and the Anti-Vaccination Movement 1853–1889." *Transactions of the Leicestershire Archaeological and Historical Society* 43 (1967–68): 35–44.

Ross, Ellen, " 'Not the Sort That Would Sit on the Doorstep': Respectability in Pre–World War I London Neighborhoods." *International Labor and Working Class History* 27 (1985): 39–59.

———. *Love and Toil: Motherhood in Outcast London, 1870–1918*. Oxford: Oxford University Press, 1993.

Roth, Phyllis A. "Suddenly Sexual Women in Bram Stoker's *Dracula*." 57–67 in *Dracula: The Vampires and the Critics*, ed. by Margaret L. Carter. Ann Arbor, Mich.: UMI Research Press, 1988.

Scarpelli, Giacomo. " 'Nothing in Nature That Is Not Useful': The Anti-Vaccination Crusade and the Idea of *Harmonia Naturae* in Alfred Russel Wallace." *Nuncius* 7(1) (1992): 109–30.

Scott, Anne L. "Physical Purity Feminism and State Medicine in Late Nineteenth-Century England." *Women's History Review* 8(4) (1999): 625–53.

Showalter, Elaine. *Sexual Anarchy: Gender and Culture at the Fin de Siècle*. Harmondsworth: Penguin, 1990.

Sigsworth, Michael, and Michael Worboys. "The Public's View of Public Health in Mid-Victorian Britain." *Urban History* 21 (1994): 237–50.

Smith, F. B. *The People's Health, 1830–1910*. New York: Holmes and Meier, 1979

Spencer, Kathleen L. "Purity and Danger: *Dracula*, the Urban Gothic, and the Late Victorian Degeneracy Crisis." *ELH* 59 (1992): 197–225.

Spongberg, Mary. *Feminizing Venereal Disease: The Body of the Prostitute in Nineteenth-Century Medical Discourse*. Houndsmills: Macmillan, 1997.

Steedman, Carolyn. *Policing the Victorian Community: The Formation of the English Provincial Police Forces, 1856–1880*. London: Routledge and Kegan Paul, 1984.

———. *Landscape for a Good Woman*. New Brunswick, N.J.: Rutgers University Press, 1992.

Stevenson, Lloyd G. "Science Down the Drain." *Bulletin of the History of Medicine* 29(1) (1955): 1–26.

Stoler, Ann Laura. *Race and the Education of Desire*. Durham, N.C.: Duke University Press, 1995.

Storch, Robert D. " 'Please to Remember the Fifth of November': Conflict, Solidarity and Public Order in Southern England, 1815–1900." 71–99 in *Popular Culture and Custom in Nineteenth-Century England*, ed. by Robert D. Storch. London: Croom Helm, 1982.

Sugg, Diana K. "Baltimore Children Getting Their Shots." *Baltimore Sun*, 20 April 1998.

Summers, Anne. "*The Constitution Violated:* The Female Body and the Female Subject in the Campaigns of Josephine Butler." *History Workshop Journal* 48 (1999): 1–15.

Sykes, Alan. *The Rise and Fall of British Liberalism, 1776–1988*. London: Longman, 1997.

Taylor, Arthur J. *Laissez-Faire and State Intervention in Nineteenth-Century Britain*. London: Macmillan, 1972.

Thompson, E. P. *The Making of the English Working Class*. New York: Vintage, 1966.

Thompson, F. M. L. *The Rise of Respectable Society: A Social History of Victorian Britain, 1830–1900*. Cambridge, Mass.: Harvard University Press, 1988.

Thorne, Susan. "'The Conversion of Englishmen and the Conversion of the World Inseparable': Missionary Imperialism and the Language of Class in Early Industrial Britain." 238–62 in *Tensions of Empire*, ed. by Frederick Cooper and Ann Laura Stoler. Berkeley: University of California Press, 1997.

Tickner, Lisa. *The Spectacle of Women: Imagery of the Suffrage Campaign, 1907–1914*. London: Chatto and Windus, 1987.

Tomes, Nancy. *The Gospel of Germs: Men, Women, and the Microbe in American Life*. Cambridge, Mass.: Harvard University Press, 1998.

Tomes, Nancy, and John Harley Warner. "Introduction to Special Issue on Rethinking the Reception of the Germ Theory of Disease: Comparative Perspectives." *Journal of the History of Medicine and Allied Sciences* 52(1) (1997): 7–16.

Tucker, Jennifer. "Science Illustrated: Photographic Evidence and Social Practice in England 1870–1920." Unpublished Ph.D. diss., Johns Hopkins University, Baltimore, 1996.

Tucker, Robert C., ed. *The Marx–Engels Reader*, 2nd ed. New York: Norton, 1978.

Turner, James. *Reckoning with the Beast: Animals, Pain, and Humanity in the Victorian Mind*. Baltimore: Johns Hopkins University Press, 1980.

Vandervelde, V. Denis. "British Anti-Vaccination Propaganda." *Postal History International* (October 1974): 376–80.

Vaughan, Megan. *Curing Their Ills: Colonial Power and African Illness*. Oxford: Polity Press, 1991.

Vernon, James. *Politics and the People*. Cambridge: Cambridge University Press, 1993.

Waddington, Ivan. "General Practitioners and Consultants in Early Nineteenth Century England: The Sociology of an Intra-Professional Conflict." 164–88 in *Health Care and Popular Medicine in Nineteenth Century Britain*, ed. by John Woodward and David Richards. London: Croom Helm, 1977.

——. *The Medical Profession in the Industrial Revolution*. Dublin: Gill and Macmillan Humanities Press, 1984.

Walkowitz, Judith R. *Prostitution and Victorian Society: Women, Class, and the State*. Cambridge: Cambridge University Press, 1980.

——. *City of Dreadful Delight: Narratives of Sexual Danger in Late-Victorian London*. Chicago: University of Chicago Press, 1992.

Warner, John Harley. "Therapeutic Explanation and the Edinburgh

Bloodletting Controversy: Two Perspectives on the Medical Meaning of Science in the Mid-Nineteenth Century." *Medical History* 24 (1980): 241–58.

Weiler, Peter. *The New Liberalism*. New York: Garland, 1982.

Weinbren, Dan. "Against *All* Cruelty: The Humanitarian League, 1891–1919." *History Workshop Journal* 38 (1994): 86–105.

Weindling, Paul. "The Immunological Tradition" 192–204 in *Companion Encyclopedia of the History of Medicine*, ed. by W. F. Bynum and Roy Porter. London: Routledge, 1993.

White, Luise. " 'They Could Make Their Victims Dull': Genders and Genres, Fantasies and Cures in Colonial Southern Uganda." *American Historical Review* (December 1995): 1379–1402.

——. "The Needle and the State: Immunization and Inoculation in Africa. Or, the Practice of Unnatural Sovereignty." Unpublished paper for the Workshop on Immunization and the State, Delhi, India, 16–17 January 1997.

Wiener, Martin J. *Reconstructing the Criminal: Culture, Law, and Policy in England, 1830–1914*. Cambridge: Cambridge University Press, 1990.

Williams, Naomi. "The Implementation of Compulsory Health Legislation: Infant Smallpox Vaccination in England and Wales, 1840–1890." *Journal of Historical Geography* 20(4) (1994): 396–412.

Winter, Alison. *Mesmerized*. Chicago: University of Chicago Press, 1998.

Wohl, Anthony. *Endangered Lives: Public Health in Victorian Britain*. Cambridge, Mass.: Harvard University Press, 1983.

Wolfe, Robert M., Lisa K. Sharp, and Martin S. Lipsky. "Content and Design Attributes of Antivaccination Web Sites." *Journal of the American Medical Association* 287(24) (2002): 3245–48.

Worboys, Michael. *Spreading Germs: Disease Theories and Medical Practice in Britain, 1865–1900*. Cambridge: Cambridge University Press, 2000.

Young, James Harvey. *The Toadstool Millionaires*. Princeton, N.J.: Princeton University Press, 1961.

Zanger, Jules. "A Sympathetic Vibration: Dracula and the Jews." *English Literature in Transition* 34(1) (1991): 33–44.

Index

Africa, 79–84

Allinson, T. R., 67, 136–38, 165, 241 n.9

Alternative medicine, 11, 13, 44, 83, 117, 121, 134, 205; anti-vaccinationism and, 32–36, 39, 41, 47; rise of, 26–32; working class and, 27–32

Anatomy, 6, 15, 95, 144, 147

Anatomy Act (1832), 6, 15, 29, 95

Animals, 124–26, 166–67. *See also* Cows; Vivisection

Anthrax, 159, 203, 205

Anti-Compulsory Vaccination and Mutual Protection Society, 39–40, 72, 120

Anti-Compulsory Vaccination League, 38

Anti-Mourning Society, 39

Antitoxins, 166–67

Anti-vaccination leagues, 38–41, 53, 92, 101, 213 n.2. *See also* Anti-Compulsory Vaccination and Mutual Protection Society; Anti-Compulsory Vaccination League; London Society for the Abolition of Compulsory Vaccination; National Anti-Compulsory Vaccination League; National Anti-Vaccination League

Anti-vaccination press, 39–40, 47–48

Aristocracy, 31, 70, 140–41

Asquith, H. H., 179

Australia, 166

Austria, 32, 78

Autopsies, 29, 147

Bacteriology, 20, 155, 158–70. *See also* Disease theories

Baker, Thomas, 160

Balfour, A. J., 179–80

Banbury, 50, 171

Bands, brass, 50, 63

Bangladesh, 201

Banners, 50, 63–64, 93, 122, 145–46, 154

Baptism, 44–45

Bayley, Thomas, 108

Bible, 62, 79, 119, 153–54

Biggs, J.T., 108, 125

Bio-weapons, 202–3

Blackface, 110–11

Blair, Tony, 204

Blood: circulation of, 4, 30, 120–21; contamination of, 34, 97–98, 114, 116–17, 121–38, 166–67; immunity and, 166–68; letting of, 13, 29, 139; purity of, 4, 30, 114, 119–23, 155; transfusion of, 139–40, 146. *See also* Vampires

Bloomsbury group, 196

Body: integrity of, 4, 107, 113, 145; violation of, 6, 46, 77, 81, 93, 112, 113–14, 119–20, 138–49; vulnerability of, 32, 46, 107–12, 114, 122

Boer War, 63, 134

Bond, Francis, 55–56

Bonner, John, 46, 63, 175–76, 200, 241 n.8

Boot clubs, 101

Bradlaugh, Charles, 101–2, 164
Branding, 111
Brazil, 5
Bright, Ursula, 46, 129
British Medical Association, 19, 124
British Medical Journal, 24, 135, 136, 200
Brown, John, 184, 199
Bulgarian Horrors, 84
Burial insurance, 101
Burns, James, 109
Burns, John, 123, 190, 193, 194–95
Butler, Josephine, 70, 90, 141

Catholicism, 45
Centers for Disease Control, 201, 203
Chadwick, Edwin, 18–19, 155
Chaplin, Henry, 177, 189, 192
Chartism, 27, 38
Child abuse, 59, 71, 104, 145, 148, 234 n.169. *See also* National Society for the Prevention of Cruelty to Children
Childhood: concept of, 118–19
Cholera, 18, 22, 211 n.37
Circumcision, 45
Citizenship, 5, 11, 75–76, 106–7, 172, 176, 196, 205–6; imperialism and, 79–84; nationalism and, 76–79, 134; parental rights and, 69, 71, 75
Cobbe, Frances Power, 144, 145
Cobbett, William, 82, 93
Coffin, Albert Isaiah, 29, 30, 139
Colley, Archdeacon, 121–22, 126, 132–33
Collins, W. J., 67, 154, 164, 167
Collinson, Joseph, 133, 155
Compulsory Vaccination Act (1853), 2, 17, 76, 96, 109, 118; origins of, 7–8, 11, 13, 19–23, 95, 152
Connell, Ira, 116–17
Conscience, 32, 34, 108, 172–75, 237 n.8
Conscience offenders, 104, 106–7

Conscientious objection to vaccination, 10, 12, 59, 102, 106, 171–97; defined, 173–75, 178–79, 181–82; gender and, 172, 191–95; working class and, 180–91
Conscription, 6, 196–97
Conservative Party, 87, 111, 177, 179–80, 197, 206
Constitutionalism, 77
Consumption. *See* Tuberculosis
Contagion: concept of, 150–52; morality and, 119, 130–33, 149. *See also* Disease theories; Smallpox
Contagious diseases acts, 7, 9, 64; repeal campaign, 38, 39, 46, 69, 111, 123, 141
Cook, Thomas, 50
Co-operative movement, 42–43
Copeman, S. Monckton, 147, 161
Corn Laws, 28
Cory, Robert, 132
Courts, 64–65, 172, 186, 187, 190
Cowpox, 20, 124, 131, 159, 161, 165
Cows, 111, 123, 124–25, 143–44
Craigen, Jessie, 46, 111, 134
Crankery, 12, 41–42, 94, 157, 242 n.9
Creighton, Charles, 131, 157
Criminals, 15, 103–4, 106, 111, 134, 138, 176, 190
Crookshank, Edgar, 157
Cross-dressing, 110
Crucifixion, 45

Darwinism, 126, 134
Defense funds, 101
Degeneration, 124, 133–38, 139, 142
Democratic epistemology, 30
Demonstrations, 1, 50–51, 62–63, 65, 68, 93, 145
Dickens, Charles, 84, 141, 152
Diphtheria, 166, 183, 205
Disease theories, 150–70; constitutional, 150–51, 158, 165–68; environmental, 150–56, 158, 162–65;

germ, 150–52, 155–70; miasmatic, 151, 152–53, 156; spontaneous generation, 153, 154, 156; zymotic, 152–53, 156, 163

Distraining of goods, 9, 51, 52–55, 60, 109

Doctors, private, 99, 127–29, 130. *See also* Medical professionalization

Domesticity, 56–57, 59–61, 68, 104–5, 186

Domestic medicine, 26

Dr. Jekyll and Mr. Hyde, 114

Dracula, 139, 140, 142–43, 149

Duncombe, Thomas Slingsby, 33

Education, compulsory, 39, 71, 88, 89, 174, 180, 194

Elmy, Elizabeth Wolstenholme, 46

Encyclopedia Britannica, 157

Enfield, 43, 100, 171–72

Epidemiological Society, 22–23

Equality under law, 86–87

Eugenics, 134, 136–38

Experimentation, human, 29, 80, 132, 143–49, 205

Factories, 43–44

Faith healing, 175

False addresses, 66, 188

Fatherhood, 9, 56–60, 68, 71, 104, 186, 191–95

Fawcett, Millicent Garrett, 46, 184–85

Femininity, 55, 56–57, 60–64

Feminism, 46–47, 60, 63, 72, 81, 122, 138, 146

Fines, 8, 51, 65, 106, 108, 171; limiting of, 177–78, 180; refusal to pay, 52, 101–2; working class and, 91, 99–102, 189

Food reform, 38, 41, 123

Foreigners, 78–97, 140

Foster, Walter, 178–79, 190

France, 78

Fraser, John, 78, 120, 173

Freeborn Englishman, 13, 32, 69, 71, 77

Friendly societies, 38, 104

Furnival, W. J., 48, 116, 123, 175

Gangrene, 4

General Board of Health, 18, 32, 33

Germ theory. *See* Disease theories

Gibbs, George, 3, 38, 135, 186

Gibbs, John, 13, 32–33, 34, 38, 73, 77, 78, 172

Gibbs, Richard Butler, 38, 122

Gladstone, William, 73, 78, 84, 86, 104

Gloucester, 55, 93, 125, 166

Gomm, Amy Frances, 125, 130

"The Good Lady Ducayne," 140

Goss, Frank, 66, 169

Gothicism, 11, 113–14, 117, 138–49

Green, T. H., 88

Gulf War syndrome, 205

Guy Fawkes, 51

Hadwen, Walter, 71, 125–26, 154, 160, 162, 167–68, 231 n.129

Hageby, Louise Lind af, 143

Harcourt, William, 72

Hayward, Charles, 101–2

Health visiting, 74, 206

Heredity, 127, 129, 130, 132, 133, 140

Heroic therapies, 28–29, 144–45

Hobhouse, L.T., 88

Hobson, J.A., 88

Holism, 27

Home: sanctity of, 73–74

Home Office, 174, 186, 188, 189

Homoeopathy, 26, 33, 34, 42

Homosexuality, 7

Horse grease, 125

Howey Foundation, 201

Hughes, Hugh Price, 45

Humanitarianism, 41, 46, 94, 133, 155

Hume, Joseph, 39, 85

Hume-Rothery, Mary, 7, 99, 119, 131, 173; blood and, 120, 142, 144; cit-

Hume-Rothery, Mary (*cont.*)
izenship and, 75–79, 84, 134; disease theory and, 153, 160, 163–64; formation of National Anti-Compulsory Vaccination League, 38–40; liberalism and, 85, 87; women's rights and, 46, 61, 64, 72
Hume-Rothery, William, 38–40, 70, 89, 133, 156–57
Hunt, Chandos Leigh, 45
Hutchinson, Jonathan, 132
Hydropathy, 26, 27, 30–34, 60, 123, 130, 172, 175
Hygieanism, 26, 29–31, 33, 121
Hyndman, Henry, 94

Immigration, 134, 143
Immunity, 4, 20, 156, 167–68, 203, 204
Imperialism, 4–6, 79–84, 111, 134, 135–36
Independent Labour Party, 94, 196
India, 4, 79, 135
Individualism, 72, 85, 87, 92, 108, 111, 122
Infanticide, 59
Infant welfare movement, 194
Inoculation. *See* Variolation
Ireland, 76, 79, 93–94, 106, 107, 109, 179, 200
The Island of Dr. Moreau, 146
Isolation, 157, 164, 169, 176

Jack the Ripper, 145
Jenner, Edward, 20, 51, 67, 115
Jervoise, Sir J. Clarke, 164
John Bull, 77
Justices of the peace, 103, 190

Keighley, 1–2, 9, 10, 93, 171, 186–87, 192, 213 n.2
Kingsford, Anna, 145
Klein, E. E., 161, 167

Labouchere, Henry, 179
Labour Party, 194, 206

Ladies' Sanitary Association, 75
Laissez-faire, 26, 28, 85, 86, 92, 111
Lamarckian evolution, 151
The Lancet, 22, 24, 25
Lancets, 3, 5, 68, 78, 144, 145, 149
Latin, 30
Leeds, 38, 65, 68
Leicester, 41, 43, 53, 74, 88, 91, 164
Leicester Demonstration, 50, 61, 63, 111, 122, 154
Levy, J. H., 87
Liberalism, 11, 69, 84–90, 92, 111
Liberal Party, 69, 85–90, 94, 111, 189–91, 194, 195, 197
Libertarianism, 72, 199
Lister, Joseph, 157
Loane, Margaret, 59, 74
Loat, Lily, 200
Local Government Board, 124, 132, 147, 161; presidents of, 123, 177, 190, 194, 197
London, 92, 95, 99, 100, 115, 126, 151, 177, 182
London County Council, 89
London Society for the Abolition of Compulsory Vaccination, 59, 70, 86, 94, 101–2, 145; leadership of, 40, 46, 123
Long, Walter, 197
Lupton, Arnold, 189
Lymph, 3, 50, 67, 97, 113, 117, 123, 124–38, 147; glycerinated, 147, 161–62, 178, 180
Lyttleton, Lord, 23, 96, 99

Magic lantern slides, 48
Magistrates 65, 68, 102, 105; conscience clause and, 171, 177, 178, 180, 181–88, 190
Magna Charta, 77
"Maiden Tribute of Modern Babylon," 146
Manchester, 42, 43, 92, 95, 117, 147
Married women's property, 46, 72
Marx, Karl, 141

Marxist International Working Men's Association, 94
Masculinity, 55, 58–60, 68, 83
Maternal and child health policies, 7
Maternalist politics, 63
Matthews, Henry, 102
Medical Act (1858), 17, 23–26
Medical botany, 26, 27, 29, 30, 33, 117, 139, 172
Medical professionalization, 11, 13, 14–17, 23–26
Mesmerism, 26, 33
Metchnikoff, Elie, 167–68
Mexico, 5
Miasma. See Disease theories
Microscope, 162
Midwives, 14, 20, 25, 26
Military Service Act (1916), 6, 197
Militia Act (1757), 174
Mill, John Stuart, 89
Milnes, Alfred, 67, 70, 72, 73, 85–86, 90, 104, 108
Miscegenation, 134, 135–36, 142
Missionaries, 80–82
MMR vaccine, 203–4
Monstrosity, 113, 114–19, 144
Montagu, Lady Mary Wortley, 19
Morison, James, 34
Morison, John, 29, 33–34, 121, 148
Morris, William, 94
Motherhood, 55–57, 60–68, 191–95
Moving house, 66, 188
Municipal socialism, 89
Murder, 143, 145

Naming children, 65–66
National Anti-Compulsory Vaccination League, 39–40, 42, 70
National Anti-Vaccination League, 46, 103, 131, 134, 200–201, 242 n.12; conscience clause and, 173, 179, 180–81, 187; defense funds and, 101; formation of, 40, 173; leadership of, 141, 148

National Health Service, 204, 206–7, 243 n.31
Nationalism, 76–79
National Society for the Prevention of Cruelty to Children, 59, 89, 145. See also Child abuse
National Vaccine Establishment, 3, 126, 147, 161
Nature, 29, 30
Newman, Francis W., 75, 90, 122–23
New Poor Law (1834). See Poor Law
Nichols, Mary, 130
Nichols, T. L., 60, 123
Nightingale, Florence, 156, 164
Noailles, countess de, 79–80
No-Conscription Fellowship, 196
Nonconformists, 44–45, 117, 174
Norman yoke, 77
Notification of infectious diseases acts, 7, 148, 176

Oastler, Richard, 82
Oaths Act (1888), 174, 179, 180
O'Brien, Bronterre, 82
Oldham, 116, 181, 186, 188, 213 n.2
Orwell, George, 42
Owenism, 27, 38, 42
Oxford English Dictionary, 173–74, 237 n.8

Pacifism, 93, 172, 196–97
Pamphlets and handbills, 47–50, 60, 63, 102, 187
Parental rights, 11, 68, 71–75, 85, 87, 108
Passive resisters, 174
Patent medicines, 159
Paupers, 98, 124, 126–31, 142, 186, 206. See also Poor Law
Peculiar People, 175
Penal Servitude Act (1891), 106
Personal Rights Association, 86–87, 148, 199
Personal Rights Journal, 45, 87, 161

Phelps, Lieutenant-General A., 141–42, 164, 231 n.129

Phonography, 43

Photography, 48, 116

Phthisis. *See* Tuberculosis

Physical Deterioration Committee, 135

Physical Puritanism, 46, 122

Pickering, John, 34, 68, 153

Picton, J.A., 74, 89, 164

Pilcher v. Stafford, 8

Pitman, Henry, 42–43, 75, 111, 117, 122, 123, 151

Pitman, Isaac, 43

Police, 1, 51–55, 78, 100, 103, 168, 216 n.55

Poor Law, 15–16, 51, 105, 206; as administrator of vaccination, 2, 8–10, 23, 94–99, 102; guardians, 1–2, 8–10, 95, 99, 102, 177, 178; medical officers, 16, 23, 25, 95; relieving officers, 95

Populism, 69–71, 122

Pornography, 146, 233 n.152

Posters and prints, 48, 53

Poverty, 153–54, 168–69. *See also* Paupers

Premature burial, 231 n.129

Preventive medicine, 17, 24, 150, 155, 159, 166

Priessnitz, Vincent, 32

Primitiveness, 80–81

Prison, 1, 9, 74, 91, 99, 101, 171, 183, 184; respectability and, 60, 102–7, 174; women and, 65, 107–8; working-class body and, 59, 107–8

Property, 72, 74, 77, 108, 111

Prosecutions, 8, 10, 65, 99–102, 177, 188

Prostitution, 7, 103, 132, 141. *See also* Contagious diseases acts

Public health, 7, 9, 75, 90, 164, 183, 201–5; medicalization of, 17–25, 166; politics of, 18–19, 155, 169

Public Health Act (1848), 18

Public Health Act (1858), 19

Quackery, 21, 27, 57, 78, 148

Quakers, 44, 174

Radicalism, 82, 93–94, 206

Rape, 146

Reading, 179–80

Reform Act (1867), 39, 76

Reform Act (1884), 39, 58, 79

Registration of birth, 8, 45, 66, 95

Religion, 44–46, 117–19, 173, 197

Respectability, 60, 63, 68, 96, 100, 102–7, 124, 131

Revolution in government, 9–10

Royal College of Physicians, 14

Royal College of Surgeons, 157

Royal Commission on Vaccination, 10, 135, 142, 177; dissenting report of, 164; final report of, 10, 40, 176, 177, 180; interim report of, 106–7; testimony before, 48, 60, 91, 99, 103, 105, 106, 108, 124, 125, 166

Rumsey, H. W., 96

Salvation Army, 44, 106, 174

Sanitary idea, 18–19, 155

Sanitation, 17–19, 89, 152–59, 162–65, 168, 169

Scotland, 76, 109, 200

Scrofula, 34, 97, 114, 127, 129, 130

Seaton, Edward, 21–23

Select Committee on the Vaccination Act of 1867, 70

Self-help, 20, 27, 30–31, 42–43

Separate spheres, 57, 68, 104, 194

Sheffield, 38, 92, 93, 119

Simon, John, 19, 22, 23, 88

Skelton, John, 27, 30, 33, 172

Slavery, 13, 82–84, 110–111; abolition of, 38, 82–84

Smallpox, 2–4, 8, 20–23, 93, 126, 136, 176, 201–3; alternative methods of preventing, 34, 121, 123; disease theories and, 150–70; epidemics, 2, 20, 115, 125, 157, 176; monstrosity and, 115. *See also* Isolation; Sanitation

Smallpox Eradication Program, 4, 201–2

Snow, John, 211 n.37

Social body, 6, 9, 23, 131, 150, 152, 205

Social Darwinism, 136

Social Democratic Federation, 94

Socialism, 94, 172, 196

Social reform movements, 41–47

Spencer, Herbert, 87

Spiritual health, 45, 113, 114, 117–19, 132–33, 149

Spiritualism, 38, 41, 45–46, 109

State intervention, 4, 6–7, 9, 11, 69, 78, 169, 191; liberalism and, 85–90; parental rights and, 71–75; working class and, 108–9

Statistics, 2–3, 47, 188

Statutory declarations, 177, 178–80, 190, 192, 196

Steedman, Carolyn, 206–7

Stevens, John, 31–32

Stoker, Bram, 142, 232 n.130

Stroud, 55, 109–111

Swedenborg, Emanuel, 40, 41, 45

Syphilis, 7, 34, 73, 97, 113, 124, 129, 131–33, 161

Taylor, P. A., 88

Tebb, William, 79, 86, 129, 146–47, 151, 162, 181; London Society of the Abolition of Compulsory Vaccination and, 40; premature burial and, 231 n.129; slavery and, 83–84

Teetotalism, 41, 93, 97, 105, 122

Temperance, 30, 38, 42, 50, 105, 122

Theosophy, 42, 45–46

Tickets of leave, 176

Tobacco, 42, 122

Toleration Act (1689), 174

Torture, 13, 31, 145, 148–49

Trade unionism, 43–44, 93, 186

Transubstantiation, 45

Tuberculosis, 158, 159; consumption 127; phthisis 125

Turner, Ben, 43, 108, 186

Uganda, 5

United Nations, 201

United States, 5, 78, 202, 203, 205

Urbanization, 19, 89, 134, 151, 153, 155

Utilitarianism, 86

Vaccination: adult, 109; arm-to-arm, 3, 97–98, 124, 126–33, 135–36, 161, 178; certificates, 9, 67, 100; definition of, 67; disease spread by, 3, 97, 124–33; efficacy of, 2; injuries from, 3–4, 114–19, 125, 135, 204; insusceptibility to, 9; invention of, 4, 19, 20; marks, 2–3; medical unfitness for, 9, 183, 188; middle-class resistance to, 38–41, 69–71, 84–90, 199; technique of, 3, 144; working-class resistance to, 39–44, 69–71, 91–112, 129–31, 144–48, 172, 180–88, 199

Vaccination Act (1840), 21, 23, 95

Vaccination Act (1853). *See* Compulsory Vaccination Act (1853)

Vaccination Act (1867), 2, 8–9, 11, 76, 85, 89, 100–101, 109, 191

Vaccination Act (1871), 2, 3, 8–9, 76, 101, 109, 191

Vaccination Act (1898), 197; calf lymph and, 126, 161; conscience clause and, 10, 12, 136, 171–72, 174, 176–88, 191–92; domiciliary vaccination and, 74, 178, 180

Vaccination Act (1907), 10, 12, 188–97, 199–200

Vaccination officers, 8–9, 51, 65–66, 74, 95–96, 100, 142, 173

Vaccination stations, 74, 92, 97–99, 100, 124, 129, 178

Vaccinators: foreign, 78; public, 3, 8,

Vaccinators: foreign (*cont.*)
24–52, 74, 95–99, 100, 126–29,
141–42, 161; vivisection and,
143–49
Vaccine: removal of, 67; substitutes
for, 67. *See also* Cowpox; Lymph
Vaccinifiers, 3, 126–31, 132, 135
Vampires, 11, 114, 138–43, 149
"The Vampyre," 139
Variolation, 4, 19–22
Varney the Vampire, 139
Vegetarianism, 38, 41–42, 94, 143,
145, 160, 241 n.9; physical purity
and, 46, 122–23, 135
Vesicles, 3, 67, 144
Victoria, 64
Violence, 51, 53–55, 59, 67–68, 90,
144. *See also* Demonstrations
Vivisection, 11, 29, 114, 138, 143–49,
160; campaign against, 38, 41,
46, 69, 94, 111

Vote, 39, 58, 68, 71, 79, 104. *See also*
Women's suffrage

Wakefield, Andrew, 203–4
Wallace, Alfred Russel, 163, 168
White, William, 40, 45
Wilkinson, J. J. Garth, 34, 45, 74, 78,
126, 143, 148; blood and, 130, 138–
39; poverty and, 153–54
Women's rights, 46–47, 60–61, 68,
179, 193
Women's suffrage, 46–47, 79, 106,
111
Workhouse, 15, 16, 18, 64, 94–95, 97,
101. *See also* Poor Law
World Health Organization, 201–2
World War I, 12, 172, 196–97
World War II, 205, 206

Young, William, 39–40, 102, 131, 154

Nadja Durbach

is an assistant professor in the

Department of History at the University

of Utah, Salt Lake City.

☞

Library of Congress Cataloging-in-Publication Data

Durbach, Nadja, 1971–

Bodily matters : the anti-vaccination movement in

England, 1853–1907 / Nadja Durbach.

p. cm. — (Radical perspectives)

Includes bibliographical references and index.

ISBN 0-8223-3412-7 (cloth : alk. paper)

ISBN 0-8223-3423-2 (pbk. : alk. paper)

1. Smallpox—Vaccination—Great Britain—History—

19th century. I. Title. II. Series.

RA644.S6D874 2005

614.5′21′0941—dc22

2004013140